A Cardiologist's Prescription for

OPTIMUM HEALTH

A Cardiologist's Prescription for
OPTIMUM HEALTH

Stephen T. Sinatra, M.D.

Prescription

- Vitamins, Minerals and Nutritionals
- Anti-Aging Strategies
- Weight Management
- Emotional Healing

- Spiritual Growth
- Preventive Medicine
- Love and Sexuality

The Lincoln-Bradley Publishing Group

New York

Memphis   *Gatlinburg*

A Cardiologist's Guide To
OPTIMUM HEALTH

The Lincoln-Bradley Publishing Group
Creative Living, Inc.
P.O. Box 808
Gatlinburg, TN 37738
(423) 436-4150

Manufactured in the United States of America

Managing Editor: Carl Mays
Project Editor: Stephen D. Williford
Interior and Exterior Design: Rick Soldin/Andrew Barnes
(Electronic Publishing Services, Inc., Jonesborough, TN 37659)
Front Dust Jacket Design: GP&P Marketing Communications,
Prospect, CT

Library of Congress Cataloging-in-Publication Data

Sinatra, Stephen T.
  A cardiologist's guide to Optimum Health / Stephen T. Sinatra.
    p. cm.
  Includes bibliography references and index.

ISBN: 1-879111-81-0

1. Health.   2. Health behavior.   I. Title.
RA776.9.S56   1996   613
                                            QBI95-20509

Library of Congress Catalog Card Number: 95-80607

Type Face: 11/13.5 Minion

1 2 3 4 5 6 7 8 9 10

DEDICATION

For my deceased father, **Salvatore Charles Sinatra**, who not only took me to church as a young boy and who taught me how to cook and dance in my adolescence, but also gave me the gift of unconditional love. For my mother, **Elizabeth Patricia Sinatra**, who loved and supported me through all my endeavors. She taught me more about health and illness than any professor, colleague or patient. Her unfortunate life-long struggle with diabetes, glaucoma, blindness, osteoporosis, fractures and chronic pain has made me look deeper into myself to become a physician who truly cares and heals from his heart.

PREFACE

I am writing this book to convey a deeper understanding of health and illness. After more than 20 years of working in a medical model and more than a decade of investigating the mind/body relationship of disease, it has become clear to me how the concepts of *dis-ease* and energy are related.

Almost 800 years earlier, in his essays on health, Maimonides, a Mid-Eastern physician, gave a similar prescription for the preservation of health and youth. This book is an up-to-the-minute update, using basic and natural concepts for an optimally healthy and happy life.

THE PRESERVATION OF YOUTH, MAIMONIDES, 1198

Avoid Oversatiety and Fatigue
Exercise Fights Illness
Fat in Meat is Bad
Avoid Milk Products
Wheat is Good for Bread
Music Distracts the Mind and Strengthens the Vital Powers
Emotional Experiences Cause Marked Changes in the Body
Meditation Decreases Evil Thoughts, Sadness and Woes

If you are a baby boomer or older, you are probably concerned about delaying aging and preventing illness. (But in the meantime, whatever you do, do not get sick in America today!)

Why? Our medical system, insurance companies and governments are soon destined to fail in providing us with quality health care. Skyrocketing health care costs can bankrupt your family and even the entire country. In today's disease-oriented society, most physicians wait until symptoms occur and then treat their patients with hospitalization, surgery and expensive drugs. The cost of this type of care is high. Who's going to pay?

There is no longer a personal interest in the individual. Practice guidelines (algorithms), computers, HMO and PSRO organizations have reduced the practice of medicine to a cookbook process. Managed competition in health care will create a system that provides low cost care for a group as if it were an individual on a budget, limiting the patients' choice of the health care providers treating them.

Where have we gone wrong? Today, we have direct contrast to 1927, when Dr. Francis W. Peabody stated in the *Journal of the American Medical Association* that the most important aspect in the care of the patient is "caring for the patient."

Today, caring for the patient is replaced by acute crisis orientations, living wills, bureaucratic control and insurance company dictates. Gone are the days of empathy, nurturing and real caring.

Today, physicians themselves are disenchanted by a system which dictates to them the guidelines for when, how and where they will care for their patients. Both physicians and their patients have become victims of the same system.

If you are an individual who wants to actively participate in your own health and healing, quality of life and longevity, read on. According to recent statistics, Americans spend over 18 billion dollars on coronary artery by-pass surgery annually. These costs can be significantly reduced.

ACKNOWLEDGMENTS

The research, writing and editing of this book and my earlier book with Lincoln-Bradley, *Lose to Win*, have consumed considerable energies over the last five years. There are several people whose contributions have assisted me in taking these books from a vision to a reality.

Steve Williford, my editor at Lincoln-Bradley, has been especially important to making this project real. His calming influence, professional direction and commitment have helped to make the reading of the books flow. His willingness to travel to my home in Manchester, Connecticut, and work for endless hours is truly appreciated. My vegetarian household was surely a shock to his meat and potato diet. Fortunately, an organic turkey was an amazing grace to his soul.

Julia Molino and *Ellen Lieberman* were instrumental in the contents of the first book. Their contributions of writing and editing were most helpful, particularly with regard to women's issues of love and sexuality.

A special thank you goes to *Jo-Anne Piazza* for her friendship, assistance and guidance in my mission. As president of Optimum Health International, L.L.C., she has endured many hours of hard work and has totally invested her "heart" in our mission. I appreciate her assistant, *Jo-Anne Renna*, who is truly a "jack of all trades." I wish to thank *Susan Graham*, LPN and massage therapist, for her creativity and editing. I also could not have completed this project without the continued support of my office staff. Thank you, *Rosemary Pontillo, Carol Gustamachio, Rebecca Dec* and *Caron Maker*. To *Sun King Wan, M.D.* and *Laurel Gay, P.A.C.*, my cardiological associates who have endured long hours of clinical work as I was preparing this book, I offer my gratitude. To *Donna Chaput* and *Lori Childers*, who assisted with the typing of this book, and to *Peggy Johnson* and *Pat Marolt*, who participated with the first edition of this book, I say "thank you."

Additional and significant thanks go to *Brendan Montano, M.D.*, my good friend, colleague and expert in depression and weight management. Your friendship and support have been instrumental in my growth. To *Jose Mullen, M.D.*, a homeopathic physician who treated my son with homeopathy and love. To *Nicholas Palermo, D.O., Anthony Posteraro, M.D., Lester Kritzer, M.D., Michael Kovalchik, M.D.*, outstanding traditional physicians with open attitudes regarding alternative care. To *Bruce Sobin, M.D.*, an internist and co-owner of my health food store, Natural Rhythms, for your assistance in editing the first book. To *Ronald Buckman, M.D., Joseph Guardino, M.D., Daniel Tardiff, M.D.*, and *Gio Hoang, M.D.*, who believe in nutritional healing, and contributed with the development of my health food store. To *Richard Delany, M.D., F.A.C.C., Harvey Zarren, M.D., F.A.C.C., Bruno Cortis, M.D., Steven Horowitz, M.D., F.A.C.C.*, and *Steven Kunkes, M.D., F.A.C.C.*, cardiological colleagues with parallel belief systems in healing the heart.

To *Arthur B. Landry, Jr., M.D., F.A.C.C.*, my former partner and perhaps the best clinical-traditional cardiologist I ever had the opportunity to work with. Your continued friendship, trust and sincerity I have always treasured.

To *Alexander Lowen, M.D.*, who touched my heart and life and to *Philip Helfaer, Ph.D.*, my bioenergetic trainer and mentor. To *Frank Hladky, M.D.*, and *Virginia Wink-Hilton, Ph.D., Joyce Bellis, John Pierrokos, M.D.*, and the late *John Bellis, M.D.*, all inspirational teachers and psychotherapists that I admire and respect.

To *Hazel Stanley*, my present spiritual guide and advisor - a wise woman with whom I can consult on matters pertaining to the spirit and soul. To my own personal healers, *Ann Dahlberg*, my rolfer, who has worked with my lower back discomfort for the past five years and continues to do so. To my physical therapist, *David Cameron*, who I can always count on when I am in trouble. To my chiropractors, *David Van Hoeyck, D.C.*, and *Sharon Vallone, D.C.*, who give me much physical comfort.

To *Holly Hatch, C.S.W.*, and *Marilyn Anderson, M.A.*, two therapists that heal from their hearts.

To my men's support group, *Bud Harris Stone, Ph.D., John Bustelos, CEO, Jerry Ainsworth, Ph.D., Rod Lane, Ph.D., Paul Nussbaum, M.D.*, and *Doug Gibson, M.D.* Thanks for all of your listening and the feedback from your hearts.

To *Sean Truman* and *George Allen, Ph.D.*, my co-investigators at the University of Connecticut studying the impact of nutritional supplementation relating to mind and body.

To pharmacists *Mel Rich* and *Raj Chopra*, two GMP manufacturers who have helped me realize my goal of developing my own antioxidant and nutritional formulas. Thanks to *Stanley Jankowitz* for pointing me in the direction of these knowledgeable men. You have been extremely supportive and helpful, especially with your knowledge of nutrition. To *Gordon Stagg*, who participated in the development of OHI. To *Fred Mendelsohn* of Environmental Lighting Concepts, Inc., who introduced me to the world of television. To *Tony Little*, a man whose mission on exercise is enhancing the lives of literally millions of people. To *Karen Berney, Marshall Hamilton* and *Dan Kagan* of Phillips Publishing Company, for believing in my mission and giving me the opportunity to write a national newsletter on "The Heart."

To my former wrestling coaches, *Donald Jackson* and the late *Ken Hunte*. Through their warrior activities, I experienced the gift of discipline with the agony and ecstasy of intensive training, hard work and winning.

To my attorneys, *Michael Darby* and *Dominic Squatrito*. Thanks for the endless hours of difficult negotiations and for protecting me in the pursuit of my vision.

Thanks to *Jeannine Cyr-Gluck* and *Elizabeth Marx*, the librarians at Manchester Memorial Hospital who provided me with vital information. To *Anna Salo*, my secretary in the Department of Medical Education.

To *Bev Grady, R.N., Mo Criascia, R.N.*, and *Lisa Holmes, R.N.*, for taking the risks in teaching alternative care.

To *Barbara Palmer* and *Kye Cohen*, who manage my health food store. Thanks for the great food prepared with love.

To my special friends, *Bill and Ursula Niarakis, Tony and Roberta Visconti, Dr. John and Mary Puskas, John and Jean Fleet* and *Drs. Bob and Kathy Lang*. Your continued support of me and my work has been so greatly appreciated.

To my ex-wife, *Suzy Sinatra,* my life-long friend and mother of my children who gave me tremendous support through my early clinical years. To my brother, *Richard,* and my sisters, *Pam* and *Maria.* Your love and encouragement have touched my heart. To my children, *March, Step* and *Drew,* who are such tremendous treasures in my life. You are all lovable "messengers" in your very own unique ways. To *Jan DeMarco, R.N.,* who has been truly helpful in the writing and the editing of both editions of this book. Your continued love and support have been valued and appreciated.

There are many other individuals who contributed to this work, particularly my patients whom I have treated for years. I have grown to love them as we all age through what, sometimes, are difficult and treacherous times. They, undoubtedly, have been my best teachers. Their struggles in battling disease have touched my heart on so many occasions.

TABLE OF CONTENTS

INTRODUCTION
- MY JOURNEY -

As a clinical cardiologist, I have worked with many cases of heart disease. And I am convinced that despite all the studies linking smoking, high levels of blood cholesterol, hypertension and adult diabetes to heart disease, these risk factors, although highly significant, do not fully explain the nature of this illness. Additional research has confirmed the dominant role of psychological, emotional and metabolic stress in heart disease as well.

To appreciate this relationship has become a major challenge for me. It is a challenge which could be understood only when I was willing to veer off the strictly conventional paths of healing. My introduction into true healing emerged during my training as a psychoanalyst. After 12 years of study in both Gestalt and bioenergetic psychotherapy, it became clear to me that pathology (becoming ill) is often a form of dis-ease that emerges from the chaotic imbalance of mind, body and spirit.

My interest in writing this book has been a slowly evolving and growing passion. Over the past 20 years, I have cared for patients struggling with heart-related disease and have come to understand some of the processes that lead to this illness.

When considering illness, diagnosis and treatment, I began to focus not only on the disease and its physical dysfunction, but also on all the human operational planes: the physical, the metabolic, the emotional, the mental and even the spiritual. I soon developed a new appreciation for conscious as well as unconscious drives. I realized that to be on such a journey, I needed to be more in touch with the body's energy systems.

The healthy operation of the human energy system involves both generative and maintenance phases. Adequate formation depends on the intake of sufficient oxygen and essential nutrients. But maintenance of balance is based on more complex variables. A deficiency or an imbalance in any part of the system may contribute, over time, to the impaired functioning of our cells, tissues, organs, and eventually, our bodies. Thus, the concept of energy is both quantitative and qualitative. A proper balance of oxygen and nutritional components, such as vitamins, minerals, enzymes and co-factors, are required for cells to function with ease.

The realization of this relationship in healing ignited my interest to explore the energetic/metabolic/nutritional constituents that make up the whole process of *Optimum Health*.

Just how important is this relationship?

Fact Coronary heart disease is the leading cause of death in the industrialized world.

Fact Cancer is the second leading cause of death.

Fact Coronary heart disease and cancer may be preventable by risk factor modification.

Fact Overweight status is a risk factor for both heart disease and cancer.

Fact The way to good health is a balanced diet, proper weight maintenance, exercise and appropriate nutritional supplementation.

Fact Prevention is easier than cure.

Fact A study recently published in *The Lancet* reported that elderly people taking multivitamins with minerals had improved immune function and had 50 percent fewer sick days.

Fact Increased intakes of antioxidant vitamins (beta carotene, vitamin C, vitamin E) could potentially prevent or postpone 50 to 70 percent of cataracts.

Fact Two studies recently conducted at the Harvard University School of Public Health and Harvard Medical School showed that taking 100 IU/day of vitamin E supplements for more than two years reduced the risk of heart disease by 26 percent in a group of more than 45,000 men, and by 41 percent in a group of more than 85,000 women.

Fact Current environmental toxins such as polluted air, radiation, chemical poisons, heavy metals, auto emissions, cigarette smoke and the increasing usage of fats in our diets boost our need for supplemental nutrients.

Fact   The Harvard Physician Study showed a 44 percent reduction in heart attacks and a 49 percent reduction in strokes for the group given 500 mg of beta carotene every other day. Similar findings in heart disease and strokes were also shown in a large study involving 87,250 nurses over a period of eight years. These studies have shown decreasing trends in the development of cancer as well.

Fact   In a California study, vitamin C intake of greater than 300-500 mg per day suggested increases in life expectancy due to a decrease in heart attacks and various forms of cancer.

Fact   In a Chinese study of 29,000 people, the ingestion of beta carotene, vitamin E and selenium showed a 13 percent reduction in esophageal and gastric cancer and a nine percent reduction in death as compared to the population not taking supplements.

Fact   Clinical research has shown that meditation and/or silent prayer have resulted in blood pressure lowering.

That's why I wrote this book. I'm convinced that life can be healthier for most people than it presently is. I think the message for how to obtain *Optimum Health* and an increased quality of life needs to be shared with as many people as possible. Unfortunately, I can't achieve this goal without some help. One way to get the message out is through this book.

In this book, I focus on how you can nurture the body with nutritional, emotional and spiritual healing. I try to provide simple answers to complex questions on gaining *Optimum Health*. Although healing is truly multifaceted, this book will provide clear guidelines about vitamins, minerals, nutritionals, fat, fiber and cholesterol. There will be valuable concepts about exercise, healing foods and the newest information about anti-aging strategies. I will also demonstrate to you how nutritional supplements can make a difference in your life.

One more thing. I realize that I provide a *lot* of information. Maybe more information than you want to know. I guess because I'm a research-based physician, I want to share as much information as possible with my peers, patients and friends. Let me suggest that you use this book as a handy health-reference. Even though you might not be immediately interested in every area I cover, chances are that one day you'll need it for yourself or someone close to you.

Why Do Some People Get Sick?

Like myself, many physicians have experienced a gradual transition in our approach to illness. We have become interested in the philosophy and psychology of healing and in complementary and alternative care techniques. Still, we need to ask ourselves the question, *What is it that makes some people ill?* For example, why do some people catch the flu in a crowd and others don't? Are there certain constitutional weaknesses in some individuals that make them more vulnerable to events?

I applied this question to the phenomenon of sudden cardiac death. Clinically, this unexpected event occurs as the first symptom of heart disease in up to 40% of the cases. This is a somber statistic for a cardiologist to deal with. As I gained more experience in treating heart disease, it became evident that heart disease is usually a slow process that evolves over time. However, a heart attack may occur at any time and may or may not lead to sudden death.

Your vulnerability to heart attack arises from a combination of traditional risk factors, including stress, emotional arousal, unexpected physical activity, intense psychological and emotional needs, depression and/or dissatisfaction with life. For many, the pathological condition of heart disease is a mosaic with variables of both controllable and uncontrollable risk factors.

The uncontrollable risk factors include family history, gender and age. The controllable risk factors include cigarette smoking, high blood pressure, high cholesterol, sedentary living, obesity, psychological stress and other variables. Many of these risk factors are actually an extension of our personalities and characters. For example, consider that high blood pressure may be related to repressed feelings, particularly anger and rage, and that cardiac arrhythmias may be related to fear, anxiety or panic.

Over the years I have come to appreciate firsthand that illness has strong emotional and psychological components. It is true that for many, coronary heart disease arises from the violation of the laws of nature. For others, however, the disease reflects the unconscious, maladaptive search for one's true self. For many of my patients, heart disease has offered them "an opportunity" to look deeper into their emotional and spiritual beings.

In addition to treating heart attacks with the traditional approach, I am now more interested in and committed to looking for the reasons why the patient developed this heart attack in the first place. I even inquire as to the specific time of the heart attack to look for contributing factors. After recovery, I attend to the patient's nutritional, emotional, psychological and physical needs. We examine together the relationship between a maladaptive lifestyle and heart disease. My role as a physician has transformed into one of seeing and treating the patient as a whole person.

Disease or catastrophic illness has the incredible potential to cause an emotional and psychological shift, bringing the individual to a new awareness of who he or she really is. For many of my patients, heart disease has enlightened them to take what Scott Peck calls *The Road Less Traveled*. Simply put, this is spirituality in the healing process. I have spent many tender moments with my patients as they gained new insights into themselves. Some even begin to see their heart disease as a "gift," moving them to a higher level.

STRESS AND ILLNESS

Is the heart just a pump to push blood around the body? Or is it a place for thoughts, emotions, passions and feelings, as the poets say? Finding the answers has been my quest now for over 20 years of medicine and 15 years of bioenergetic analysis.

Early in my practice, I noticed that many of my patients experienced high levels of stress. I began to research this correlation. Later, I published some of my findings on the relationship between stress and disease, with particular application to the heart, in medical journals.

I have found my patients to be my best teachers. As a result, I realized that I needed to pursue specialized training in the field of psychotherapy. The more I read, the more I wanted to know. The connection between mind, emotion and heart became more clear to me, but I still needed to put it all together. The missing piece was the study of one's character, including my own.

My investigation further convinced me that the power of emotions is directly related to health and illness. The study of the relationship between the mind and body is so vast and intricate that the more I pursued these relationships, the more inadequate I felt. The subject was broad, unexplored and, at the time, relatively untapped.

Although initial research discussed the relationship between stress and illness, and personality and heart disease, there was little data available on the development of character and its effect on subsequent cardiac illness. I wanted to know if there was something beyond Type-A behavior.

Was Type-A behavior just a symptom of one's personality? Was there something more profound, undiscovered and worthy of further analysis? Might this be the missing link?

I had begun my search for causative factors that may have the potential to render one vulnerable to heart disease. The identification and modification of these character traits for enhancing and prolonging life became my purpose. This is why, as a traditionally trained cardiologist, I decided to later become a psychotherapist as well. (To my knowledge, I am the only certified Cardiologist and certified Bioenergetic Psychotherapist in the world.)

Bioenergetic therapy is a psychoanalytically-based therapy originating from the works of Wilhelm Reich. Reich, an Austrian psychiatrist and a student of Freud, proposed that love and a healthy sexuality could cure the ills of mankind. Reich was known for his writings on the "relationship of disease, emotions and the denial or absence of pleasure." He described cancer as a resignation from life. He believed that cancer originates because of the unreleased feelings of sadness and anger that cause depression.

Recently, it has been verified that emotions do play a major role in cancer. Bernie Siegel, in his book, *Love, Medicine, and Miracles*, discusses the cancer personality as being one who is stuck and unwilling to give up. Siegel says that "fighting back" through releasing anger and suppressed feeling, as well as forgiving and loving the self, visualizing the self overcoming the enemy cancer within, is the way to heal.

Alexander Lowen has spent a lifetime expanding Reich's theory and developing his own. As a student of Reich's, Lowen created the therapy called bioenergetics, a body-oriented analytic therapy focusing on the muscular tensions in the body that are the physical counterparts of the emotional conflict in the personality.

In bioenergetic analysis, the therapist can determine where tension is located and where energy is blocked. By utilizing various techniques and exercises to charge and discharge the body, the bioenergetic therapist can release trapped energy, which allows for dissipation of tension.

Lowen's theory incorporating emotional conflict and physical expression in the disease model so appealed to me that I decided to study under him in a program of self-exploration and psychotherapy. I was particularly struck by Lowen's focus on breathing in his approach to body therapy. It became more apparent to me that energy and breathing were related to heart disease. I have seen the "inability to breathe" and restricted breathing patterns in many of my coronary patients. For example, many of us have noticed aggressive, coronary-prone individuals suck in air during conversations (even while continuing to speak) and exhale brief sighs and/or muffled grunts when breathing out. This disturbance in respiration becomes a charged, nonpulsating energetic cycle which makes it hard to relax while breathing. Many of these patients also tend to hold their breath as well. Such respiratory motility problems cause rigidity and chest wall tension.

Thus, learning to breathe is an essential ingredient in obtaining *Optimum Health*. Why? Because deeper, fuller breathing not only increases the physical amount of oxygen needed to drive the body's metabolic processes, but it also assuages tissue spasticities and releases tension. By freeing up blocked feelings and emotions, breathing gets the body in touch with feeling. As a psychotherapist, I have seen many patients perform deep breathing exercises and experience more feeling with subsequent emotional release and crying. This, in itself, is healing. Breathing is thus the focus of any body-oriented therapy. Personally, I learned the value of deep and fuller respirations both in my own bioenergetic therapy with Lowen and in a program of rolfing. I decided to enter a rolfing program to further my healing after my father died of a ruptured aorta.

Rolfing is an intense body therapy aimed at loosening up deep tissue spasticities by direct myofacial massage. Rolfing, deep tissue work and massage are all excellent therapies designed to get you in touch with your body and its feelings. I still continue to have monthly rolfing sessions. In addition to loosening up the spasticities in my lower back and pelvis, rolfing also assuages the sympathetic nervous system. Like meditation, yoga, tai-chi, and qi-gong, rolfing is an alternative therapy with considerable merit in healing the body.

Alternative medical care is in direct contrast to allopathic care, or traditional care, which relies on acute crisis intervention, pharmacology, surgery and other various "cookbook" approaches to treat the underlying disorder. For example, the cardiologist treats an acute heart attack with a multitude of drugs and invasive interventions. In an emergency, such traditional therapies are life-saving for the patient. However, in non-emergency situations, you have many options from which to choose.

The Allopathic Medical Model

The standard allopathic model is crisis-oriented or, in simple terms, a Band-Aid fix. Consider the use of aspirin for a headache. Although aspirin may give you some relief for the headache, why the headache occurred or how to prevent the headache, in most cases, is not really examined. The typical model of medicine in this country is based on fixing and administering relief with pharmacological, surgical and other interventions.

For example, many heart patients rely on bypass or angioplasty alone to prevent further attacks. Although these treatments may buy time for the patient to heal himself or herself, *bypass and angioplasty procedures are not cures.* They are only "aspirin for a headache." In heart disease, the real healing needs to take place after the bypass or angioplasty. Unfortunately, many patients do not understand preventive medicine and are not coached properly by their physicians.

Even with physicians' advice, patients must assume personal responsibility for healing. Many of my patients put considerable pressure on me, requesting an "instant cure." They rely on my knowledge and experience in the use of pharmacological agents and want the "magic bullet" to end their suffering. In these instances, my patients wish to relinquish their power to me. Although this is an adequate system for some, for many, this medical model simply does not work.

I had my own family experience of how a straightforward medical model can be insufficient. Both of my sons have struggled with asthma since they were six years old. I noted, at times, that their asthmatic attacks were precipitated by emotional stress. They were often most vulnerable when there was no outlet for their frustration, hurt or anger. At other times, there were obvious infectious or environmental precipitants that triggered what was often an emotionally terrifying experience for them, the abrupt inability to breathe.

My oldest son, Step, had asthma from age six to 14. His condition was treated with traditional medicine, i.e., occasional antibiotics, steroids and various sprays to open up his airways. Although his health care providers performed skin tests and allergy shots, there was no investigation of nutritional, emotional or psychological concerns. When he could not breathe, he became powerless. He was totally reliant on allopathic techniques to improve his breathing.

One day, my son had a powerful realization while sitting in the doctor's office. He looked around the room, observing other children clinging onto their parents' arms as they awaited their turn to see the physician. I am sure these children must have been fearful of the many needle procedures they would have to endure. But Step, as a 14-year old, interpreted these behaviors in a different light. Step said he "made a decision that day." He came to the realization that he did not want to be "like those other kids . . . victims, scared, weak and dependent on everyone else." I believe my son had a major "aha" that day in his own personal growth. He made a decision that he was not going to use his sprays, pills or even obtain any further allergy shots. When he discussed this with me, I offered him my whole-hearted support.

Step made a conscious decision, and with it he changed his life. Following this internal commitment to be well, he had perhaps one or two minor flare-ups of his condition. To this day, he has been completely free of any asthmatic bronchitis. My son was able to cure himself by accessing his own inner healing ability. Recently, Step discussed this experience with Drew, my youngest son. Drew motivated his own inner healer in a similar way, using his power to promote healing. He, like Step, found the courage to heal himself.

HEALING AND EMPOWERMENT

Getting well requires a mobilization of man's intrinsic forces against disease. We must remember the great physicians of history: nature, time and patience. Paracelsus, a physician during the reformation, stated, "Nature cures; the doctor only nurses." The physician and the patient must share in the healing process. Patients have the power to enhance healing, but it is the role of the physician to help stimulate and nurture the power that the patient possesses.

Learning how to empower others is a process I learned in athletics. One powerful experience comes to mind. It was the last wrestling dual meet during my senior year in high school. Although I was undefeated in dual meet competitions, my opponent from our rival high school was not only undefeated, but was also the team's best wrestler and team captain. During this school year, we both had combined records of 26 and 0.

I can remember my fellow high school classmates anticipating and talking about this match for weeks. For three days prior to the competition, I couldn't sleep. My fear of losing was overwhelming. After the weigh-in and just prior to the start of the meet, my coach called me over. He said, "Sinatra, you are the captain for this meet."

A chill ran through my body. I knew the coach had his favorites which he placed in the awesome position of captain for a dual meet. Perhaps I had not yet been worthy of leading our team into battle. But after he chose me, my excitement peaked. Just prior to the introductions, my opponent and I walked out on the mat, shook hands and looked eyeball to eyeball.

For the first time, I felt that I was on his level. Now we were on equal footing: both captains, both undefeated and both highly motivated to win. My coach had empowered me with this small but extremely important gesture. He gave me that little extra confidence I needed to win and remain undefeated.

Although later in Division I Collegiate Wrestling I defeated nationally ranked opponents, my last high school wrestling match was my greatest and most difficult. After the referee raised my hand in a 7-5 decision, I was so exhausted and "out-of-my-head," I actually walked over to the wrong bench and sat down! I really didn't know where I was. It was probably embarrassing, but I didn't care. I had given 110% of myself and stretched my exhaustion and fatigue to the utmost limit. After I returned to my own bench, my coach just smiled and told me to sit down.

Just as a good coach can take an athlete to a higher level in self-confidence and achievement, a good physician can help a patient to regain balance, health and life. Like a coach, a physician has to believe in the patient and make the patient believe that the opponent, heart disease, can be defeated. You, and only you, can make it happen. My 20 years of medicine have reinforced one thing more than anything else - it takes a combination of nature and the patient's inner healer to win, or cure the heart. A good physician will promote the power inherent in every patient to regain his own balance to health.

Unfortunately, the sick person may not perceive it this way. The difficult reality to the physician is that the patients often feel that the sickness or discomfort come only from the outside. The more sick they become, the more they believe the sickness is caused by external forces. In this belief system, patients are vulnerable to becoming victims of the illness; stuck, fearful, confused, withdrawn, upset and even despairing. They can't figure out why they cannot get "fixed." In this desperation, patients unconsciously seek out physicians, hoping the doctors will agree with their conclusions . Sometimes, a "magic bullet" like Penicillin works for a strep throat or pneumonia, and real healing does take place.

It is almost mandatory and essential to choose such a "bullet" to help ease the patient's suffering. If the patient has a positive expectation and faith in the physician's remedy, often more positive results will occur. This may be due to a combination of choosing the right agent, and the optimistic charge of both the patient and the doctor. Sometimes, remedies also work as a "placebo effect." Regardless of how the healing takes place, both the patient and the physician are satisfied.

However, if the remedy fails, patients will often blame their health providers for failing to "cure." Sometimes, patients will go to multiple physicians, or "doctor shop," hoping that someone will find the solution and save him or her. Such recurrent failures set the stage for total dependence and powerlessness. The power of the patient to heal himself or herself is soon lost to the perceived power of others.

In this disturbed co-dependency, energy grows stagnant. Thinking becomes limited. A division occurs between thinking and feeling, mind and body. The natural pulsatile flow of energy is disrupted. Although the healer may have some influence over the disease the patient is confronting, it is the patient's willingness to take responsibility for his own healing that is crucial. The physician and the patient must share and collaborate in the healing process. Patients, indeed, have within themselves the power to enhance healing. Physicians must help the patients find, stimulate and nurture that power.

IMPORTANCE OF MULTIPLE HEALING TECHNIQUES

Physicians, in general, have large egos. It takes a strong ego to survive medical school and vigorous post graduate training. But sometimes our greatest confidence can be our greatest weakness. The need for the physician to "be right" may get in the way of healing. I have a problem with doctors who tell their patients "vitamins are worthless," "therapy does not work" or "cardiac rehabilitation is a waste of time." I have heard these scenarios over and over from my patients. I have even seen cardiologists "fire" their patients for taking nutritional supplements. On the other hand, it is genuinely touching when a physician approaches me to inquire about targeted nutritional supplementation, supportive psychotherapy and emotional release.

Many times, my journey has been a lonely one. I often face rejection from my peers, antagonism and even criticism for "not following the standard of care." At times, I have felt hurt, shamed and even humiliated by these remarks. And yet, I believe that I have offered my patients treatment that goes far beyond the traditional standard of care. When necessary, I recommend cardiac catheterization, angioplasty and even bypass surgery for my patients - often, as much as my colleagues. But I firmly believe that complementary therapies - vitamins, antioxidants, nutritionals, psychotherapy, mental imagery, rolfing, martial arts, meditation, etc., when combined with traditional medicine, go well beyond what has been established as the standard of care.

After all my years of study and personal experience, I believe I would be doing my patients a disservice not to offer them the opportunity to select from all that I have learned. Not to recommend alternative therapies, for me, would be to offer less than what I know might be the best potential standard of care.

But although I have had some sadness and despair during my journey, I still have much hope and optimism about my profession. Some physicians are remarkable in their continued openness and desire to keep learning new things. As physicians, we must be open to the metaphor, "Lose to Win," by giving up some of the old while being vulnerable enough to go out on a limb and consider some of the not so "sophisticated" healing therapies.

Therefore, as a cardiologist, I use multiple healing techniques. When catastrophic illness has become a major threat, mobilizing the patient's inner healer is of critical importance. Consider, for example, the traditional treatment of cancer.

Radiation and chemotherapy are not magical cures; their justification is that they kill cancer cells. The physician must continually balance potential gain (death of cancer cells) with potential loss (killing of normal cells). The negative side of chemotherapy is that it damages our working immune system, the body's own method for combating cancer cells, infections and other diseases. This additional burden on the body's own defense system can indirectly leave the patient vulnerable to secondary infections, illnesses and rapidly multiplying cancer cells. Such a case comes to mind from my internship at Albany Medical Center in 1972.

I was treating a middle-aged male in his early 50s who had been recently diagnosed with lung cancer. Previously a heavy smoker, he unfortunately developed a large unresectible tumor in his right lung. His prognosis was grim to say the least. I remember the oncologist's instructions to give him a powerful but toxic chemotherapy agent called Cytoxin. After the administration of the anti-cancer drug, the patient died within 36 hours due to overwhelming infection and shock. Although this gentleman would have ultimately succumbed to the invasion of cancer, the fact remains that the antidote used in this case hastened his death.

Fortunately, many patients experience life-extensions through the use of chemotherapeutic agents. But oftentimes with exhausting and debilitating side effects. Like chemotherapy, radiation also destroys normal tissue adjacent to cancer cells with the same undirected voracity that it attacks cancer cells. The body is left with the monumental task of repairing healthy as well as diseased tissue. It is the wise physician who recognizes the need to counteract the negative impact of traditional medicines, chemotherapy and radiation by strengthening the body and its immune system. This necessitates a high level of nutrition as well as freedom from stress, tension and depression.

In addition, mobilizing the patient's will to live and inspiring hope are critical strategies in combating catastrophic illness. Techniques integrated in the field of alternative medicine offer the physician an array of tools to engage the body's inner healer in a mind/body and spirit approach to illness.

Recent studies performed at Ohio State University found that highly depressed, nonpsychotic patients had significantly poorer DNA repair in immune cells exposed to radiation than their less depressed counterparts. Both depressed groups fared significantly poorer in DNA repair than the psychologically healthy nondepressed group. These findings suggest that depression or emotional stress may contribute to the incidence of cancer by directly diminishing immune surveillance and integrity. Lifting the patient out of depression is not easy, but neither is it beyond reach. Again, healing requires a totally integrated approach to the mind, body and spirit.

Researchers are now acknowledging that the mental processes that can cause disease may be redirected for healing. Jean Achterberg, a pioneer in mental imagery, believes that nature has created few one-way processes. If we can become ill through mental stress in our lives, we must also have the inherent power to improve health with the use of purposeful and positive mental processes. Positive imagery has been shown to stimulate lymphocytes, T-cells (natural killer cells) and neutrophils. According to research, imagery can also help reduce levels of adrenal corticosteroids in high-stress individuals. It alleviates emotional strain and reduces physical pain while altering the course of disease and improving the individual's outlook on his or her illness.

As a cardiologist, I rarely treat cases of cancer. However, some cancer patients have approached me, requesting my assistance in participating in their healing. In addition to the emotional support that I can give, I recommend a broad nutritional approach which includes elimination of long-chained fatty acids, i.e., arachidonic acid. I also recommend a Vegan diet of no animal proteins or dairy products. A great fuel for cancer cells are the long-chained fatty acids found in animal protein and dairy products. If you can eliminate the fuel, you may stifle the cancer growth. I also recommend vitamins, minerals, Co Enzyme Q_{10} and glutathione, which I will discuss in a subsequent analysis. For example, L-Arginine, which will be discussed in the section on aging, has been used with success in breast cancer.

Because L-Arginine stimulates T lymphocytes and enhances the body's natural killing mechanisms, this simple nutritional approach may be used as adjuvant therapy in breast cancer when used with traditional approaches. When the body's own responses are mobilized together with the cancer-fighting techniques of modern medicine, the combination can frequently bring about remarkable results.

Treating an illness or dysfunction is not just treating a part of the body. In other types of healing, such as alternative, naturopathic or homeopathic care, the healer involves the patient with a holistic approach. For example, the healer may investigate not only the physical expression of the illness, but also the emotional, psychological, nutritional, metabolic and in some cases, the spiritual ramifications of it. Thus, a holistic approach provides an understanding of the patient and his or her illness in terms of the whole patient.

Nowadays, the treatment of dysfunction requires an investigation of mind, body and spirit. For example, consider my own medical school training.

In the 1970s, the training of physicians focused on pathology, illness and treatment. "Preventive medicine" had no place in medical schools at that time. Interactions between the psyche (the mind) and the soma (the body) were yet to be considered. Our course work on nutrition included minimal instruction on fat, fiber and cholesterol in heart disease and cancer. We also studied the harmful effects of alcohol in the body, and some instruction included B vitamin supplementation.

However, there was no education about processed foods, environmental toxins, the impact of polluted water, the health hazards of heavy metal toxicity and the treacherous leakage of radiation poisoning the environment. There was minimal education about the perils of vitamin and mineral deficiency. As a young physician, my own understanding of nutrition was very little. It received no emphasis at medical school, internship, medical residency or even my fellowship in cardiology. It became a big void in my training as a physician. Not until the latter part of the 1970s, when the Framingham data was released, was high cholesterol recognized as a major contributor to heart disease.

Since preventive medicine was not taught, my traditional medical training in the early 70s was consumed with struggles of health and illness. There was also very little time for the investigation of why people became sick. I focused on comforting the sick and attempting to slow down or terminate the diseases they already had. Pharmacological agents became my first line of treatment. After all, the medical profession became drug-oriented after the discovery of Penicillin in the 1940s. My training emphasized disease models and treatment plans with the multitude of pharmacological agents that were available to me.

I trained extensively in a traditional Western medical model of health and disease. I studied hard, worked long hours and often played the "midnight hero" in many highly charged medical dramas. Although I enjoyed my work and felt highly competent in what I was doing, I was somehow not fulfilled. Something was missing in my role of a physician and healer. As battling illness began to take its toll, I searched for missing links in the quest for healing. In my studies as a psychotherapist, I began to appreciate the deeper process in which health is maintained, lost, regained and often lost again. I began to direct my energies more toward preventative medicine, looking deeper into lifestyle, eating habits, emotional factors, nutritional needs and relationship needs. Over time, I began to realize that I was becoming an allopathic physician in recovery.

Obesity and Heart Disease

Similarly, I have experienced a transformation in my work with overweight patients. As a director of a weight loss program at Manchester (CT) Memorial Hospital, I have worked as both a physician and pyschotherapist with many obese individuals on a long-term basis. In this program, the overweight individuals fasted on liquids for several weeks.

Juicing, vitamins and minerals and behavioral modification were all components of the program. Exercise was also a vital component in weight reduction. As a therapist for a group of 21 participants, I witnessed first-hand that weight loss is more than just a physical struggle.

Obesity often has its roots in emotional issues. Eating disorders are critically linked to the emotions involving self-esteem, love, acceptance and even sexuality. I was indeed fortunate to be the leader of a courageous group of men and women. We spent six months together for three-hour sessions on a weekly basis. They taught me invaluable lessons about the emotional and psychological issues behind weight loss and weight gain. I also learned that obesity is a very common metabolic disturbance in humans.

I noticed that many of my participants oftentimes became "stuck" when they lost 30, 40 or 50 pounds. If the patient was not stuck emotionally on a sexual or relationship issue, the halt was frequently due to a metabolic condition. These individuals needed an additional boost or "jump start" in their body. Frequently, I used nutritional interventions, such as zinc, vitamin B-6, Co Enzyme Q_{10}, chromium picolinate and other herbs and supplements. Although some individuals needed more intense psychological counseling and/or an advanced exercise program, many needed only a simple metabolic adjustment. As in heart disease, the approach to obesity includes a dietary/nutritional approach, as well as an approach involving emotional, psychological and physical factors.

There is absolutely no reason for people to develop heart disease or other illnesses due to an overweight condition. Unfortunately, overweight status is still a primary contributor to major diseases such as high blood pressure, diabetes, heart disease and even some cancers. A healthy diet not only will improve weight status, but also will protect you as well.

IMPROVING DAILY NUTRITION

Changing your lifestyle can add years to your life, prevent illness and lower the cost of medical care. Improving daily nutrition, exercise and a well-planned program of targeted nutritional supplementation can prevent illness and improve quality of life. There is an information explosion about the healing properties of naturally occurring elements in vegetables, fresh fruits and fish. God nurtures us with foods that heal.

Phytonutrients stimulate healing. The following food healing information is of critical concern to every human being alive on the planet.

Onions contain quercetin, which prevents bad cholesterol from harming our bodies as well as being an excellent natural antihistamine, which I've used in the treatment of my child's asthma.

Broccoli contains sulphoraphane which helps prevent cancer.

Similarly, **cabbage** has isothiocyanates, which also help prevent cancer.

Mackerel, sardines and salmon are abundant in Co Enzyme Q_{10}, a miracle nutrient for the heart.

Anchovies and fish foods have DMAE, a substance known to improve one's memory. For years, folklore has touted fish as a brain food. Now we learn that folklore was fact instead of myth.

Asparagus contains folic acid, a vital nutrient for young women anticipating getting pregnant. Folic acid has also been discovered to prevent heart disease, especially in the elderly.

There are literally thousands of **flavonoids** and hundreds of **carotenoids** that will prevent and even cure illnesses and diseases. Popeye didn't know it, but **spinach** contains lutein, a bioflavonoid that's vital in healing advanced macular degeneration of the retina, which is the leading cause of blindness in the United States.

It is so important for us to learn from the nutritional secrets hidden in common foods and become aware of the dangers of preservatives and additives in processed products. A diet rich in foods and nutrients that heal may well be our best line of defense against the country's environmental and degenerative killers, such as cancer, heart disease and autoimmune disorders. In an age where our bodies are ravaged by the effects of environmental toxins, stress, cancer-causing chemicals and the passage of time, how can we defend ourselves? Our diet is one of the most powerful weapons in our arsenal. As trite as it sounds - you *really* are what you eat!

NUTRITIONAL SUPPLEMENTATION

After my previous book on nutrition, my path took me into another area of growth - targeted nutritional supplementation. Nutritional health can be deceptive.

Consider that many of us lack such necessary natural nutrients as magnesium, Co Enzyme Q_{10}, B vitamins, flavonoids, etc. A deficiency of any of these components will impair the healthy functioning of the cell, resulting in disrupted pulsation and, ultimately, disease. Such a deficiency, often undetected or unsuspected in many of us, contributes year after year, to the impaired functioning of our cells/bodies.

Consider, for example, the treatment of depression. We all know how valuable cognitive and body-oriented psychotherapy are in mobilizing both insight and energy. However, many cases of depression require additional neurotransmitters that can be supplied by specific types of psychotropic medicines.

A large majority of cases (up to 70%) are deficient in magnesium. Therefore, without this type of cellular support, standard psychotherapy alone would obviously be inadequate in the approach to the whole person. It would be like treating only one-half of the problem. Again, it is this comprehensive mind/body approach in realizing the full potential of healing that continues to ignite my interest in investigating the metabolic and nutritional constituents that together integrate the process of *Optimal Health.*

Many people have asked me why I took on the overwhelming project of designing vitamin and mineral formulas. Actually, during the writing of my book, *Lose to Win,* in the late 1980s-early 1990s, I became a firm believer in vitamins, minerals and antioxidants. Previously, my traditional, allopathic thinking inclined me to have a strong negative bias against these essentials; however, when I researched the sound scientific principles behind vitamins, minerals and antioxidants, I started taking preparations myself. I tried many combinations. I started taking beta carotene, vitamin E, selenium, Co Enzyme Q_{10}, chromium, L-Carnitine, quercetin, bromelain and various herbs.

In fact, I counted at least 12 to 15 bottles on my shelf, and was literally taking between 25 and 30 pills a day. "This is crazy!" I thought. There had to be a better method, preferably one in which all those ingredients were integrated into one combination.

In addition, I began to recommend these same nutrients to my patients. The complexity and expense were more than most of them could tolerate. Many of them asked if there wasn't just one pill that contained all these ingredients. Again, with my patients as my motivators and my messengers, I began another search. After finding the right chemists, pharmacists and GMP Manufacturers with outstanding delivery systems, I developed several state of the art formulas with variations.

Although I felt confident about taking vitamin and mineral supplements, I was amazed to find that there were many preparations that contained ingredients that would not enhance health and healing. Some, I believe, were even dangerous. The formulas I developed contain no iron or copper. There are also no preservatives, fillers, hydrogenated oils, dyes or harmful substances that could disrupt cellular functions.

In addition to supplementation we must also keep in mind the recommendations made by the National Cancer Institute, such as consuming five to nine fresh fruits and vegetables a day. Although I try to do this on a daily basis, sometimes I find eating this many fruits and vegetables is absolutely impossible. Therefore, I take my daily vitamin and mineral supplement that makes up for this deficit.

I began to read everything I could get my hands on. I became intrigued with the healing properties of bioflavonoids, carotenoids and a multitude of vital nutrients found in fresh fruits and vegetables. These nutrients not only enhance healing, but also prevent diseases. I felt the need to incorporate such nutrients into my own formulas. I was learning new things at a remarkable rate. The more I learned, the more inadequate I felt. I began to do computer searches into the medical literature, discovering literally hundreds of articles dealing with targeted nutritional aspects of health and healing, as I continue to do today. Sometimes when my eyes were tired, I would reach for more spinach, hoping to revitalize the energy in my eyes!

ANTI-AGING

As I progressed in my research, I became so excited about my growth that I found myself breaking out of the constraints of private practice. So little was understood by my peers, I felt responsible and enthusiastic to make myself more available for teaching other health professionals about nutritional, metabolic and emotional healing. Consequently, I lectured frequently throughout the U.S. and Europe, instructing physicians over the last ten years. In December of 1994, I experienced a new level of awe and education.

I was lecturing in Las Vegas, Nevada, at the second annual Anti-Aging Conference with Dr. Bob Goldman and Dr. Ronald Klatz, two prolific pioneers in anti-aging medicine. My contribution was on *Aging, Exercise, Nutrition and the Heart.* Attending other talks and meeting with researchers, I developed a new excitement. This conference was indeed provocative! It opened my eyes to new developments in aging, health and healing. Although I have been very comfortable with taking vitamins, minerals, antioxidants and Co Enzyme Q_{10} for years, I had never really investigated the anti-aging supplements such as DHEA (dehydroepiandosterone sulphate), melatonin, DMAE, etc.

I was shocked to find that many university professors were not only taking vitamins and minerals, but also consuming these anti-aging supplements as well. I also met researchers who presented well substantiated data and insights into anti-aging technologies. I became excited about nutritional and metabolic approaches to aging. After all, aren't the degenerative diseases of the this century really forms of premature aging?

I now know, for example, that premature heart disease and various forms of cancer, autoimmune diseases and Alzheimer's are really entities of premature aging. As I again began to reconsider my patient population in the light of my new understanding of aging, this experience re-emphasized that specific nutritional and dietary deficiencies are rampant in our population.

There are very serious, yet preventable, health problems in this country. However, in today's existing medical system, the prevention of disease and health problems continues to take a back seat to the treatment of existing diseases. My mission and my path is to make people aware of how they can directly optimize their health, ward off disease and live a healthier life. By raising consciousness and initiating a healthy preventive lifestyle, individuals can literally prevent premature aging and the diseases of this century.

CONTINUING HEART EDUCATION

After lecturing to health professionals during the winter of 1994, I was approached by Phillips Publishing Company in Potomac, Maryland. I was recruited as an editor for a national newsletter, *HeartSense,* that incorporates traditional, complementary and alternative methods in healing the heart. I had previously been impressed with the impact of Dr. Julian Whitaker's newsletter, *Health & Healing.* Whitaker's innovative approach to preventative medicine had reached hundreds of thousands of readers across the country. I believe that he made a difference in many of their lives. He probably even reduced the cost of health care as well. I decided to author the Phillip's newsletter. I can only hope that this opportunity will enable me, like Whitaker, to provide readers with monthly, up-to-date information about healing the heart and discovering *Optimum Health.*

This book focuses on nurturing the body with nutritional, emotional and spiritual healing. It provides simple answers to complex questions to lead the reader to *Optimum Health*. Although healing is truly multifaceted, this book will provide clear guidelines about vitamins, minerals, nutritionals, fat, fiber and cholesterol. There are valuable concepts about exercise, healing foods and the newest information about anti-aging strategies. I will also demonstrate to you how nutritional supplements can make a difference in your life, and also include a special section regarding women and children.

You will investigate the nuts and bolts of nutrition as well as the real reasons behind obesity and why we can't lose weight. Excess weight is on the surface, manifesting itself in a "body armor," but being overweight is just another way that the body sends a signal to the mind for the need to heal itself emotionally, physically and spiritually. The emotional issues of obesity are indeed deep and buried in the personality. Some portions of the text will elicit an emotional response from you: hope, inspiration, sadness, fear or anger. The content may challenge you to seek the core of your weight problem.

This book is not merely a self-help manual; it is about expanding one's consciousness. Today is a time of awareness, of taking responsibility for one's self and living in harmony with one's body.

Although you can lead a horse to water, the rest is up to the horse. Similarly, I believe this book can lead you to a new consciousness and awareness that will make a difference in the quality and even longevity of your life. Take this journey with me to an exciting new plateau of awareness and health. The rest is up to you!

Chapter One

EIGHT SIMPLE RULES FOR OPTIMUM HEALTH

Roger Buffaloe is a man who several years ago, while only in his mid-30s, weighed nearly 400 pounds. Roger Buffaloe is now a man who weighs 186 pounds, as he has for the past several years. How did he come to weigh so much and how is it that after years of dieting (and failing) he finally lost over 200 pounds? What caused Roger to become obese and why couldn't he stop eating excessively? Roger is an example of many overweight people in our society who are morbidly obese (40 percent or more above desirable weight). Four out of every ten Americans are overweight (20 percent or more above desired weight), and one out of five, or 34 million adults, is obese. There has been much discussion about obesity among the medical community. Books have been written on the psychological, the behavioral and the systemic causes of obesity.

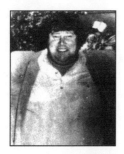 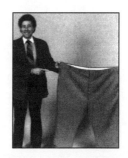

I can't say there is not a comprehensive program that addresses all of these concerns—there are many. You may have tried some of them. But if they haven't worked for you in the past, read on. Let's review the contributing factors to overeating so we all can have an understanding of the basis of eating disorders and begin at the same point. First of all, *stop feeling guilty*. Regardless of whether you are ten pounds or 200 pounds overweight, don't beat yourself up saying, "I shouldn't have; I must stop myself; I must have control; I must deny myself pleasure in the short term in order to gain long-term results."

RULE NUMBER ONE: DENIAL OF PLEASURE CAN LEAD TO OBESITY AND EARLY DEATH

"Well," you might say, "I can understand how eating disorders can lead to early death, but how can denial of pleasure?" As a cardiologist and psychotherapist, it is easy for me to see that self-denial can cause extreme unhappiness that sets up stress and heartbreak that lead to heart disease and, frequently, death. *Denial of love, denial of human contact, and denial of emotional outlets clog the system just as surely as do fats and cholesterol!*

Always doing what we "think" is best, not acting on what we truly feel, stopping ourselves from doing what we always wanted because of fear of rejection or loss, or denying ourselves the simple sensual pleasures of life that came so easily in childhood stops the natural flow of energy that we depend on as our very life force. Just as stagnant water can become poisonous and toxic, blocking our intentions, feelings, intuition, pleasures and desires can be equally as toxic, leading to frustration, unhappiness, despair and, eventually, denial.

When we approach weight loss, one of two things usually happens:

1. We deny ourselves the pleasures of eating, and through a series of small victories and perhaps one or two slip ups, we lose weight. Great! But denial of pleasure breeds resentment and resentment harbors contempt, fostering feelings of guilt and frustration.

2. Because our view of food is seen as friend or enemy, small setbacks are seen as failures. We give up in defeat vowing to start anew tomorrow or we binge and cry that we might as well be fat and fulfilled. Wrong. We might be physically full, but we are not emotionally fulfilled. We are

guilty and self-loathing and these unforgiving feelings start the cycle of denial all over again.

This is what happened to Roger Buffaloe at nearly 400 pounds. How could he possibly feel anything but absolute denial? He also learned that complete denial leads to complete failure. We must allow ourselves foods that we enjoy, but in a manner that is reasonable. Less can be more. I suggest *awareness* over denial. As Roger now realizes, if he eats a piece of bread without butter, he can have more bread than if he eats it with butter. This is awareness. This is choice. And it's not deprivation. He can still eat bread, preferably a high-fiber, textured, whole-grain variety that will give him a satisfied, full feeling without doing damage to the body.

Weight loss and healthy eating require a true commitment to awareness and reaching a level of consciousness that supports self-nurturance. This can be done without denial of pleasure. People who gain weight and then lose the weight, only to regain it back again develop a yo-yo syndrome that does not work. The approach to weight loss is finding foods that not only taste good, but also are nurturing to your body.

Recently, my friends and I had a celebratory dinner that was entirely low-fat, yet as delicious as any Thanksgiving dinner I've had. The menu consisted of roasted turkey, fresh green and yellow beans, a pasta salad, a salad of cucumbers and tomatoes and bread. We ended the meal with fresh fruit pies. Because the rest of the meal was low-fat, I chose not to deprive myself and to have a small piece of pie, though I realized that the crust of the pie was probably made with lard, a pure animal fat frequently used in baking. A two-inch piece of pie contains ten to 15 grams of fat, which was more than the entire meal I just consumed. The American Heart Association recommends a daily diet of no more than 65 grams of fat a day for an average sized man such as myself. Since the meal contained minimal fat, I was able not to deprive myself, with the awareness that the total fat content for this meal, including the "forbidden" pie, was only about 20 grams! This is eating with awareness. This is curative. And this is healing.

On the other hand, a typical fast-food meal, including a double cheeseburger, french fries, a shake, and an apple pie, contains an alarming 70-80 grams of fat! And this is only one meal. If this lifestyle were continued, one could conceivably eat 200–225 grams of fat a day! This is not only "fattening," but dangerous!

RULE NUMBER TWO: FORGIVE YOURSELF

If we allow ourselves a little bit of what we are being denied, in a program of awareness we can become masters of our own enjoyment and be fulfilled. (More on this later as we get into "how." For now, let's stick with "why.") If we are unable to stay within the contained means and do indeed overeat, and we continue to berate ourselves, we only add to feelings of failure and self-doubt. On the other hand, if we can allow some leeway for human frailty, we can begin anew.

Let's not kid ourselves, though. Eating our favorite foods in a contained environment isn't always easy. A taste of ice cream may lead to an entire bowl. But rather than requiring willpower or discipline, Roger found the key was forgiving himself and getting support from others. Roger was, and is, extremely disciplined in many ways. He overcame a learning disability to teach himself how to read after quitting high school because he was labeled "fat and stupid." Having managed a business at only 16 years old and turning it from a Mom and Pop shop into a very profitable venture, he received his high school equivalency degree and later became a highly successful businessman. Roger never lacked willpower. But he did lack support. His teachers thought he was dumb and lazy. His father criticized him for making poor grades and his mother just didn't understand what could be the problem with his weight and lack of control over his appetite.

Frequently, overweight adults come from families where achieving was more important than being - where there was little acceptance of the children as they really were because they were not as their parents wanted them to be. Does this mean we should blame our parents for not giving us unconditional love? Not necessarily. They probably received similar treatment from their parents, or from a society that encouraged them to believe that this is the way to instill success into their children. On the contrary, too much pressure (even for adults), only tempts us to rebel or to loath our shortcomings—what we have come to call failure.

RULE NUMBER THREE: GET SUPPORT

On top of trying to lose weight, we have work pressures, family pressures, and if overweight, perhaps sexual issues begging to be resolved. Where does one "problem" stop and the other begin? We have a bad day at work and so follow it up with a cocktail or two. Our libidos get activated and rather than risk rejection, or worse yet, nudity, we try satisfying it with creamy ice cream. Of course, the cycle goes on and on. In an *aware* consciousness, however, we can direct our energies. We can call or meet with others who know our struggles and who can encourage us to come over for a glass of juice instead of a cocktail, or who can talk us through our work frustrations and then help us to plan dinner. With this type of understanding, planning social occasions and meals can truly be rewarding rather than dreaded.

As Roger neared the 400 pound mark, he lost more and more friends. Not because they thought Roger was any less interesting or amusing than he was before, but because *Roger* felt too vulnerable to accept their invitations. He became more and more isolated, even from his wife, literally barricading himself with fat and cutting off the very support that is necessary for achieving any goal. Just as Roger was carrying nearly 400 pounds of physical weight, he was also carrying about 400 pounds of emotional burden. His psychic pain was devastating - he thought of himself as an outcast and acted it, becoming lonely and alone. How many of us, when in pain, turn away from those who love us, those who could help us most? And as friends, how many of us refuse to support another in a similar situation? What is not needed is, "Are you eating again? You are just going to get fatter and fatter." But rather, "Instead of eating that bag of potato chips, can I fix you a crunchy bowl of popcorn?"

RULE NUMBER FOUR: EAT HIGH-FIBER AND LOW-FAT FOODS

One of the things Roger learned while dieting is that texture is frequently as satisfying as flavor. When craving ice cream, the creaminess of a low-fat frozen yogurt can usually fulfill the urge. And today there are new products on the market that allow the taste of ice cream without the fat or sugar. While I personally prefer and recommend food in its most natural form, recent food engineering has made possible tasty "diet" foods. The creation of Nutrasweet, the sugar substitute, has enabled people who are resistant to natural-food eating to be able to watch their sugar intake while still enjoying the foods they like. (Remember, however, that food substitutes are not natural ingredients and while they may have been approved by the FDA as being non-harmful, they are not a natural approach to weight loss, which is what this book encourages.) This is why I suggest having a small portion of frozen yogurt to stop a craving for a creamy comfort food. But ultimately, you know what type of eater you are and what you are willing and unwilling to try. I am writing this book, however, to encourage you at least to try this approach: *Awareness over denial.*

High-fiber and low-fat choices will allow you to lose weight without giving up naturally good-tasting food. This has been substantiated by many of my patients. They started out using my dietary recommendations for a high-fiber/low-fat diet in order to heal their hearts. A diet low in saturated fats reduces the level of "bad" cholesterol that contributes to hardening of the arteries and heart attacks. A diet high in fiber keeps the body and appetite nourished while allowing most of the refuse of the digested food to be flushed away by the intestines. While my patients started on this diet to heal their hearts, they ended up losing weight! This is why *pasta is now considered a healthy food for dieters*, especially if it is a *pasta made from whole-wheat or semolina flour.* As we now know, these are complex carbohydrates. Since they are not made with refined sugars, any increases in blood sugar that occur after eating is gradual and healthy. Add a simple sauce of vegetables, for which I give many recipes later, and you have a perfect "diet" meal. Of course, we must return to the idea of eating with *awareness.* One plate of pasta will more often leave us feeling full and "rewarded" than two or three plates of large curd cottage cheese - a typical "diet" food - and with fewer calories!

When Roger was losing weight, many of the newly engineered diet foods were unavailable, but this is not what caused him to turn to a high-fiber/low-fat diet. He tried every diet available: The Scarsdale Diet, The Grapefruit Diet, The Aviator's Diet and protein drinks. With none of them, however, could he keep the weight off when he returned to "normal" eating. Obviously, it was the "normal" eating that needed to be changed. Fifteen years ago the public was just learning about the benefits of fiber. Roger took this information to heart. He would carry with him pure fiber crackers that even he says did not have a good taste, which he would snack on when needed, and he would eat fruit, a source of natural sugar, when he felt his energy was low. Being a steak lover, Roger didn't eliminate red meat from his diet, but he did cut it back significantly, and he would always remove all the visible fat before taking even one bite. In this way he didn't feel deprived, yet his eating was *contained.* He was aware that if he ate the steak, he could not follow it with bread, butter and salty french fries.

RULE NUMBER FIVE: AVOID SALT, SUGAR AND CAFFEINE WHILE CONSUMING AS MUCH WATER AS POSSIBLE

Now, this may sound like denial, but let me explain. Salt, sugar and caffeine do not need to be avoided altogether, but they should be used in moderation for both improved health and weight loss. You see, there is a direct relationship between caffeine intake and sugar cravings. It works like this: Sugar intake quickly boosts the blood sugar and just as quickly lowers it, thereby causing a sugar craving in order to boost energy again. Caffeine works in a similar manner: It boosts our energy level and drops again, thus causing a craving for a sweet or another cup of coffee to keep us going. While increasing sugar consumption increases energy and staves off hunger pangs induced by the dropping of blood sugar from a previous sweet or cup of coffee, it creates a cycle of eating sugar and/or drinking coffee as often as every two hours! Such increased sugar intake can obviously lead to an increase in accumulated fat.

The way to prevent or even to stop this cycle is to begin your day with a complex carbohydrate that will slowly be converted to blood sugar. Instead of the quick boost that a sweet roll gives, a bowl of oatmeal, for example, will allow a more gradual increase and subsequent decrease in blood sugar and, therefore, will prolong the time of satiety. Eating a complex carbohydrate that also has high amounts of fiber, such as shredded wheat with blueberries or strawberries, will control hunger even longer because fiber taken with water or another liquid will bulk in the gastrointestinal tract, thus creating a feeling of fullness.

If you choose a high-fiber, complex carbohydrate for breakfast, you may safely have a cup of coffee (without added sugar) without beginning the sugar/caffeine cycle. While the caffeine may cause a food craving, it will be satisfied by the gradual release of energy caused by the slow burning of the complex carbohydrate as opposed to the need of a quick fix with a processed sugar item. Remember, anything that is sugary tasting or sticky feeling is probably made with processed sugar, such as the table sugar found in commercially packaged breads and cereals; so *read labels*! The ingredients are listed in order of the highest quantities of ingredients. Therefore, if sugar is the first or second ingredient, it may comprise the majority of the product.

Breakfast may begin or prevent a day of overeating, so choose wisely. Try to replace the tempting foods on the left with the tasty alternatives on the right.

Avoid	Replace with
Sugared cereals	Whole grain cereals, oatmeal
White bread	Wholewheat bread
Commercial pancakes	Buckwheat cakes
with processed syrup	with honey or natural maple syrup
Belgian waffles	Whole grain waffles
with whipped cream	with spreadable fruit
Sweet rolls	Rolled oats
Blueberry muffins	Bran muffins

When making food choices, invoke the general rule of thumb that is easy to remember: The closer the food is to its natural original form, the better. In other words, whenever possible, buy wholewheat bread from your local baker instead of white bread from the grocery market. While you can still use "convenience foods," choose frozen waffles from a health food store instead of packaged toaster waffles. You can make a batch of buckwheat pancakes by merely adding water to a mix available at many of the farm stores that sell fresh produce, instead of using a processed biscuit or pancake mix.

Even my 15-year old son prefers multi-grain pancakes (my recipe follows in the *Recipes For Life* section) to those he gets in his friends' homes, because my pancakes have a chewier texture and a fuller flavor. And I serve them to him with pure maple syrup tapped from the trees around a cabin I have in Vermont. Okay, okay. You don't have to tap your own trees, but if you can splurge for a jug of pure maple syrup instead of the commercially packaged brands, not only will the flavor be more robust, but it will be healthier as well. Another healthy choice is to spread a layer of honey on the pancakes. While dousing them in either syrup or honey is not advised, a small amount gives flavor and satisfaction.

I also recommend the consumption of generous quantities of fluids at breakfast whether in juice, decaffeinated beverages or even just plain water—a cardinal ingredient in health. Water consumption cleanses the organs of excess sodium that is often hidden in many of today's foods, especially commercially packaged convenience foods such as canned soups, boxed mixes and sauces, and even sweets. *Selected foods especially high in sodium include pickles, ketchup, mustard, soy sauce and pickled fish,* to mention a few. *Sodas* can be one of the worst offenders of a low sodium diet. Even some low-calorie carbonated soft drinks have sodium in them. So if you are in the habit of drinking a diet beverage instead of water with a meal or to quench thirst, it will not only prevent a good opportunity to cleanse the system, but will also add to its contamination.

Remember that a high sodium intake also contributes to high blood pressure and heart disease, so *it's wise to replace all sodas with water,* tap or bottled, and to drink as much water as possible throughout the day. In addition to sodium and sugar content, *many soft drinks contain emulsifiers, artificial coloring, phosphoric acid, and antifoaming agents.* These chemicals cause metabolic stress to our body as do other additives, preservatives and synthetic agents commonly used in processed foods— setting up our next rule: Read Labels and Eat Natural.

RULE NUMBER SIX: READ LABELS AND EAT NATURAL

Controversies regarding nutrition seem to be on the news almost nightly. For example, *60 Minutes* ran a program regarding the pros and cons of the new proposals for food labeling. Consumers in the past who have relied heavily on food labels for nutritional information have now been rescued by the FDA with their recent policies for clearing up misleading advertising information. They are tackling such dilemmas as how much fat is low-fat? What does low-sodium mean? Or for that matter, what does low-calorie mean? Manufacturers in the past have boasted that a product can be "cholesterol-free," yet it may contain large amounts of saturated fat which is eventually *turned* into cholesterol in the body. With the new definition, cholesterol-free will be legally defined as less than two milligrams of cholesterol per serving. Likewise, "low-cholesterol" will be less than 20 mg of cholesterol.

"High-fiber" is another term that is frequently unregulated, but the new legislation will require specific grams of fiber per serving to be labeled high-fiber. New FDA standardizations will make it easier for consumers to rely on factual nutritional information. Not only will consumers be able to determine the amount of calories in a particular item, they will also be given information about the number of calories from fat, the amount of saturated fatty acids (SFAs), cholesterol, fiber, carbohydrate, protein, sodium, potassium and even information regarding vitamins and minerals.

Okay. Enough about the good news. What about the bad? What are the Feds doing about the chemicals, preservatives and other harmful ingredients that are added to commercially packaged foods? Although the FDA has issued formal regulations on literally hundreds of food additives, these are agents that are still listed as GRAS (Generally Regarded As Safe). These food additives are chemicals used in artificial flavors, colors, bleaches, emulsifiers, softeners, thickeners, hydrogenators, deodorizers, conditioners, fortifiers, driers, alkalizers, firming agents, stabilizers and buffers. They will add color and eye appeal to food that does not need refrigeration, but for all practical purposes, these agents are literally "dead;" that is, they do nothing useful but extend shelf life. And are they *really* safe?

Don't Become a Garbage Dump!

Two commonly used GRAS additives, butylated hydroxyanisole and butylated hydroxytoluene, frequently referred to as BHA and BHT, are antioxidants made from *petroleum*. BHA and BHT are found in almost every processed food, including cereals, shortening, ice cream, dairy foods, peanut butter, potato chips, meats, dressings, snacks, etc. They do indeed give foods an extended shelf life and also prevent rancidity. However, these additives have been reported as having a casual relationship to allergies and nervous system disorders.

Monosodium glutamate (MSG) is also considered a food enhancer in thousands of foods. "Convenience foods," such as TV dinners, processed meats, tenderizers and dressings, contain considerable quantities of MSG. In fact, industry officials indicate that MSG is the most widely utilized chemical flavoring agent. Considering that MSG has been utilized since 1907, it has a long history of use and has been closely scrutinized. It has been proven to show some side effects such as asthma, palpitations, chest pain, weakness and heartburn that may occur in both children and adults. In experimental animals, MSG has also been shown to cause permanent brain damage.

Headache is probably the leading symptom of MSG intake, frequently sending patients to their doctors for unnecessary evaluations and interventions when a good nutritional history and diet change would suffice. What does all this mean to the consumer? Unfortunately, the average consumer takes in thousands of chemical additives in his food. But we cannot blame it all on the food industry. We really do want convenience, speedy preparations, a longer shelf life and quick and easy menus. Major food companies take advantage of the consumer by advertising campaigns that are impressive but sometimes misleading. Although processed foods may be inexpensive, the consumer does pay a price in terms of physical symptoms and perhaps increased susceptibility to illness.

We need to become more discriminating shoppers. Read labels and look for ones that say "no preservatives" and "free from additives." But do not be seduced by reading "no preservatives;" also look to see if artificial flavorings or colorings have been added. Watch out for the camouflage labels which list "natural flavoring, hydrolyzed protein, sodium caseinate and autolyzed yeast." These are used frequently to disguise MSG. We need to be suspicious of chemical names and ingredient abbreviations.

Avoid BHA, BHT, sodium nitrate, sodium nitrite, caffeine, sulfur dioxide, butyric acid, diethylene glycol, sodium benzoate, and amyl acetate. If you do not understand the language, or feel you need a Ph.D. or an M.D. degree to figure out the contents, then the product should be avoided. Be aware of the toxic ingredient *aluminum,* and be particularly cognizant of the use of *white flour additives.* Additives such as *ammonium chloride, potassium bromate and propionic acid* (sodium or calcium propionate) are all unnatural to living organisms. Just as industrial chemicals can pollute the environment, these chemicals, added to breads, pollute the body. We need to realize that additives and chemicals actually add nothing to the nutritional value of foods. They are frequently added to make inferior substances taste better.

But, the far better option is to consider natural and organically grown foods. Try to learn about and seek out organic foods which are free of pesticides and chemical fertilizers.

Recent surveys have indicated that 55 percent of pesticide residues in the U.S. diet are supplied by meat! Dairy products contain 23 percent pesticides, and pesticide residues in the U.S. diet supplied by U.S. vegetables, fruits and grains are 11 percent. As a matter of fact, an alarming 94 percent of chlorinated hydrocarbon pesticide residues in the American diet are attributable to meats, dairy products, fish and eggs.

In the last few years, numerous studies have indicated that women on high fat diets increase their risk of breast cancer. Although their diet may be a factor, new research indicates that it may not be the fat itself, but rather the toxins and pesticides contained in the fats which are causing the problem. Studies have determined that breast tissue from cancer patients had higher levels of DDT and higher concentration of PCBs (polycholorinated biphenyls).

Man-made pollutants such as DDT and PCBs are chemicals which react with estrogen receptor cells in human breast tissue. As these deadly environmental pollutants mimic estrogen, they are absorbed into the woman's body and stored in human fat. DDT is the most notorious pesticide linked to breast cancer and is part of the class called organochlorides. Although DDT is banned in the U.S., it is still produced in third world countries, particularly Central and Latin America, China and India. In a study involving Israeli women, the banning of organochlorine pesticides, resulted in a cancer decline of 20 percent. Prior to the ban of DDT in Israel, Israeli women had one of the highest breast cancer mortality rates in the world. PCBs are by-products of petroleum. But these two environmental toxins are just the tip of the iceberg.

Presently in the U.S., there are over 75,000 different industrial chemicals which are utilized for agricultural and commercial uses. Minimizing or eliminating pesticide use around the home, avoiding air pollution and drinking purified water are some ways you can reduce your risk of exposure. I would also recommend eating as many organic foods as possible.

Organic gardening indicates that the soil has been free of any artificially produced fertilizers for several years or even decades. Natural foods are gradually becoming more and more popular with consumers. Although the consumer may pay a few pennies more and may have to accept shorter shelf lives, the dividend can be a healthier body and mind. We have to be willing to *give up precooked, instant, refined and chemically treated foods.* If you want good health, you need to compromise and take more responsibility for the ingredients you put into your body. Go out and be a detective and guard your body since this is the only one you will ever have.

RULE NUMBER SEVEN: MOVE!

The definition of a calorie is a unit for measuring energy. This means that for every calorie that we take in, we must expend an equal amount of energy in order to remain at a balanced weight. When we take in more calories than we expend, we gain weight. When we expend more energy than we take in, we lose weight. And when the two are balanced, we can remain at a constant weight.

Okay, so you know this already. You may even feel hopeless that you could ever expend more energy than you take in because you are not an athletic person. Don't believe it. Any little activity greater than you are doing now will burn more calories. So even if you are consuming the same amount of food today as you were yesterday, but you add a bit more movement to your day, you will lose weight slowly. Now, add to today's diet some foods less dense in calories than yesterday and you are losing weight twice as fast.

Notice that I say "movement," not exercise. I think exercise can sometimes be a scary word. People visualize running down the road in sweaty shorts and sneakers or pumping iron. Professionally speaking, I must say I don't recommend either. Both put a tremendous amount of stress on the heart muscle and other muscles and tendons that pop and burst because of overzealous or incorrect use. Let's take it easy.

Remember, this is a program of non-denial and enjoyment.

Let's start out *walking*. The evening breeze is cool and spring or fall crispness might be in the air. Or perhaps there is a beautiful red August moon that you can see from your window. Get up. Walk outdoors. Enjoy nature. This is a holistic way of living. Mind and body are one. Human life and wildlife are on the same planet. Let's enjoy each other as we are all part of the same universe. Even if you can't find time to walk every day (though I think you might, once you get used to the beauty of the landscape), think of every little movement you make and take it one step beyond. Walk out to the driveway to get the mail instead of picking it up in your car on the way home. Walk around the bed to make up the other side rather than reaching over. While watching television, my daughter does leg lifts. Think of this not as strenuous exercise, but as an efficient use of exercise time!

When Roger first started losing weight, he couldn't even reach over to tie his shoes. He couldn't walk more than a few yards. Four hundred pounds is a lot of weight to move around. So he started walking out for the newspaper each morning and taking out the trash. He even began cleaning out closets. Roger was a successful businessman who, if he wanted, could hire a housekeeper to clean closets. But Roger knew that each added movement would add to his successful weight loss. Every little movement counts. Like a savings account, Roger added more and more movement to his daily regimen until he accumulated the lifestyle he has today. Now he plays racquetball three times a week and even won his division in the North Carolina State Championship. He was one of the oldest men to win this title in the United States - and to think that only six years previously he could barely walk far enough to take the trash out.

RULE NUMBER EIGHT: ADD VITAMINS AND MINERALS TO YOUR DIET

Taking vitamins and minerals will help protect your body. While you are going through the strenuous shifts and changes that occur with weight loss, targeted nutritionals are especially important. Remember that your metabolism is going to change. And if you are replacing high fat and sugary foods in your diet with natural foods, you are going to have some noticeable physical differences. For example, you may have larger bowel movements, but this may remove important minerals as well. While hair and eyes may become shinier, your skin may at first break out and then clear to a creamy complexion. We call this process elimination and purification. The old "garbage" that is in your body is being flushed out and replaced with healthier natural foods. Taking various vitamins and minerals, or foods high in content of these, will aid in this transition.

Once you are on a balanced diet, you can decide if you want to take supplements or choose to get your vitamins and minerals through your food. I suggest a combination of fresh fruits and vegetables, and nutritional supplements.

Some people question why they need to take vitamins and minerals in a supplemental form when they can get them in the foods they eat. Unfortunately, the "apple a day" principle does not hold true today as it did a century ago. In this day and age, the need for vitamin and mineral supplementation is critical. Why?

Few adults (nine percent) eat a balanced diet containing at least five to nine fresh fruits or vegetables per day. Even when eating such a balanced diet, most people are unlikely to get the larger amounts of certain vitamins (especially beta carotene, vitamin C and vitamin E) which have been effective in clinical trials. Although you may consider vitamins in foods the best way to stay healthy, the foods we eat today may not be as rich in nutrients as they were years ago. Also, food processing frequently strips our foods of many of the most important nutrients, leaving the less important ingredients for your table.

We need a wide assortment of vitamins, minerals and accessory nutrients to stay healthy and to help prevent disease in a way that satisfies our hunger, but will not make us fat. You may not be getting everything you need from the food you eat, even with my recommended menu! Why?

Because food doesn't come with a label that specifies how much of each nutrient is in the portion you eat. Your brain tells you when you're hungry, but your brain can't tell you if it needs a particular vitamin or mineral. It can't say, "I need a magnesium fix today and I'm running short on iron. Go out and buy some pumpkin seeds and add them to the menu." Your brain can only tell you, "Eat something," and will continue to fuel your appetite until satisfaction is achieved.

Our need for supplemental nutrients is also due to the increase in environmental toxins such as polluted air, radiation, chemical poisons, heavy metals and other man-made risk factors such as auto emissions, cigarette smoke and the increasing usage of fats in our diets. These environmental factors affect biochemical reactions that cause dangerous free radical formations in our bodies, causing premature aging and disease.

Now That's Fat!

Roger tells the story of the time he and another 400-pound friend got into Roger's Corvette in front of his luxury auto dealership. With much effort, they struggled into the low-slung car and, once seated, attempted to shut the doors simultaneously. But neither could. Between them, there was just too much man inside the little car. With his employees watching, Roger didn't want to bear further humiliation by getting out and admitting defeat, so he became determined to get the doors shut. First he leaned outward and told his friend to pull his door shut, then to reverse the action while Roger pulled his shut. Since their first attempts were not successful, their repeated efforts created a rocking motion and the two 400-pound men swayed from side to side as they tried to physically reposition, and figuratively remold, their huge bodies into ones that would fit into a svelte Corvette. As the car rocked from side to side, Roger admits it must have been a funny sight. His employees began gathering at the windows of the dealership and laughing hysterically. Roger waved to them, smiling and encouraging their fun while pushing down his true feelings of hurt and shame. Finally, they got the doors shut and left behind the embarrassing situation.

It was with the same single-minded resolve that Roger finally decided to lose weight. Not long after becoming stuck in the chair of a shoe store and dumping an unsuspecting lady on the floor when he stood up and took a row of connected seats with him, he was rushed to the hospital with an inability to breathe. Roger had been feeling some discomfort sleeping and breathing, he was running a slight temperature and his head felt stuffy. His doctor examined him, listened to his chest, and could find nothing more. He diagnosed a cold. After almost a month the symptoms got worse, so Roger saw another physician. Again, the doctor could not hear congestion in Roger's chest when he listened with a stethoscope. Again, a cold was the diagnosis. Because Roger felt so terrible, he was sure there was something more. He asked for a chest x-ray. And when it was returned, the doctor suggested Roger be immediately hospitalized. Roger had a severe case of pneumonia, which couldn't be detected with a stethoscope through the layers of fat around his 60-inch chest.

When Roger was checked into the hospital, they took his vital signs and wanted to check his weight. However, the nurses feared he was too large for even medical scales, which went up to only 300 pounds, and told him he might have to go to their laundry room to be weighed. His shame and humiliation were intense. Luckily, they brought in a special scale that saved him the further pain of being weighed as cargo. As he was waiting for the process to be over, he saw a cadaver being wheeled out of a room. When Roger learned that the man had died from complications of pneumonia, a "click" went off in his head. Roger had an advanced case of pneumonia, resulting from difficulty diagnosing the disease because of his weight. Roger suddenly realized - and believed - that one way or another his overeating was going to kill him. This was Roger's spiritual message, "That perhaps now he had an opportunity in this crisis."

I see many overweight people who end up as cardiac deaths. Clinical studies show that obese people move less than thinner people and many heart attacks occur within a short time after a high-fat meal. Movement and light, low-fat meals are two ways of contributing to a healthy heart. If it hadn't been the pneumonia that scared Roger into the realization that his weight was dangerous, it might have been a heart attack, and he might not have been as lucky. As it was, Roger left the hospital cured of his pneumonia and determined to lose weight. The energy he used in building his businesses and hiding the pain of his fat he would now channel into losing weight. Just as he previously gave his entire attention to work and food, Roger made losing weight his new obsession.

Roger got the message. And listened.

As a cardiologist, I have seen many cases of heart attacks, near death experiences and, unfortunately, death itself. Some of my survivors got the transformational message. Some patients believed that their heart attacks were really spiritual gifts that would make them change their lives. They, indeed, reframed their illnesses and found opportunities in these crises. Frequently, when one gets severely ill, or experiences a near death, a spiritual and/or emotional growth may occur. I have seen many patients dig deeper into themselves as a result of developing catastrophic illnesses. For some of these fortunate people, they had a gift in disguise. I believe this was the case for Roger Buffaloe.

While in the hospital, Roger had time to analyze his eating habits. He had been dieting for at least 20 years and nothing had worked, so he concluded that diets don't work. The only "diet" he could count on was the age-old way of eating less and eating lighter. He didn't just worry about counting calories. Instead, he focused on lowering his fat intake. If he reduced the amount of red meats and oily foods he was consuming, he would need to increase fiber foods in order to eat less and yet feel full. It just made sense.

So Roger set a reasonable goal. Once he achieved his goal, however, he then started to "play games" with his diet. He would allow himself bread without butter except for the last bite, on which he would smear just enough to get the full taste. After a short time, he surprisingly learned that he no longer liked the taste of butter. It was too heavy, too oily, too strong.

Roger lost weight. The people who had known him his whole life didn't recognize him, and others whom he didn't know well would say, "I heard you lost weight, but I couldn't imagine losing this much! How did you do it?" Word spread and everywhere Roger went, people asked him for weight-loss advice. He explained to them the concept of eating low-fat and high-fiber foods, but many of them didn't understand about whole grains and fiber. He was thrilled about his own success in losing weight and wanted to help others. Just as he shed his fat and his fat lifestyle, Roger sold his grocery markets and opened a weight-loss center where he could teach people about fat, fiber, and vitamins. Like Roger, I believe in eating with awareness. The rest of this book will teach you how awareness, in itself, is the most important step in achieving *Optimum Health.*

Chapter Two

FAT IN AMERICA

A recent article in the Journal of the American Medical Association (JAMA) declared a "Fattening of America." Obesity is a major problem for our society, with now an alarming 30% of our population being obese.

Most researchers would agree that extreme degrees of obesity increase the risk of cancer and heart disease in both men and women. The health consequences of weight gain in women has recently been validated and is quite disturbing. In the February 8, 1995 edition of the *Journal of the American Medical Association*, data clearly indicates that even a modest weight gain during adult life is associated with the increasing risk of developing coronary heart disease. This recent information is especially germane to women who generally consider themselves to be "not too" overweight. Even being mildly overweight is a real problem.

The United States population is never at a loss to find new ways to lose weight. We all know there is an abundance of diets available. Although some are more successful than others, any diet will work for a motivated individual. The odds of maintaining weight loss, however, are discouraging. Most diets result in the majority of individuals regaining their weight when they resume "normal" eating patterns. Studies show that only a small fraction of overweight people who succeed in weight loss are able to keep the weight off for more than a short period of time.

As we saw in the story of Roger Buffaloe, diets don't work. Dieting in general implies a temporary change in the way we eat, instead of a permanent shift in the way we perceive ourselves in our relationship with food. Diet also implies deprivation. When one utilizes deprivation, food is not a friend, but rather an enemy. Typically, people think that self-sacrifice is the only way to achieve success, and that the enjoyment of food is a sin that leads to an overpowering sense of frustration and failure. This emotional roller coaster can be quite disturbing. An ideal diet comes from one's own consciousness and individualization. Such insight and awareness of what is healthy and what is unhealthy, what you can live with and live without, is really the key to losing weight.

For example, people who starve themselves or force themselves to eat unusual or unpalatable foods are bound to fail in the long run. Clinical studies have demonstrated that people who participate in these diets fail to achieve long-term weight loss and may often end up weighing *more*. A more practical approach would be to *gradually increase and improve the quality of one's diet by eating a variety of healthy low-fat/high-fiber foods that taste good.* Just as most people can change from whole milk to two-percent milk and eventually lose their taste for whole milk, similar changes may take place with just a little experimentation. We all have food preferences. The secret is to utilize our favorite foods, making adjustments to balance them with less caloric or healthier choices.

For example, one serving of premium ice cream contains two to three times the calories of a serving of frozen yogurt. Therefore, the choice is to eat more frozen yogurt or less ice cream. This awareness is a small but crucial step in *nutritional healing.* A long-term weight loss program, therefore, is really a lifestyle that is palatable and somewhat calorie-deficient but enjoyable. Over time, the brain makes the gradual switch into believing that frozen yogurt is the same as ice cream.

Calorie is a word that frequently comes up in daily conversations but not everyone knows its definition. A calorie is a measure of energy. When we speak about food, we give it a number, reflecting the amount of energy it yields when it burns. It takes energy to perform activities. If the body needs a steady supply of calories to fuel it with energy, any food supply will do. But if we supply our body with an overabundance of energy in the form of calories, this creates weight gain. In simple terms, the problem with being overweight is a problem of energy balance. Energy balance is the relationship between energy intake and energy expenditure. For example, it takes approximately 100 calories of energy to walk one mile. If we walk a mile and then drink a 200 calorie frosted shake, we will not lose weight but only add to it. When the energy balance is positive, the extra calories are stored as fat. When the energy balance is negative, fat is broken down to provide the necessary energy the body needs. This simple fact is a cardinal ingredient in weight loss.

OFF THE COUCH AND MOVE ANYTHING!

Keeping this energetic point of view in mind, we need to ask how the body conserves and expends energy. The body is utilizing energy at rest as well as during exercise. This is reflected in one's basal metabolic rate (BMR) or the energy required to sustain the basic functions of life (breathing, heart rate, organic functions, etc.). The BMR may vary from one individual to another as well as from one activity to another.

For example, an athlete may have a higher metabolic rate than a sedentary person, thereby resulting in a higher utilization of energy. The active person may have a higher resting metabolism as well, which means that he or she may be able to consume just as many calories as an inactive person and not gain weight when the other does. This is sometimes referred to as a fast or high metabolism. The resting metabolic rate is also related to the surface area of the body. As weight increases, the amount of energy needed to keep basic bodily functions running increases. This means that an overweight person's body perceives that he or she needs more energy and thereby conserves it. The way to change the metabolic rate is to become more active.

Unfortunately, many obese people do not expend much energy. In fact, you may notice a slow-motion quality about them that looks even restful, without much twitching and fidgeting. Even these tiny movements, however, burn energy. Exercise, a word that conjures up intense fear and revulsion in many, is one of the most crucial ingredients in weight loss. Frequently, the overweight individual detests exercise, but *any* movement is precisely what is necessary for long-term success of weight loss.

Metabolic requirements also vary with age. The highest rate of energy intake per body weight in humans is required by infants. There is a gradual decline in childhood and further decline in adult life. Metabolic rates for women are usually lower than those for men, so women may need to consume less calories, except during pregnancy and lactation, when energy demands increase. Although there are calorie charts available for review, there is considerable variation in these energy requirements, even for individuals of the same size, age and sex. For example, for a 130 pound, moderately active woman, the caloric requirement is approximately 2,000 calories. However, there may be as much as a 20 percent variation for women with the same activity level and body size.

Recent findings in the medical literature on mechanisms in the development and maintenance of obesity have focused not on just the consequence of eating too much, but also on expending too little energy. Two recent medical studies on the development of obesity in infancy and adulthood suggest that differences in activity may be the key point in obesity. In one study, clinical investigators measured the total seven-day energy intake and energy expenditure of a group of infants, aged three months, and related their results to weight gain during the first year of life. The data indicates that infants who are overweight on their first birthday have a 20.7 percent lower expenditure of energy than infants who are of normal weight. The two groups do not differ significantly in energy intake. These findings suggest that both activity level and food intake are critical in determining weight gain at an early age, but the former appears to be more significant. *An increase in physical activity will expend more energy and is probably more important in weight reduction than caloric intake.* So the first awareness in losing weight is to think in terms of achieving a negative energy balance.

SOLVING THE WEIGHT-GAIN MYSTERY

It was once believed that the major cause for obesity was overeating. But if this were true, the easiest way to lose weight would be to eat less. As this is not so easy, it is clearly not the whole story. The causes of weight gain are numerous, multi-faceted and complex. These include genetic, environmental and psychosocial factors, as well as individual differences in eating patterns, resting metabolic rate, biochemical shifts and the unusual phenomenon of "brown fat."

Brown fat is more metabolically active than stored fat and actually has the ability to burn energy, turning excess calories into heat production. This is believed, for example, to be a major factor in the dissipation of heat in hibernating animals. Some researchers believe that thin people who eat excessively and yet are not overly active may have a larger quantity of brown fat in proportion to stored fat, resulting in a greater expenditure of energy. We all know individuals who seemingly "eat all they want" and yet remain thin despite the fact that they are not overly active. Brown fat may be the secret to this mystery. (Many people, however, do not have much brown fat and, instead, have an undesirable storage of adipose tissue or body fat.) Overwhelming research indicates that all of these factors, in combination with a lifestyle of inactivity, appear to be the core factors in weight gain.

Consider the fact as we have mentioned previously, that it takes approximately 100 calories of energy to walk one mile. If we walk one mile a day, we will have an energy output of 700 calories per week. Multiply this times 52 weeks and our calorie expenditure per year will equal 36,400 calories. Since a pound of fat contains approximately 3,500 calories, this daily one mile walk is equivalent to the loss of approximately ten pounds of fat in one year if all other factors remain equal. Thus, by simple mathematics, it becomes clear how this whole energetic concept works in obesity and weight gain.

Caloric intake (what you eat) is another major consideration in weight loss. When the caloric intake is below the daily energy require-ment, the initial loss in body weight results primarily from a depletion in the body's carbohydrate stores. In continued weight loss, body fat is metabolized and, therefore, required to supply the caloric deficiency. In other words, by *restricting food intake and/or by increasing physical activity, the body burns up fat.* Fad diets, however, are the opposite. These are diets that tend to fool the body's biochemistry by manipulating proteins, car-bohydrates or fat. These types of diets are nutritionally unbalanced, usu-ally advocating levels of high protein, with and without high fat intake, and low carbohydrate consumption. In the late 1970s, such diets were found to be associated with cardiac arrhythmias and even sudden death.

The once popular ketogenic diets, such as the Atkins diet, employed a high-protein, high-fat/low-carbohydrate regimen to achieve rapid weight loss. Since these diets are largely composed of eating fat with very little glucose, the body relies on the breakdown of fat for its metabolic func-tion. This results in a high blood level of free fatty acids which are insuffi-ciently burned, thus producing ketones. Ketones make the blood more acidic, resulting in loss of appetite.

The Scarsdale Diet is based on eating a diet high in protein and low in fat. In this case the body metabolizes its own fat, not only from adipose (fat) tissue, but other tissues as well. If you consume excessive protein, however, especially while not exercising, this can be converted to fat, and may actually work against your weight-loss goals.

Although these diets may cause initial weight loss, it is done at the expense of the body. Besides, these diets are unnatural and cannot be tol-erated for long. The most effective nutritional programs are those that are balanced with proper amounts of carbohydrates and proteins. A low-fat/high-fiber concept is the most scientifically sound concept.

Obesity—Futuristic Medicine

An interesting way of looking at obesity includes the advances in biotechnology and engineering. Is obesity related to the genes? Recently, researchers from Rockefeller University reported that they had identified and actually cloned an obesity gene found in mice. It is thought that the gene directs fat cells in the body to produce a hormone that tells the brain to suppress the appetite. Thus, if the hormonal protein is absent, deficient or abnormal, no regulation of the appetite occurs. Although more research is needed in this field, it is conceivable that some individuals do have a defective "fat gene." For now, there is nothing we can do but wait for more investigations to be done. In the meantime, it is important to follow the rules of a healthy lifestyle and, for the very obese, consider some of the medically managed fasting programs in process at many hospitals in the country.

While this may be a good way to start weight loss, I believe such an involvement requires close medical supervision with continual follow-up investigation while evaluating sound nutritional principles. In addition, a long-term involvement with behavioral modification is still necessary to prevent the old patterns from re-emerging. This was the case in our hospital-based program. Although most participants lost more than 40 pounds of weight, some of them regained the weight. Weight reduction needs long-term commitment, emotional support and psychological awareness.

Three

LOVE, SEX AND YOUR WEIGHT

This book is designed to give you valuable tools to effectively and permanently transform your relationship with your body. Of course, a beneficial result is that you will have a trimmer, more physically fit, healthier body. But the deeper, more profound transformation is about your relationship with yourself. This requires a physical, mental and emotional shift. If you now find yourself criticizing your body, condemning yourself, feeling self-hate or hurting yourself, working through these core emotional issues and getting to the heart of the matter will free you.

Weight loss comes out of healing the relationship between the body and the mind. The results of healing your inner conflicts will be self-acceptance, self-love and a sense of truly honoring your body. Using a holistic approach to weight loss prevents using dieting as yet another unhealthy neurotic expression of an unresolved self. The vicious cycle of hating your body, going on a diet, losing weight, gaining the weight back, hating yourself and your body must be interrupted and healed. These are habits disrespectful to yourself.

A holistic approach does not mean you have to go on a vegetarian diet or become spiritual. It simply means that the approach to a permanent body change is multi-level: emotional, behavioral, physical and nutritional. In the overweight syndrome, we create negative feelings about ourselves and our bodies. Emotional factors such as depression, helplessness, guilt, loneliness, boredom, self-hate, denial of anger, fear and hopelessness are meshed in this cycle.

IT'S TIME TO REFRAME

But let's reframe your attitude toward your body and weight loss. The concept of "reframing" is to reshape negative attitudes and beliefs, some of which we learned as young children, in a more positive light. Reframing results in seeing the good aspect of any given situation or person, including ourselves. For example, let's reframe your attitude toward your body and weight loss. Let's see your overweight condition as a gift because it is now the impetus for you to delve deeper into your psyche and into the blocks that have hampered your self-image and self-esteem. You can use it as a motivating force to heal deep emotional issues, become more alive, and live a more pleasurable, fulfilling life free of obsessive-compulsive behavior.

What a joy life can be when your thought process is free from a preoccupation with your body and/or your food. After all, what we think, we can internalize and begin to believe. What we believe, we become. If we think we have an unattractive body, for example, and think it often, we believe we are unattractive, and thus, may act in an unattractive manner. This negativity limits the vast possibilities of experience. If we reframe this view, we will consciously look at ourselves in a constructive, not destructive, way. In other words, we can now look at our beautiful hair or bright eyes and see ourselves attractively. This does not mean we should stay stuck in fat bodies, but we should use positive reframing as a tool to get past this unconscious block.

For people who are chronically overweight, food becomes a vehicle with which to block the emotions. In their book, *Overcoming Overeating*, Jane R. Hirschmann and Carol H. Munter make a distinction between stomach hunger and mouth hunger. When you eat in order to fill your body because your stomach is hungry, you are in a healthy relationship with food. If you find yourself wanting food out of mouth hunger, even when you are not hungry, you are experiencing something emotional, an anxiety out of conscious awareness; that is, you are using food to try to assuage, hide or substitute for the feeling. I agree with this theory. For example, perhaps we are feeling deep despair or intense rage, but these feelings do not feel safe. We then feel anxiety about having these feelings. If we are not getting in touch with our true feelings and expressing them, overeating may be a futile attempt to sublimate whatever the true feeling is.

Another example might be love. A lot of us can give but cannot receive. We may not be able to take in love, but we can take in food. Therefore, we use food as a substitute for emotional and spiritual hunger. Afterwards, we get upset and scold ourselves for binging and being fat, though it is not the food that is the problem but what it represents. It is what the food substitutes for that people *really* need to examine. Food may be used as a drug. Like alcohol, we medicate ourselves with it, especially sugar, but it never cures the problem. It exacerbates it. It continues. And the reality is that we physically feed ourselves to death while we *emotionally starve* ourselves to death. What a paradox!

The cause of eating disorders, addictive behavior and obsessive-compulsive patterns often stem from a variety of painful experiences in childhood, frequently combined with bad habits that were taught in the family system. Unless we are actively involved (through support groups and workshops, therapy or a personal search) in uncovering the causes, the core issues remain, although unconscious. A powerful beginning is to get in touch with our own experience; that is, to bring out of darkness and into the light our own unconscious motivations for overeating.

WORMS ARE GOOD!

You may be thinking, "I don't need to do that. My body may be a problem, but not my mind. Why open a can of worms?" However, as a physician, I know that the body speaks the truth and the mind can be deceived. I choose to trust the body. The body reacts to repressed emotions. Unfortunately, most parents do not teach children to honor or express their emotions, and they give many mixed messages about the very natural human aspects of their physical being. Children are told, "Stop crying," when they are hurt and have a need to cry. They are told that anger is not ladylike or that men should not be afraid. Many people have been treated disrespectfully and abusively (physically or emotionally) through the years and have come to view this treatment as normal, acceptable and to be expected, even deserved. As children, some would even get hit, emotionally abused, reprimanded or abandoned when they expressed certain emotions such as anger, sadness or fear. Alice Miller, author of *The Drama of the Gifted Child*, tells us that parents unknowingly have the power to form and deform the emotional and physical lives of their children.

We were all born with the natural ability to release emotion. If we watch a baby who is upset, we will see that he or she will cry or scream and that when finished, the body softens and the baby is peaceful and smiling again. However, if the baby is misdirected from its natural pattern, this may result in lifelong repression of feelings. Where does all this repressed emotional energy go? It becomes an unresolved memory in the unconscious. The energy actually gets stuck in the body, in the muscles and in the cells. This unreleased energy becomes the seat of "dis-ease" and "dis-harmony" inside of us.

DOWN MEMORY LANE

For you to begin to lose weight, it is very important to take an honest look at how your parents related to you in terms of food, diet, your emotional needs and your self-image. This may be a painful look. Be aware that you might have some denial systems blocking you from seeing the truth, but it is worth a try. This is why support groups can be so helpful when attempting to lose weight. What feelings were you not allowed to have as a child? Were you told to stop crying when you were sad? Did you get punished? Were you taught to control yourself, control your feelings? Were your parents controlling about what you ate and how much you ate? Did they force you to eat everything that was on your plate, even if you were full?

Take some time to look back at their belief systems about food and about body size. Did your parents believe that "a fat baby is a healthy baby?" Were you ever given the message that if you didn't eat, you would get sick? Were there reward systems set up around food? If you were hungry and wanted to eat, did you ever hear the familiar phrase, "don't spoil your appetite"?

What does it mean? How can anyone "spoil" an appetite by eating? Appetite is an internal signal; hunger pangs indicate a need for food. Eating satisfies, not spoils an appetite. What parents really mean when they say this is that the child should stifle his or her appetite, or natural feelings of hunger, in order to please the parent. They mean, "Don't eat when and what you want to eat, but eat when and what I want you to eat."

A powerful way to heal the wounds that we all carry from childhood is to be able to now express what we wanted to express back then, but couldn't. This is best done in therapy or in some other safe environment. In this way, we will be able to diffuse the old feelings that we have about past events and not apply them to current situations. In other words, once an old feeling is released, when a new experience causes us to react emotionally, it won't contain the charge or the excess baggage of all the other past repressed feelings. Therefore, the present feeling will be more manageable, the anxiety lessened, and your need to turn to food will be considerably assuaged.

It is important to allow negative emotions to come up so they can be released and yet it is also important to reframe them. This may sound like a contradiction. How do you know when to do what? The rule is to first EXPERIENCE the feeling without judgment or self-editorialization, and then to investigate it once it has been discharged. For example, let's say you constantly insult your body. You can feel how angry you really are at yourself. You have been feeling these particular feelings for quite some time and the intense emotional charge must be expressed and released. Take some time privately or perhaps in a therapy session to vent this anger.

Once you do this, (perhaps you'll need to do this every so often for a while) you can eventually try to understand the roots of this behavior. It will then be easier to catch yourself saying or thinking something self-destructive so you can reframe it in a positive light. This process can be particularly effective in losing weight. When you find yourself reaching for food when you are not hungry, rather than eating right away, sit down with a pen and a pad and write what you are feeling or immediately express these feelings verbally. In this way, you derail the maladaptive motivation behind the mouth hunger.

TAKE SUCCESSFUL SMALL STEPS

It is important to point out here the need for patience. If you want to successfully change your patterns, it will take time, repetition and a tremendous amount of patience. Realize that you are taking a totally new approach to reshaping your body. Let go of any sense of time and urgency. Relax. Pushing too hard and forcing the flow will create a destructive, frenetic energy with this process. People want fast results, fast cures and immediate gratification, but I am a firm believer in taking out the struggle and in not driving ourselves beyond normal capacity. Healing unhealthy and destructive patterns requires focus, time and energy; so patience, lots of nurturing self-love and self-support are necessary here. It is healthful to let go of preconceived notions of how much weight you have to lose and in what span of time. Expectations, after all, can lead to disappointments. They can trigger a sense of failure and a vicious cycle of obsessive eating.

A major pitfall in losing weight is creating an unattainable goal. Our society has placed a tremendous pressure on us to be beautiful. The model we have been given for beauty is a thin body. But we must all get to a place where we feel a sense of peace about our particular body types. There is indeed a danger in seeking total perfection, as it is truly an unattainable goal. Perhaps you are bottom heavy and overweight, but you begin to make changes in your lifestyle and you start to reduce. You are exercising and firming up and looking much slimmer, much better. If you continue to focus on your heavy thighs, however, you create a counter productive attitude. Instead of feeling and expressing a tremendous gratitude toward yourself for reshaping your body, an expression which will encourage your entire being to continue to change your patterns, you are busy putting yourself down for "heavy thighs." This creates a futile, rebellious feeling inside. A part of you will be feeling, "Why bother? No matter what I do, it's never enough."

SEX?

In this multi-level approach to creating and maintaining a new body, it is very important to establish a beneficial goal. If you want to change your body in order to have a healthy body/mind connection, your focus is in the right place. If your reasons for losing weight are that you think if you do so you will get love, or so-and-so will want you or envy you, or you'll get that job or someone to pay attention to you, etc., you are setting yourself up to fail. This can be an unfulfilled expectation. What if you lose the weight and it doesn't happen? Or, what if you lose the weight and it does happen, but you still feel unfulfilled? The way to protect yourself from an unfulfilled prophecy is to set your sights on a beneficial intention. "When my lifestyle patterns change, when I have a healthier relationship to myself and my body, I will feel more alive, more at peace and, therefore, I will experience more pleasure." If you can begin to see yourself in a healing process and feel a sense of hope and excitement about it, you can begin to enjoy the process rather than being caught up in the end result. Let go of the struggle, or the "I'll be happy when . . . " syndrome.

Liken this venture to reprogramming a computer. There are many circuits. Some circuits are emotional blocks, some are faulty belief systems, some are negative family patterns, some are your own destructive habits, and on and on. Where have you been short-circuited? What experiences have caused you to cut off from yourself? All this must be worked on in order to heal yourself and your unconscious obsession with food. The unconscious drives are stronger than the conscious drives. It is frequently the unconscious desires that direct us. Thus, to begin to enjoy food and feel we have permission to eat, we must be at peace with ourselves emotionally. There is often a direct correlation between anxiety and overeating. If understanding ourselves better and feeling that we are actively involved in our own healing reduces anxiety, it will have a positive effect on healing the eating compulsion. When we bring aspects of our unconsciousness into the light of awareness, they are no longer hidden forces and we begin to have a greater ability to not let them control and harm us. If overeating is a negative way to cope with feelings, especially feelings of fear or powerlessness, then creating a better relationship with the emotional self will significantly support the healing of this compulsion.

This was probably the case with Roger Buffaloe, who must have had feelings of powerlessness, most likely rooted in his childhood. By becoming a successful businessman, he established the *Image* of success, which gave him a sense of control. He obviously did not have this in his eating habits. The truth is, he was out of control. This is a typical scenario of many obese individuals, male and female. With women, there may be even a greater risk of obesity because of their lack of early support to express themselves emotionally and physically, and particularly because of their feelings of vulnerability.

What I want to help you get in touch with now is the fearful side of weight loss. Both men and women have concerns about this deep core issue, sexual vulnerability. To get in touch with your own feelings about this, write or say aloud the following, and take your time to fill in the blanks:

"If I lose weight, I'm afraid . . . will happen."

"If I lose weight, I'm afraid . . . (who) will pull away from me."

"If I lose weight, I'm afraid I'll hurt . . . "

"By being overweight, I feel protected from . . . ."

"By being overweight, I don't have to deal with . . . ."

"If I have a sexier body, I'm afraid . . . ."

While I was a therapist in the hospital-based weight loss program at Manchester Memorial Hospital in Connecticut, it became increasingly clear to me that the issue of sexuality was a major factor in the overweight syndrome. Many of my OptiFast weight-loss clients communicated their intense fears regarding weight loss. There were also issues of love and relationship. For example, one of my clients said, "By eating, I will make myself so unlovable that I will never get hurt again." She had deep, painful issues regarding love and sexuality. For some of my clients, losing weight was like shedding "suits of armor." The physical padding that being overweight provides can be viewed as a protective armor. This maladaptive defense mechanism, unconsciously created to avoid pain, actually holds past pain deep inside your tissues.

Are you unconsciously or consciously holding on to the weight to protect yourself sexually? Do you use the weight to avoid other forms of intimacy? It is important to honestly delve into these possibilities because unless they are uncovered and dealt with emotionally, it will be very difficult to reduce and keep the weight off. To shed the armor makes us vulnerable. It is this shedding of armor and the ensuing vulnerability that is for some a major cause of resistance in losing further weight. Let me give you an example.

SEXUAL VIOLATION MAY CAUSE WEIGHT GAIN

One of the ladies in my program lost 30-40 pounds. She was quite intuitive about herself, particularly since she had been in psychotherapy. After the miraculous weight loss, however, she became blocked and actually started to gain weight. She told us she was "sick of the diet." She was putting up tremendous resistance. I asked her if anything was wrong and she said she had no problems. But there was a problem. The body told the truth in that she started to put on weight. So I asked again what was going on with her. She told me she wanted to go back to her old manner of eating. Then I asked her what was going on with her relationship with her husband.

At that point she froze. She looked at me and she started to cry and then said, "I'm very scared." She communicated to me that her husband was looking at her with a new energy. It was an energy that she did not feel comfortable with and yet did not know why. As he approached her with this new energy, she became more and more frightened and was afraid of his sexual advances. She remembered these looks from when she was a little girl. Although she had been in therapy before, she had not worked on sexual issues.

For some reason both she and her therapist did not feel that this was important. Unfortunately, sexual issues are frequently avoided by the client as well as the therapist. Frequently, in therapy, there is a taboo on working on issues of sexuality. The therapist, experiencing some counter-transference here, may unconsciously move away from the real issues that both the therapist and client are confronted with.

In this case, this woman had been wounded as a child. She indeed had a history of subtle sexual violation. Although this did not appear to be overt; that is, she did not appear to have recollection of any childhood abuse or molestation, she did feel an uneasiness about a masculine drive and an energy suggesting sexual advances.

Previously, I quoted Alice Miller's work in discussing how parents unknowingly, and the key word here is *unknowingly*, cross a boundary that has a sexual connotation. A five-year-old child cannot distinguish between love and sexuality. Love and sexuality are the same thing for a five-year-old child. When a child sits on her father's lap, for example, and enjoys the warmth and love of cuddling and then wants to leave, this is a way of satisfying her need for simple contact and then her need for separation. This is a common phenomenon in children. However, if the father frequently uses his daughter as an object for his own need for contact, this is crossing a boundary. The child feels this intrusion energetically, which is also transferred into the unconscious and later experienced as a sexual taboo or a fear of subsequent sexual contact. But where does one leave off and the other begin? Aren't fathers naturally loving toward their children, some more enthusiastically than others?

I believe incest issues nowadays can be seen as fashionable and over-played, but crossing boundaries can be very subtle and, in most cases, unconscious. Loving and genuine affectionate feelings for a child are the reality of human nature. The trap for both the parents and the child is that the unfulfilled need for contact in the adult is acted out on the child rather than the parents finding it in their own relationships.

Of course, there are also more overt cases of sexual abuse which include not only seduction but molestation, incest and rape. While not all overweight people have been sexually abused as children, abundant medical literature indicates that eating disorders are a frequent result of sexual abuse. Symptoms found in incest and rape victims include fear, sleeping and eating disturbances, as well as sexual dysfunction. Obesity and compulsive eating are ways that survivors of childhood abuse protect themselves. Overeating and putting on weight as body armor can be a way to avoid unwanted sexual advances and thus become less vulnerable.

Although many clients in psychotherapy do not remember overt or covert sexual abuse, the body does remember. For example, a powerful female colleague of mine told me that several years ago she had a severe weight problem. While today she is an attractive women at 5 feet, 7 inches, weighing approximately 125 pounds, she used to weigh 180 pounds. She communicated to me that in her college days and particularly in graduate school when she was training to become a massage therapist, she was very heavy and heavily armored. She did not know why. She had an obsession with food that she did not understand. She also related to me that she had the feeling that she was molested as a child, although she didn't know how, nor could she remember the circumstances.

When she was working on her own body as a massage therapist, the memories began to come back. She saw a counselor and she reconstructed some of the forgotten memories of childhood. Although she could not put it completely together, she said that there was a feeling of aggressive male energy that was sexual in nature when she was a young girl. When she went to college, she got involved in a very passionate relationship, and this brought up the previous unpleasant experience of male energy coming toward her as a defenseless young child. At that point she started to put on weight. She gained approximately 50 pounds, becoming less attractive. After she gained her insight and the awareness that her sexuality was the key to her obesity, she began to cry and cry and cry. She grieved for months. She knew how important crying was and used it as a healing modality. After this long process of grieving, she became in touch with her true self and began to lose the weight in an easy and timely manner. She now is able to help others who have been in similar situations.

In addition to sadness and anger, unrecognized fear creates forces in our personality that unconsciously make us eat. It is not uncommon to find that the root of an individual's weight problem is prior sexual abuse, which may be obvious in some and not so obvious in others. It is also a simple fact that some people just like to eat. Not everyone has a hidden sexual issue as an origin to their weight problem. As a matter of fact, the converse was true in another of my clients. Jean had a strong sexual desire that she found imprisoned in her body.

After losing approximately 40 pounds, however, she developed a feeling of freedom about her sexuality. This realization occurred in one of her dreams. She dreamed that her whole body was encased in an orthopedic cast. It suddenly started to crack from the front to the back. As her body armor was falling apart, she found herself in the bathroom with a naked man - a symbol of sexuality. She communicated that she had good feelings in the dream. She in fact liked the dream. She did not experience fear. What she was experiencing was a new emergence of feelings of aliveness and vitality. She was excited about her new body and the way she looked. Her self-image was improving, and she was looking forward to experiencing her new awareness of sexuality. Jean's dream was indeed a signal of emotional healing.

The need for emotional healing is a global one. In our particular society, we have not been given tools with which to understand our emotions. On the contrary, our society has negated the value of emotions and judged certain emotions as weak or inappropriate. It considers strength to be holding yourself up and being strong. This is not true strength if we are "just acting" strong while inside we don't feel strong at all. People have become afraid of emotions and tend to feel uncomfortable when around someone who is crying deeply. It is felt as dangerous and threatening. We have all been taught to cut off from and repress our feelings and have not been given healthy ways to release pent-up emotional energy. The following are a *few tools that will help bring about the emotional healing that will aid in developing greater self-esteem and subsequent weight loss.*

BREATHING

When we are afraid, anxious or nervous, we hold our breath. Due to the high level of stress in living, unfortunately, most people don't breathe deeply enough. Faced with a fight or flight trauma, a simple deep breath can sometimes save lives. It brings our focus of attention back to the immediate and grounds us in our bodies. The best way to become aware of our own need to breathe is to watch for signs of anxiety. Wanting to eat, even though we are not hungry, may be an overt sign of an unconscious motivation that deep breathing could assuage. Some of us may reach for a cigarette or an alcoholic drink. Again, deep breathing can sometimes get us through the crucial point when we are about to do something self-destructive. A more prolonged form of breathing is meditation. If you are not ready to meditate, or don't feel it is for you, however, you will benefit by simply taking time out of each day to sit quietly and breathe deeply and slowly. Making contact with your body through breath is an important part of reconnecting with yourself.

Meditation

Meditation is easy to learn. The most difficult part may be finding the time. But creating the time, whether it be every day or three times a week, can be rewarding, offering you growth and insight. You might feel tremendous resistance or fear of doing it wrong, but there is no one set way to meditate. Often, the biggest obstacle is our own judgment that we are not really in a meditative state. The mere fact that we have taken five minutes or 45 minutes to sit or lie quietly and breathe, however, is meditative in itself. Don't compare yourself to others' accounts of their meditations. If your quiet time doesn't measure up to how you perceive meditation to be, you run the risk of thinking you failed. As you practice it more and more, you will find that your body quiets down more easily.

In order to do this, you must go to a room where you won't be interrupted. Put the answering machine on. Sit in a comfortable chair or lie down on a carpet with a small pillow (optional) under your head. If this is the first time you are attempting meditation, your body might find five reasons why you have to pop up and do something. You might lie down and feel very fidgety. Close your eyes. Start by taking five slow breaths in and out through the mouth. Tell yourself to relax. Continue to breathe slowly and deeply, either in through the nose and out the mouth, or in and out through the nose, whichever is more comfortable. Feel your body. Put your consciousness in your head and, slowly, as you breathe, run your consciousness down your body. If you are having trouble relaxing, tell each part of your body to relax by saying, "My head is relaxed, my legs are relaxed, etc."

Many thoughts might run through your head. Don't resist them, but don't focus on them. Merely note them and let them pass. You may imagine opening a door and saying to all these thoughts, "I know you're there, but I don't want to let you in." See or feel these thoughts going out the door and close the door behind them. You may need to do this a few times.

When you feel you are relaxed enough, you will begin breathing naturally. Take in slow deep breaths every so often, and remember to let the air out slowly. Imagine that you have an inner physician. This inner healer is very wise and loving and may be called upon for a vast supply of ideas and information. Tell it all about your pain, particularly about your body. Let yourself flow with this process. See what you need to express to this inner healer and then ask it for help or guidance. State, for example, that you want to attract the perfect support system. Know that you have a right to ask for this. If you feel sadness, let yourself cry. Whatever you feel, allow it completely. Stay open to receive insights, but don't struggle. Just trust that guidance will come in various ways. For example, you might be in the shower later and feel inspired to call someone to establish a connection. Einstein supposedly got his best ideas while in the shower and relaxing. Follow whatever instincts you may have. When you feel complete, take a few more breaths. Slowly open your eyes.

You can also use meditation to reframe your self-image. If you have been overweight for many years, you may be holding onto a self-defeating image as a "fat person" who is doomed to a lifetime of being fat and/or struggling with fat. Go into a deep relaxation and remember to breathe deeply and take your time. When you are deep in relaxation, start to ask yourself to bring forth all your fears about your own body image. For example, you may fear that you will never have the pleasure of a thinner body. But affirm to yourself that you will by saying, "I am becoming thin." Take deep breaths as you do this. When you feel complete, start to work on the self-image you would like to have.

Tell yourself that you can indeed change your body. You can change destructive patterns. Remind yourself that other people have done it, and you can too! Take some time to visualize yourself feeling healthier, lighter, stronger and filled with vitality. Remember, repetition is very important in shifting your belief systems and your attitude. Working your mind on a deep level will aid the momentum of this reprogramming process.

EMOTIONAL EXERCISES

Another essential door to unlock is getting in touch with the various conflicts you may be holding onto unconsciously in terms of having a trimmer body. You can either do this sitting down with a paper and pen or by releasing them verbally or physically, as I will describe. There are many different exercises you can do. For example, when you feel very sad, try to lie down, tilt your head back, and let down into the feelings. Get deep into sobbing. The more you cry from your abdomen, the better the release. As you are in this state, try to get in touch with the grieving you have had during your struggle. Crying is the most healing of all the emotions. Crying will release the heartbreak, which will help prevent the possibility of real heart disease.

If you feel angry, however, or enraged, try yelling or screaming while in your car. Remember to roll up the windows so you feel private and safe. Or, go out to the woods or a secluded beach and scream at the person whom you are feeling angry toward. Get it all out. Say everything you feel without editing your language. Because he or she is not present, this is your opportunity to release the energy. You could also take a tennis racket and physically hit your bed and scream.

Another good exercise is to lie on your bed and just kick. By kicking and screaming and shaking your head, you can simulate a temper tantrum. Other forms of anger-release work include making a fist and jutting out your jaw in defiance or protest. Another way is to twist a towel and release a sound while your are doing it. There are forms of therapy that teach you how to release your negative emotions using safe, private, effective and beneficial techniques.

Getting in touch with your negativity and learning about your "dark side" can be the most healing aspects of therapy. For example, in our "Healing the Heart Workshops," exploring the dark side is absolutely essential and crucial in the healing process. This is particularly important for those with heart disease who have obvious issues of heartbreak, taking in love and expressions of intimacy and sexuality. Many people may find it difficult, however, to start to release the years of pent-up emotional energy alone.

It is a sign of great strength to realize you want to help yourself. This may include doing emotional release work alone at home or in a safe place such as a therapist's office. It is important to release the core of your sadness, your anger and your fears one way or another. When this happens, we begin to get in touch with our true needs and really experience our true selves. This is a significant step in the right direction, and a profound step in obtaining *Optimum Health*.

BASIC NUTRITION—BACK TO SCHOOL

In order to eat nutritionally, it's important that you understand some basics about how food affects your body. Although some of this information may be more than you care to know right now, I hope you'll find yourself referring back to this chapter again and again.

Remember that the loss of excess fat results from a negative energy balance and that energy is derived from calories. Food calories can be divided into three major components: proteins, carbohydrates, and fats, with alcohol being a fourth less important contributor. When counting calories we need to consider the percentages that come from proteins, carbohydrates or fats in any given serving.

Each of these nutrients provides different amounts of energy (calories per gram or per ounce) measured through sophisticated clinical studies. The following provides useful values for comparison:

- Carbohydrates contain four calories per gram or 112 calories per ounce;
- Fats contain nine calories per gram or 252 calories per ounce;
- Proteins contain four calories per gram or 112 calories per ounce.

From this brief analysis, one can easily see that an individual can eat over twice as many carbohydrates or proteins as fats and still have the same caloric intake. Alcohol has seven calories per gram or 196 calories per ounce, which is usually only one cocktail.

Foods are classified according to their calorie density. For example, three ounces of fish contains approximately 150 calories, which is less than three ounces of beef chuck which contains approximately 300 calories. Such caloric densities are usually related to the amount of fat in the food. Fish contains relatively less fat than beef. Therefore, more fish can be eaten than beef for the same amount of calories. But more fish may not be needed to satisfy hunger, so one can reduce total intake and, therefore, lose weight.

We can see that it is important to know the fat content in food. Being nutritionally aware is to choose foods that provide the most nutrition with the fewest fats and calories. For example, the calories in whole milk are approximately 50 percent fat while the calories in one-percent milk are approximately 18 percent fat. If most of us can make the gradual transition from whole milk to one-percent milk, the amount of calories is reduced by nearly half. One-percent milk is less calorie-dense, and therefore, more healthy. And remember the cardinal rule: *No deprivation and no loss of pleasure.*

Such a weight-loss program may not only be one that is calorie-dilute but also one that contains healthy amounts of carbohydrates, proteins and fats. In considering a healthy diet or a healthy lifestyle, we again have to remember that deprivation is the oppositional force. When putting our meals together we strive for a reasonable balance of carbohydrates, proteins and fats, but do we know how to do this properly? The rule of thumb is surprisingly simple: *Approximately 65 to 70 percent of your diet should be complex carbohydrates, while 10 to 15 percent of the daily intake should include proteins, with the remaining calories coming from fat.* But why eat fat at all?

The body requires essential fatty acids for normal functioning, and most foods, including some vegetables, have at least 15 percent of their total calories in fat. The American Heart Association recommends 30 percent of the dietary intake from fats, but I think 15 to 20 percent is adequate. The real problem in lowering fat content in the diet is that fat simply tastes good. Although many Americans are now fat-conscious, most of our diets still approach a fat content making up approximately 40 to 50 percent of our daily intake. Considering that the American Heart Association recommends that fat intake be less than 30 percent of the total calories, and the famous Pritikin diet, which some cardiologists endorse, only has five to ten percent of the total calories coming from fat, I think we can find a reasonable balance that is neither too strict nor depriving of pleasure.

NUTRITIONAL AWARENESS KEEPS POUNDS OFF, FAT OUT

Medical research indicates that weight gain is not only related to the total number of calories but also to the total number of grams of fat in the diet. Reducing our intake of fat is a cardinal ingredient in weight loss and good health. Generally, people have considerable resistance to reducing the fat intake in their diets. However, it is crucial to point out that fat intake should be kept to a minimum to maximize weight loss and ensure a health conscious lifestyle. In considering a nutritional awareness program, and particularly in losing weight, it is important to focus our attention on the number of grams of fat in our daily consumption. This can be done by reading labels and avoiding various cooking techniques that result in excess fat content.

Mushrooms, for example, contain approximately less than ten percent of their calories in fat, but if they are deep fried in oil or if they are broiled in butter, the calorie content is considerably higher. Onions are approximately three to five percent fat, but fried as onion rings, the fat content approaches 90 percent. Again, this is calorie-dense and a poor choice when seeking a healthy, nutritional balance.

In calculating the percentage of fat in a particular product, you must know the calories per serving and the number of grams of fat per serving. The calculation process goes something like this: Multiply the number of grams of fat by nine (remember there are nine calories per gram of fat) to determine the total number of fat calories in a food product. Next, divide the number of fat calories by the number of total calories in the serving. Now convert this to a percentage by multiplying by 100 (grams fat $\times$ 9 divided by cal/serving $\times$ 100 =). The goal in losing weight and staying healthy is to primarily choose foods that are approximately less than 20 percent fat.

Let's now focus attention on the calculations of carbohydrates and proteins. One has to keep in mind that each gram of protein or carbohydrate has four calories. The calculation for caloric value in proteins and carbohydrates is similar to fat content, but then we need to multiply by four instead of nine. Then divide the number of protein or carbohydrate calories by the number of calories per serving and again convert this to a percentage (multiply by 100). With simple arithmetic one can determine the percent of calories of protein, carbohydrate and fat in a particular food. For example, potato chips are approximately 60 percent fat. For the usual serving of ten potato chips there is approximately 115 calories, one gram of protein, ten grams of carbohydrates and eight grams of fat per serving.

To determine the percentage of fat, remember our formula requiring two crucial pieces of information: (1) The total number of calories per serving; (2) The grams of fat per serving. Therefore, multiply eight grams of fat by nine calories per gram and this equals 72 calories. Next, divide the number of fat calories by the number of total calories, which is 72 over 115. Now convert this to a percentage by multiplying by 100. The figure comes out to 62.6 percent of its calories from fat. Since potato chips contain such a considerable quantity of fat, in this case even a small portion is detrimental to diet and health. At 115 calories and eight grams of fat for ten chips, just imagine *how many calories you can consume sitting with a bowl of chips watching television and not even feel satisfied.* It is important to understand that substituting foods that give us the same satisfaction but less fat content and consequently, less weight gain will alleviate the feelings of hunger. Again, our most important tool in losing weight is knowledge and awareness of the fat content in our diets.

Protein and carbohydrate awareness is equally important. The American population is highly preoccupied with the seeming need for protein. Meat and potatoes for most of us was our typical diet growing up. We all have heard the stories of how meat is necessary for protein in our diet and for strong and healthy bodies. Yes, it is true that meat provides a major source of protein, but how much protein do we really need?

Ordinarily, most scientists are in agreement that approximately one gram of protein is necessary per kilogram (2.2 pounds) of body weight per day. Therefore, a 150 pound sedentary man needs approximately 55 to 65 grams of protein per day. If we consume enough calories, however, excess proteins will be converted to fat and stored in the body to be burned later for energy. Since a man of this size consumes approximately 2,400 calories per day, the recommended protein consumption should approximate 12 percent of his dietary calories. But if this individual were to eat more protein as opposed to carbohydrates, much of the excess protein would be stored as fat. Since most Americans consume approximately one and a half to two times as much protein as they need, this is an easy and often overlooked source of weight gain.

YOU AND YOUR BUN

The process of converting protein (amino acids) into fat is called deamination. This can cause considerable metabolic stress to the body. During this process the nitrogen that is released from the amino acids is quickly converted into ammonia. Since ammonia is toxic to the body, it is changed into the breakdown product called urea. Blood urea nitrogen, or BUN, is a measure of the kidney function and really is a product of the breakdown of nitrogen waste products in the body. In a normal balanced diet where protein consists of approximately ten to 15 percent of the total caloric intake, our bodies can easily dispose of the urea through the normal functioning of the kidneys. However, taking excess quantities of protein, such as 20 to 25 percent, will cause a buildup of urea, which needs water for metabolism. If we do not drink enough water, our body takes it from our tissues to dilute the urea, placing an enormous burden on the kidneys.

Such a scenario occurs in individuals on very high protein diets. Wrestlers trying to "make weight" frequently use this destructive technique. I did this during my college career, when as a wrestler I needed to maintain a weight approximately 10 to 12 pounds lighter than my natural and healthy weight. Our coaches recommended a high protein diet - and we wondered why we were continuously "dying of thirst!" Yes, I was able to make the weight on every occasion, but at the expense of my renal or kidney function. After nine years of wrestling through high school and college, my kidney function was slightly abnormal when I entered medical school. The excess toxicities induced by high protein metabolism, coupled with a poor intake of fluid, probably affected the status of my kidneys. Unknowingly I caused renal dysfunction in myself, which could have been extremely hazardous. Luckily for me, I stopped the "protein diet" before it had the time to do lasting damage. Protein, though, has many important functions in the body. It makes up the muscles, ligaments, tendons, organs, glands, nails, hair and some body fluids. Proteins are also essential for growth. Amino acids are essential in building healthy muscles.

Amino acids are the building blocks of protein. Because protein is composed of different acids, each amino acid has a specific function. There are two types of amino acids - the essential and the nonessential. The nonessential amino acids can be produced by the liver, and include approximately 80 percent of the amino acids we need. The remaining 20 percent must be obtained from outside sources. There are nine essential amino acids. If we do not consume foods with enough of the essential amino acids, the body may be unable to produce the protein it requires for healthy functioning. We all have read signs, particularly in elementary school cafeterias, with statements such as, "Eating meat builds strong muscles." This is because meat sources are considered to contain the highest sources of protein. Unfortunately, meats also contain considerable quantities of hidden fat. Other complete protein sources include dairy products, eggs, fish and fowl.

Although the need for protein in the United States is grossly exaggerated, the proper amount of amino acids is indeed crucial. For example, some individuals on weight loss programs, particularly fasting programs, do not consume enough protein. This can be injurious to their health. If the body does not take in the proper amount of amino acids and grams of protein per day, then it will take the protein from its own muscles. Yes, the body will find a way to produce protein. Unfortunately, it does not distinguish skeletal muscle from heart muscle. Therefore, overzealous fasting and dieting may lead to deterioration of the heart muscle, making a person susceptible to arrhythmias and perhaps even sudden death events. In our hospital weight-loss program, for example, we were particularly careful to maintain the minimal daily protein requirement for each individual. We frequently performed electrocardiograms on these participants to ensure a proper functioning of the heart.

We all need a basic minimum of protein. We need to keep ourselves in a "positive nitrogen balance." If the body results in a negative nitrogen balance, we lose protein from our own muscles. Therefore, it is important to select foods that are good sources of protein. Proteins may come from animal sources such as meat, fish, eggs and milk; but also from grains, vegetables and fruits. Most of us now know that animal proteins such as fish, turkey and white meat chicken offer complete proteins and are lower in fat than red meats. Eggs contain protein and some fat, but do have high quantities of cholesterol. One egg contains 225 mg of cholesterol which is almost the maximum daily requirement as well. The American Heart Association recommends that most people should limit their cholesterol intake to less than 300 mg per day. Most overweight individuals should keep their meat and egg consumption to a minimum. Vegetable sources of protein, though highly desirable, are often deficient in one or more of the essential amino acids. Thus, vegetarians may need to supplement their diets with dairy products or combine other foods to make complete proteins. Excellent sources of vegetable proteins as well as carbohydrates include beans, peas, grains and lentils to mention a few.

Carbohydrates make up the most calories in our foods and should be the major source of nutrients in our diet. They are the primary energy storage molecules found in most living organisms. Carbohydrates come from the plant kingdom. The edible portion of plants is called starch. The walls of most young plants are frequently made up of cellulose and starch, containing many sugar molecules linked together. These are called polysaccharides, groups of complex sugars that are found in most of the complex carbohydrates or "starchy foods" in our diets such as peas, beans, potatoes and corn. Disaccharides consist of two sugar molecules, with the familiar names being sucrose (table sugar), maltose (malt sugar) and lactose (milk sugar). Monosaccharides are the simple sugars such as glucose and fructose and contain only one sugar molecule.

Complex carbohydrates are the predominant feature of a healthy diet. It is important to remember that complex carbohydrates should make up at least 65 to 70 percent of our caloric intake. The American Heart Association recommends at least 50 percent of calories from complex carbohydrates; however, I prefer more calories from complex carbohydrates and less calories from fats. Complex carbohydrates cannot be absorbed quickly into the bloodstream though, unless they are broken down by the digestive process. Once they are digested, the breakdown products from polysaccharides are commonly referred to as glucose. Fructose, a monosaccharide, is found naturally in fruit and honey and is easily converted to glucose. Sucrose (table sugar), which eventually breaks down into glucose, makes up approximately 25 percent of the total carbohydrates we eat and occurs naturally in most carbohydrates, especially in beet or cane sugar and maple syrup.

The primary function of carbohydrates is to provide energy for the body. If there is a positive balance of carbohydrates, the glucose may be stored as glycogen in the liver. Our body needs this glucose to maintain its normal function. While the liver can breakdown glycogen in situations where glucose is needed but not consumed, it is best to consume carbohydrates on a daily basis to provide a continual energy source.

GUESS HOW MUCH SUGAR YOU EAT?

Simple carbohydrates are most often found in sweet foods such as pastries, cakes and cookies, which are usually made with refined sugar, particularly cane sugar. The problem with eating large quantities of sucrose is that it contains calories but no vitamins, minerals or fiber. Simply stated, although such sugar provides energy, it really has no positive effects except satisfying our craving for sweets. *Sugar will increase calories and will cause weight gain.* Such simple carbohydrates should be kept to a minimum as they add nothing to the body but calories.

One of our goals in carbohydrate awareness is to increase your consumption of nutrient-dense foods and decrease your consumption of calorie-dense foods. Most Americans are unaware that three-fourths of all the sugar we eat comes in processed foods. Although some of us still continue to use a little white sugar in our coffee, tea or on our cereal, the amount of "hidden" sugar in breads, soft drinks, candies, cakes and donuts is extremely high. *The average American, for example, consumes approximately 100 pounds of sugar per year!*

Consuming simple carbohydrates also causes a metabolic stress to the body. Simple sugars require less digestion and so when ingested, the sugar molecules enter the vascular system more quickly than other nutrients. This causes stress on the pancreas, resulting in high insulin releases. Such high amounts of insulin are required to metabolize the sugar. This may result in metabolic swings in our body, alternating between periods of high blood sugar and then low blood sugar.

These periods are experienced as mood swings, manifesting both high and low energy. After a high-insulin surge, for example, low blood sugar may cause fatigue and light-headedness. This frequently occurs after the "coffee break." During the coffee break we may consume coffee with simple white sugar added and perhaps a donut. Such an increase in simple sugar results in an increase in insulin. After the initial surge of insulin, the blood sugar usually drops. For this reason, we may be hungry again not long after our coffee break. This sets up a vicious cycle resulting in the need of stimulation, that is taking another cup of coffee and donut followed by a very high-calorie lunch. Caffeine, which we will discuss in a subsequent analysis, is yet another ugly player in this game.

Since glucose is the brain's only food, the brain utilizes a considerable portion of the glucose in the body. Unlike other muscles and organs, the brain can burn neither fat nor protein except in situations of a very prolonged fast. Therefore, low blood sugar affects the brain. Symptoms of fatigue, light-headedness and dizziness easily occur.

The advantage of eating more complex carbohydrates is not only for their additional vitamin, mineral and fiber content, but also in time required for metabolism. The more unrefined the carbohydrate, the slower the release of glucose into the blood stream. The more refined the sugar, the more quickly glucose is placed into the bloodstream, resulting in higher surges of insulin and possible later symptoms of hypoglycemia. Thus, simple carbohydrates should be kept to a minimum at all times, whereas complex carbohydrates should make up not only the majority of our total carbohydrate intake but also the majority of our diet. Diets high in complex carbohydrates include fruits, vegetables and grains, providing large amounts of fiber as well as nutrients. This is a key factor in any discussion on nutrition and health.

Five

FIBER CAN BE FUN

This chapter could save your life.

Most doctors would agree that a diet high in fiber results in a reduced risk of developing many chronic diseases. The importance of fiber in human health has been demonstrated by large population studies. African people on high-fiber diets have a very low incidence of coronary artery disease, colon-rectal cancer, diverticulosis, gallbladder disease or constipation. The African Bantu population, for example, has an average cholesterol of 90 to 100. In this culture, coronary artery disease is practically nonexistent. Primitive cultures tend to rely on wheat, corn, rice and grain.

These complex carbohydrates that we mentioned in the previous analysis are exceedingly more productive for the body than the refined carbohydrates and simple sugars that are found in processed Westernized foods. The harvesting of meat for slaughter is also a relatively recent addition to civilization. Was man ever meant to eat meat? If we compare the teeth of man to the teeth of a dog or a cat, we can easily distinguish the absence of carnivorous incisors in man's mouth. Carnivorous animals, those relying on flesh in the diet, generally do not succumb to coronary artery disease. They have genetic protection, as they were intended to eat meat.

Civilized man, on the other hand, has a diet composed of meats and fats and yet has a vascular system that is not accustomed to such abuse.

Such a drastic change in Western man's diet has been associated with a multitude of diseases, including dental caries, diverticular disease, large bowel cancer, hiatal hernia, coronary heart disease, diabetes, gallstones and obesity. Over the last two centuries there has been a profound change in man's diet. Although hunter/gatherers did consume animal protein, they were dependent upon seasonal migratory habits of herds. Therefore, their meat intake was limited. The most drastic changes in Western man's diet have included an increase in meat, fat and sugar, and a decrease in coarse carbohydrates and dietary fiber (Table 1).

Dietary fiber is the part of the plant food that our systems cannot digest and, when ingested, passes through the small intestine unchanged. How many of us, for example, have changed a baby's diaper only to find the outer shells of corn kernels are still intact even though their nutrients had been absorbed? The absorbable portion of corn is starch. The insoluble or undigested fiber increases the speed of transit through the intestines. Insoluble fiber includes cellulose, heavy cellulose and lignin - the supportive skeleton of plants and the fiber found in most fruits and vegetables. Soluble fiber, on the other hand, includes pectins, gums and mucilages. These entities make up the intracellular cement of plants and have several positive effects on the body that promote health and help prevent various disease states. Soluble fibers form a gel-like material that inhibits cholesterol and LDL absorption. Gums are effective in reducing blood glucose levels and in addition may prohibit cholesterol absorption. Pectins, likewise, have been shown to reduce blood lipids as well. *The familiar phrase, "An apple a day keeps the doctor away," is well spoken.* Apples are a good source of pectin, as is the white pulp of grapefruit. If you want to lower your cholesterol, eating pectin is very healthy. I will show you in a subsequent analysis, my natural cholesterol lowering approach, which does incorporate natural soluble and insoluble fibers.

Most complex carbohydrates contain both types of fiber. The predominant type of fiber depends upon the plant species. Wheat bran, for example, contains more insoluble fiber than soluble or viscous fiber. Oat bran, rich in gums, is considered a better source of viscous fiber. Insoluble fiber is also found in cabbage, broccoli, turnips, Brussels sprouts, kidney beans, green beans, chick peas, nuts, cereals, breads made from whole grain wheat, rye, oats, barley and corn. Fruits, especially the skins, are also an excellent source of insoluble fiber. Soluble fiber is found in specific fruits such as strawberries, peaches, apple pulp, and citrus. Berries and seeds of fruit are especially rich in soluble fiber.

TABLE 1

Changes in Food

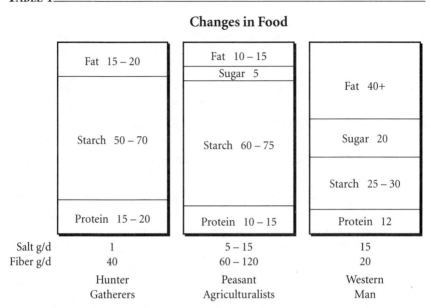

	Hunter Gatherers	Peasant Agriculturalists	Western Man
	Fat 15 – 20	Fat 10 – 15	Fat 40+
		Sugar 5	
	Starch 50 – 70	Starch 60 – 75	Sugar 20
			Starch 25 – 30
	Protein 15 – 20	Protein 10 – 15	Protein 12
Salt g/d	1	5 – 15	15
Fiber g/d	40	60 – 120	20

FIBER HELPS PREVENT COLON CANCER

The physiological effects of dietary fiber occur from our first mouthful of food. High-fiber foods are "chewy." Chewing stimulates the flow of saliva and secretion of gastric juices. Such prolonged chewing also gives the brain a message of satiety. For example, if we chew coarse brown rice, or a high-fiber cookie for that matter, the increased time it takes for swallowing creates a conversation between the brain and the stomach. Since it may take several seconds to perhaps several minutes to ingest such high-fiber foods, the stomach has more time to register the feeling of fullness. Such high-fiber meals fill the stomach and provide a feeling of fullness, particularly when ingested with generous quantities of water. The combination of water and fiber swell the stomach, satisfying hunger quickly. Soluble fiber also delays gastric emptying.

In the small intestine, insoluble fiber reduces the rate of digestion and nutrient absorption. In the large intestine, dietary fiber, particularly the insoluble form, increases the bulk of stools. Fiber has a water holding capacity that prevents water from being absorbed through the colonic mucosa in the large intestine. This helps prevent dry, hard stools, thereby alleviating constipation. In general, cereal grains containing cellulose and fruits and vegetables containing pectin serve as excellent bulk-forming natural laxatives. Fiber, as we previously stated, increases fecal transit rate. *Therefore, it may protect us against colon cancer because of its laxative effect.* The quicker the waste is eliminated, the less time is allowed for carcinogens to be formed by bacteria and possible chemical reactions in the bowel.

Statistics from population studies all over the world suggest that a high-fiber diet is protective while a high-fat diet may enhance the risk of colon cancer. Consider the United States and Finland, two countries that have a high incidence of colon cancer. Both of these populations consume high-fat diets, but colon cancer mortality is significantly lower among the Finns who consume a much greater amount of cereal fiber than the Americans. The problem with the "normal" American diet is that it contains too much fat and not enough fiber. The average American consumes between 11 and 17 grams of fiber. The National Cancer Institute recommends at least a daily consumption of 20 to 30 grams of fiber (Table 2). *I recommend 30, with 35 being the maximum.* This is essentially twice the daily intake of a typical American, estimated at 11 grams for women and 17 for men. *Diet, therefore, is an important contributing factor in colon cancer. It has also been estimated that 35 percent of all cancers in the country are caused by improper diet.* Since colon cancer, in general, is more prevalent in obese persons, a high-fiber diet is especially essential for this group.

As fiber gives bulk to food without providing additional energy, fiber-rich foods offer excellent advantages to the obese population. It is also an important consideration in the diabetic population as well. A diet rich in complex carbohydrates including fiber may improve blood sugar by offering a large continuous supply of energy rather than short bursts, thus perhaps reducing the amount of medication required. The American Diabetic Association suggests that patients who have diabetes mellitus should double their fiber intake. It is important to consider that diets rich in fiber also contain less fat and cholesterol and fewer calories. This too is as beneficial as weight reduction is in treating the diabetic condition.

FIBER HELPS THE HEART

These implications are also exceedingly important when one considers the causes of coronary heart disease. In experimental studies, soluble fiber

TABLE 2

Recommended Daily Fiber Intake Compared with Current Intake

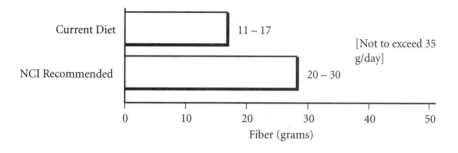

Reprinted with permission from ©1990 Health Learning Systems, Inc.

sources (pectin, guar gum, barley and oat bran) have been shown to reduce blood cholesterol levels when taken in generous amounts. We have all heard of the cholesterol-lowering effects of oats and oat bran. As little as two ounces of oat bran per day can reduce your cholesterol seven to ten percent. Actually, any oat product, i.e., oat bran, oatmeal or even Cheerios for that matter, is effective as a cholesterol-lowering agent.

Recently the media has questioned the validity of oat bran, indicating that larger amounts may be needed to lower one's cholesterol. While this may be true, if oat bran is supplemented with other fiber-rich foods it creates an additive or synergistic effect on the body. As little as one to one and one-half cups of beans in one's diet, with some oat bran, can lower cholesterol by 60 points. I personally favor oat bran and oat products, particularly since they are excellent sources of soluble fiber and in clinical studies have demonstrated definite reduction in LDL cholesterols in many people.

Wheat bran, on the other hand, has a less significant effect on cholesterol because it is an insoluble fiber. However, wheat bran is considered by some to be the best bran to eat in reducing the risk of colon cancer. As previously mentioned, it helps to sweep away the possible cancer producing substances from the intestines by enhancing fecal bulk and increasing transit rate. Insoluble fiber acts in several ways to reduce blood cholesterol as well. This type of fiber may prevent the absorption of many chemicals into the intestines, particularly the bile acids. Bile acids are necessary to form cholesterol in the body.

If there is a restriction of bile acids because of altered absorption and greater secretion, this results in the continuous drain of the natural body stores of cholesterol. By the same token, cholesterol may also be trapped by fiber and lost through the stools rather than be absorbed. Pharmaceutical companies in this country have created substances that act in a similar way, but doesn't it just make sense to increase our intake of dietary fiber? Why take a synthetic drug if we don't have to? In addition, fiber-rich complex carbohydrates serve as a good alternative to foods high in fat, as recently published in the *New England Journal of Medicine*; people who eat more fiber foods eat less fat foods. Therefore, it makes sense to increase the fiber in our diet. Western diets are too high in fats, sugar and salt, and too low in fiber and starch. To put it simply, *Americans need to eat more like the inhabitants of some of the undeveloped countries in the world.*

Increasing our starch and fiber, reducing our sugar and salt and omitting as much fat as possible should not present any major difficulties. We do not deprive ourselves if we consume fiber. The risk/benefit ratio is exceedingly high. Although there are some potential adverse effects such as bloating, cramps or flatulence, these symptoms are only fleeting and will disappear when our own intestinal flora adjusts to the change in the nutritional environment. One drawback of fiber-rich foods may be that they inhibit the absorption of minerals, including calcium and iron. But vitamin and mineral supplementation, or the increased consumption of yellow and green vegetables and fruits, will help to replenish such minerals. Other rare potential hazards of fiber include the remote possibility of obstruction of the GI tract, particularly occurring in individuals who have undergone surgical procedures for peptic ulcer, stomach cancer or ulcerative colitis. These individuals should consult their physicians when utilizing high-fiber diets.

Remember, however, most diseases are helped or prevented by fiber, including not only diabetes, diverticulitis and colon cancer, as we mentioned, but also coronary heart disease. The risk/benefit ratio of fiber is overwhelming on the side of benefit. By increasing the amount of fiber in diet, we can gradually enhance the quality of our health, feel better and help to prevent many of the illnesses of modern man (Table 3).

TABLE 3

REPORTED HEALTH BENEFITS OF DIETARY FIBER

- Improvement in bowel function
- Reduction of serum cholesterol levels in hypercholesterolemic patients
- Displacement of fat, saturated fat and cholesterol from the diet
- Improvement of glycemic control among patients with type II diabetes mellitus
- Treatment and prevention of diverticulosis
- Reduction of colon cancer risk

Reprinted with permission from © 1990, *Health Learning Systems, Inc.*

In the following table (Table 4), you will find some quick and easy fiber foods that I recommend.

TABLE 4

QUICK AND EASY   *Fast Fiber Combinations*

Food Combinations	Grams of Dietary Fiber	Total Combined Fiber
1 raw carrot with	2.4	7.3 grams
½ cup raisins	4.9	
1 pear with	5.0	7.1 grams
2 graham crackers	2.1	
3 cups popcorn with	3.0	6.7 grams
1 cup dried figs	3.7	
½ cup cantaloupe with	2.7	6.6 grams
3 dried prunes	3.9	
½ cup blueberries with	2.5	5.8 grams
⅔ cup Shredded Wheat	3.3	
1 baked potato with	3.7	5.7 grams
½ cup apple sauce	2.0	
¾ cup oatmeal	2.8	5.7 grams
1 mango	2.9	
⅔ cup Raisin Bran with	3.6	5.3 grams
½ cup apple sauce	1.7	
½ cup brown rice with	2.4	5.3 grams
1 apple	2.9	
½ cup corn (cooked) with	3.9	5.3 grams
1 slice whole-wheat bread	1.4	

CHOLESTEROL—MYTH, FACT AND FICTION

Cholesterol is a topic of much conversation these days. The public is so frequently inundated by media and advertising regarding the health hazards of high cholesterol that this topic is of interest to both the healthy and the unhealthy alike. Almost every patient I have in my practice wants to know his or her cholesterol level, the young and the old, those with and without heart disease. But what is cholesterol? And why is there so much conversation regarding it?

Cholesterol is a fatty, wax-like substance that is both manufactured by the body and taken in through foods. It is needed in the production of hormones, cells and bile salts. (For example, cholesterol is a source of the adrenal steroid hormone cortisone, as well as the sex hormones.) Since our liver manufactures cholesterol, it would reserve enough to support the daily functioning of the body, even if we did not eat any cholesterol at all. Without cholesterol, our cells could not function. We need cholesterol for membrane synthesis, particularly in the stabilization of our cells. In small amounts, therefore, cholesterol is vital to our health and survival. But whenever a person eats beyond his energy requirements, a surplus amount of cholesterol accumulates in the blood. In addition, the liver feeds on the saturated fat to produce even more cholesterol.

It is this gradual buildup of white fat and cholesterol that increases the risk of atherosclerosis, which consequently increases the risk of coronary heart disease and stroke, as well as peripheral vascular disease. When too much cholesterol gets into the blood, it may become sticky or sequestered in vessel walls resulting in a gradual hardening and narrowing of the arteries. This hardening of the arteries is known as atherosclerosis. This artery-clogging action of cholesterol creates plaque in the vascular channels and heightens the risk of cardiac illness. There are many large population studies which indicate that as one's cholesterol rises, one's risk of coronary artery disease also rises.

LOWER YOUR CHOLESTEROL AND LIVE!

Consider the Japanese, whose diet mainly consists of rice, fish, and sea vegetables. This culture has the lowest incidence of coronary heart disease in the world. The American diet, on the other hand, consists of considerable quantities of saturated fat found in meats, oils, nuts and dairy products. The Americans have one of the highest rates of coronary heart disease in the world. The well known Framingham Study, for example, clearly demonstrated that there is a direct relationship between coronary heart disease and a typical American diet. This study began in 1948 and utilized more than 5,000 subjects from Framingham, Massachusetts. The subjects were analyzed in regard to health habits such as diet, smoking and high blood pressure. The results indicate that the higher the cholesterol intake, the greater the probability in developing heart disease. Currently, approximately one in four Americans has a high blood cholesterol. *The good news, however, is that if your blood cholesterol is high, you can reduce your risk of heart disease by simply lowering it.*

A landmark study (Coronary Primary Prevention Trial) by the National Heart, Lung and Blood Institute showed the benefit from lowering cholesterol is considerable. In this trial, each one percent reduction in blood cholesterol was associated with a two percent reduction in coronary heart disease risk. Thus, participants who reduced their cholesterol by 25 percent, reduced their risk of heart attack by almost one-half. Other studies have also demonstrated that *lowering cholesterol levels actually can reverse the buildup of blockages in coronary vessels, resulting in a regression of atherosclerosis.* Since the medical literature is so overwhelmingly supportive in the direct relationship between cholesterol and coronary heart disease, all reputable physicians should counsel their patients about the potential hazards of cholesterol. In fact, physicians do frequently recommend that patients know their cholesterol levels and take a more active role in healing themselves, particularly through dietary choices.

I have found that patients nowadays have become so aware and so knowledgeable about cholesterol that they not only want to know their total numbers, but also ask questions regarding HDL and LDL, lipoproteins that carry cholesterol in the blood. The blood is like sea water and cholesterol is a fat. Since water and fat do not mix, cholesterol is carried in the blood in combination with a protein, referred to as high-density lipoproteins (HDL) and low-density lipoproteins (LDL). HDL cholesterol, commonly called "good" cholesterol, is considered to be a type of cholesterol scavenger in the body. HDL picks up cholesterol from blood vessels and transports them back to the liver. LDL, on the other hand, infiltrates the blood vessel walls, thus increasing the risk of "plaque" buildup in the vessels. If the plaque buildup occurs in the coronary vessels, this could render an individual susceptible to heart disease. LDL is a noxious substance by itself. When combined with the toxic effects of cigarette smoking or the membrane-tearing effects of high blood pressure, it results in a gradual inflammatory process that invades the blood vessel wall, causing a buildup or a proliferation of the vessel which leads to gradual closure. Thus, the higher the LDL, the more one is at risk for heart disease. Conversely, the higher the HDL, the more protection one has from heart disease.

Cardiologists frequently not only look at total cholesterol, but also at the cholesterol fractions of LDL and HDL. Individuals who are at the most serious risk for developing coronary heart disease include those people with a low HDL and a high LDL. So, doesn't it make sense to increase your HDL and lower your LDL? One way to increase HDL is by *losing weight*, as studies prove they have an inverse relationship. *Vigorous exercise* is another effective way to raise the HDL. Effective ways of lowering LDL also include weight loss, as well as *reduction of fat in the diet*, utilization of more *dietary fiber and cessation of cigarette smoking*. Cigarette smoking is indeed a major cardiovascular risk factor, not only because of the toxic effects of tar and nicotine, but also because cigarette smoking enhances the effect LDL has on the vascular wall. In a recent European study, smoking was found to increase the total cholesterol and cause a reduction in the HDL, particularly in women.

EMOTIONS AFFECT CHOLESTEROL

In addition to smoking and diet, there are many other factors known to affect cholesterol. For example, *emotions* are a major consideration.

Calming touch has been shown to actually lower blood cholesterol while stress increases it. Yes, it is true that excessive stress and tension can affect the regulation of cholesterol in your body, regardless of the intake through diet. Scientific studies have shown that accountants during tax season who are under severe deadlines to perform have considerable elevations in their blood cholesterol during the months of January through April. Following the tax season deadline of April 15, their cholesterol levels fall.

Perhaps one of the most interesting studies comes from the race car study done in England. Race car drivers take many chances and probably have an unconscious fear of death. In this particular study, drivers who raced on the circuit had alarming increases in both cholesterol and triglycerides. Thus, the fear of the death is perhaps the strongest emotional factor one can endure, which was reflected in the high metabolic constituents of blood cholesterol. But what about positive feelings such as love? Can they influence cholesterol?

LOVE

Feelings have been shown to have a major effect on cholesterol. This was seen in an animal study of rabbits. Rabbits who received preferential care from their trainers had lower cholesterol levels and less significant plaques in their arteries than rabbits who were not cuddled. Thus, touching and cuddling proved to enhance *Optimum Health* in these animals. Humans are no exceptions to this rule either. *As* simple as it sounds, love indeed heals. In our workshops on Healing the Heart, we clearly demonstrated profound cholesterol lowering when one experiences contact, connectedness and feelings. In these four to seven day workshops, cholesterol lowering was reported in every one of our participants, with some participants losing as much as 100 mg/dL of cholesterol in a mere four to five days of group support. Although these participants were given low-fat, high-fiber diets, the sudden drastic reduction in cholesterol supports the notion of how emotional discharge can positively impact our health.

When we hold in our emotions and feelings, we create undesirable biochemical situations in our bodies that can render our blood more susceptible to cholesterol elevation. Unfortunately, most of us are unaware of these factors. In our Healing the Heart seminars, people are nurtured by a supporting environment, one feels connected to others and cholesterol levels fall.

TABLE 5

NATIONAL CHOLESTEROL EDUCATION PROGRAM

Blood Cholesterol	Level	Recommended Action
Greater than 240	High	Refer to physician
Between 200-239	Borderline High	Refer to physician
Less than 200	Desirable	Repeat in five years

Although digging into emotions and opening a can of worms can have tremendous positive impact on our emotional and physical health, the commitment and vulnerability can be difficult for many of us. But I invite every one of you to consider looking into your emotional self. Growth is painful, but well worth it in the long run.

CHECKING YOUR CHOLESTEROL

Levels of blood cholesterol can vary considerably among different individuals. How do you know if your cholesterol is too high? Recently the National Heart, Lung and Blood Institute panel of experts has advised standard guidelines for doctors and their patients (Table 5). Individuals with total cholesterols below 200 mg per deciliter appear to have a more favorable profile than individuals with cholesterols greater than 240. Patients at serious risk for coronary heart disease also include those with HDL levels less than 35 and LDL fractions greater than 160 (Table 5A). LDL levels below 130 mg per deciliter are considered desirable. HDL greater than 60 mg per deciliter are also considered protective. (Thus, most doctors and patients would agree that it is necessary not only to know your total cholesterol, but also to know the fractions of LDL and HDL.)

Although HDL can be modified by exercise and weight reduction, most doctors would agree that the reduction of saturated fat is the most important way to lower the LDL in your diet. Saturated fatty acids increase plasma cholesterol levels. It is a simple fact that cholesterol in the blood increases as a result of taking not only cholesterol in the diet, but also saturated fats. Approximately fifteen percent of total calories in the typical American diet comes from saturated fatty acids, which is one reason Americans have such high serum cholesterol levels. Saturated fatty acids that have the greatest impact on raising cholesterol include lauric acid, myristic acid, and palmitic acid. Other nutrients, particularly

TABLE 5A
CLASSIFICATION OF HDL, LDL, TRIGLYCERIDES

HDL Cholesterol

More than 60 mg/dL	Protective
Less than 35 mg/dL	High Risk

LDL Cholesterol

Less than 130 mg/dL	Desirable (for heart patients)
Greater than 160 mg/dL	High Risk

Triglycerides (Fat Storage)

Less than 200 mg/dL	Desirable
200 - 399 mg/dL	Borderline - High
400 - 1,000 mg/dL	High
More than 1,000 mg/dL	Very High (Dangerous)

linolenic acid (polyunsaturated fatty acid) and oleic acid (a monounsaturated fatty acid), may reduce LDL concentrations and its bad effects.

While there is some controversy about the mechanism of LDL reduction, it is undisputed that using polyunsaturated and monounsaturated fats, such as olive and canola oils, instead of saturated fats, such as butter, will reduce LDL levels. When the body takes in saturated fatty acids, the liver transforms them into blood cholesterol. Butter, for example, has little cholesterol, but has 99 percent fat, so when it is ingested, the liver converts a portion of it to cholesterol.

CHOLESTEROL CULPRITS

Another way in which our diet choices can increase our cholesterol levels is simply through an increased intake of total calories. Obesity commonly associated with an increased caloric intake, for example, increases serum cholesterol simply on the basis of more ingested calories. Obesity can also result in lowering the HDL (good cholesterol). Weight loss, on the other hand, will help to reduce the LDL levels.

A major recommendation for lowering cholesterol is to reduce the intake of total calories. Again, this means reducing our total fat intake in grams. Reducing the level of saturated fatty acids and replacing them with monounsaturated fatty acids and small quantities of polyunsaturated fatty acids is also recommended. Recently, however, it was suggested that one should utilize more polyunsaturated fatty acids in the diet, but investigations have indicated that such an increase in polyunsaturated fatty acids may actually result in lowering of the HDL. This is an undesirable effect that we wish to avoid. A better alternative is to use more monounsaturated fats, such as *olive oil* and *canola oil*. A more detailed description of polyunsaturated and monounsaturated fats will be given in the subsequent analysis on fatty acids. For now, I ask you to focus your attention on the cholesterol effects of saturated fat.

Saturated fats are found predominantly in foods of animal origin such as meats, organs, butter, cream, cheese and most other dairy products. Very high amounts of saturated fats are also found in chicken fat, beef fat and particularly in organ meats such as heart, kidney and sweetbreads. Other saturated fats include coconut oil and palm oil, frequently used by manufacturers in processed foods and packaged baked goods. *Coconut oil is approximately 99 percent saturated fat,* actually containing higher percentages of saturated fat than butter or meat. It is important to recognize these oils that are used in nondairy creamers as well as commercially prepared whipped creams and vegetable shortenings to prolong shelf life and prevent rancidity. A good rule of thumb is to *limit our intake of commercially prepared baked goods, meats, saturated fats and oils.*

We should also lessen the intake of dairy products and eggs. Did you know that *one of the most cholesterol-producing items in the American diet comes from milk?* Milk fat found in dairy products, including milk, butter, cheese, cream and ice cream, not only contains high amounts of cholesterol, but also saturated fats. It is essential for weight loss and lowering cholesterol levels to reduce these items in the diet. For example, approximately 50 percent of whole milk's total calories are from fat. Thus, it is best to gradually shift to two-percent milk, which is preferable to whole milk but still contains about 36 percent of calories from fat, down to one-percent fat milk, which contains about 18 percent of calories from fat. Skim milk is the most preferred. Skim milk and one-percent milk really do not contain excessive amounts of fat and they are also rich in protein and calcium, so it is not necessary to totally eliminate dairy from the diet. It is strongly recommended, however, that individuals with high serum cholesterol and those who want to lose weight use either very low-fat or skim milk whenever possible. Butter, cream, cheese and ice cream should be eaten infrequently and only in small quantities, as they contain both high levels of saturated fat and cholesterol. Low-fat substitutes are also available for all of these items.

Eggs are another culprit. Each egg yolk contains approximately 225 mg of cholesterol. Since the recommended intake of cholesterol is less than 300 mg per day, it is suggested that eggs be cut to a minimum. Egg whites, on the other hand, contain no cholesterol and are also an excellent source of protein. Egg substitutes contain no cholesterol but some researchers say that they contain saturated fats. Since eggs contain considerable quantities of protein and particularly important minerals such as magnesium and sulfur, I am not recommending that we discard eggs completely from our diet. Eggs are perhaps the best source of sulphur that we can obtain in our diet. Sulphur is an extremely important mineral and antioxidizing agent. If you do like to eat eggs, my recommendation would be to try poached eggs since they are not laced with excessive oils and fats that are commonly used in the preparation of fried and/or scrambled eggs.

To consider eggs, we simply need to be more prudent and aware of other components in our diet. For example, the average American consumes approximately 500 mg of cholesterol per day as opposed to the recommended less than 300 mg. Unfortunately, the egg industry has taken a beating in this regard. The "all American" breakfast of two eggs, bacon or sausage, buttered toast and sweetened coffee has approximately 800 mg of cholesterol. Since two eggs contain approximately 450 mg of cholesterol, it is no wonder that the egg industry and the Heart Association are at variance with one another.

In Montauk, at Gurney's Inn, on the tip of Long Island, I did the major writing of the first edition of this book. I preferred Gurney's because of its seaside atmosphere, healthy spa diet and its accessibility to a multitude of alternative care techniques that I suggest, such as yoga and massage. The beach and dune walks, led by Susan Yunker, were particularly enjoyable. Their spa menu was also very low in fats and cholesterol.

At Gurney's, I met a surf fisherman named Bob. He was a successful contractor, only in his mid forties, who recently sought advice from his physician for atypical chest discomfort. During the evaluation, his cholesterol was 275 (undesirable) and his triglycerides, another measure of fat in the blood, were 900, which is extremely undesirable. He told me that for 30 years his early morning breakfast was two eggs, bacon *and* sausage with toast and coffee. After seeing his physician, who recommended a prudent diet, his cholesterol came down to 180 and his triglycerides to 260. Incidentally, after six months of choosing the proper foods he lost 12 pounds! With such metabolic improvements, his risk of coronary disease is considerably lower. Whole eggs are an excellent choice for nutrition. They are a poor choice for cholesterol.

SOME HEALTHY SUGGESTIONS

Organ meats have the highest cholesterol of all known tissues. Three ounces of sweetbreads, for example, contain approximately 2,600 mg of cholesterol! This is one item that should be absolutely forbidden to any health-conscious individual. *Other items that I recommend be forbidden to people who want to stay healthy include processed meats such as bacon, salami, sausage, hot dogs, and bologna.* These items should be avoided because of their high content of saturated fatty acids and calories, not to mention harmful nitrites and sodium levels. *Most hamburgers are 50 percent fat.* All of these meats mentioned above are also high in cholesterol. Preferable meat choices would include chicken and turkey (without skin), although dark meat chicken contains similar amounts of cholesterol to beef. White meat turkey, on the other hand, has lower amounts of cholesterol and saturated fatty acids than chicken and is recommended as a preferred meat substitute. Wild goose is another good alternative.

Although trimming the fat from meats and removing chicken skins does reduce the amount of fat and cholesterol, frequently the ingested cholesterol goes unnoticed, as in marbled meats. Such marbling in the meat contains high quantities of fat later converted to cholesterol and, therefore, should be avoided. *If you insist on red meat, however, the best cuts are London broil or top round steak,* particularly if used in hamburgers. If you ask the butcher to trim all the excess fat and grind the meat for hamburgers, they will have approximately four to five grams of fat per serving as opposed to 20 grams found in chuck burgers. For my cardiology patients who like red meat I frequently recommend a recipe (included in this book) for an eye of round. Again, this is what nutritional awareness is all about.

Another alternative to meat is fish. Cardiologists usually recommend two to three helpings of fish per week to their patients. Fish is rich in the Omega-3 fatty acids that are beneficial to the cardiac patient. Omega-3 type fatty acids, or fish oils, are not found in significant quantities in most foods other than small amounts in soy beans, walnut oils and flax linseed oil. Most researchers agree that *Omega-3 fatty acids have the favorable effect of making the blood less sticky.* Alterations in platelet function may help you live longer. This was recently shown in a two-year study in male survivors of heart attacks in which a moderate intake of fatty fish and fish oil decreased total mortality by 29 percent. While this effect occurred without any reduction in serum cholesterol levels (in this study), Omega-3 fatty acids in cold-water fish or shellfish can cause slight lowering in lipids and small decreases in LDL cholesterol without affecting HDL cholesterol.

Population studies, particularly from the Netherlands, Japan and the Greenland Eskimos, seem to indicate that diets rich in fish products lower the incidence of coronary disease. A typical Eskimo diet, for example, has about 40 percent fat calories coming from whale, seal and fish.

Despite this high percent of dietary fat, the incidence of coronary heart disease in Eskimo men is extremely low. Like the Japanese, who also ingest large quantities of fish, the Eskimos are protected from the epidemic of coronary heart disease that plague the Western societies. Perhaps the cod liver oil that your mother used to give you as a young child really was good for you! Fish oil in small quantities is acceptable. Although it makes sense to avoid as much oil as possible, fish, flax, olive and canola are the ones I recommend most.

Shellfish is considered by many nutritionists to be taboo because of its high content of cholesterol. In reality, however, most shellfish do have acceptable levels of cholesterol with the exception of squid. Squid contains approximately 250 mg of cholesterol per 100 grams. Crab, lobster, oysters and clams have lower levels. It is true that shellfish do contain more cholesterol by weight than poultry and even some red meats, but it is lower in saturated fats. As a clinical cardiologist, keeping this data in mind, I would not restrict the amount of shellfish in the diet. It would be prudent, however, to use less squid and shellfish and more fresh fish.

A word of caution, however, about fish, shellfish and fish oils: Fish caught in coastal waters may be contaminated with pesticides, heavy metals and PCBS. As a striped bass and bluefish fisherman, I can attest to my concern about this problem. It is true that fish can be easily contaminated, as heavy metals and PCBS may reside in their fat. The recommendation here is to *cut out as much of the dark meat from the fish as possible, as this is the fatty part.* It usually occurs in the center of the fish and toward the tail. With careful dissection, many of the pollutants found in this heavily oiled section can be eliminated. It is important to note the data on increased mercury levels found in deep water fish such as tuna and swordfish. Although fish is an excellent source of protein as well as

Omega-3 fatty acids, one should use caution about the possibility of heavy metal toxicity. Although I do not restrict Omega-3 fatty acids from fish, I do prefer a combination of grain and vegetable oil sources of Omega-3 fatty acids, such as found in flax seed.

The grain and vegetable oil sources of Omega-3 fatty acids already mentioned are also beneficial. Pumpkin seeds and soy beans supply small amounts of Omega-3 fatty acids as well. Cholesterol is not found in these oils nor in grains, fruits and most vegetables, but olives and avocados are particularly high in total saturated fat and should be limited. Coconut, coconut oil and palm oil should also be avoided for this reason. Most processed foods or preserved foods contain coconut oil and/or palm oil, so be sure to read labels! Processed foods reporting palm or coconut oil should be absolutely avoided. In the next chapter we will discuss the issue of fat, and both the hazards and potential benefits, of most oils.

DR. SINATRA'S NATURAL CHOLESTEROL LOWERING PLAN

A Simple High-Fiber Nutritional Approach to Cardiac Health

Many of my patients have come to me about a natural cholesterol lowering plan. Although I still consider using drugs for cholesterol lowering, the side-effects of these drugs are quite disturbing. For example, there is one class of cholesterol-lowering agents called HMG co Reductace Inhibitors that are indeed terrific cholesterol killers, but in the process, these agents disturb 20 biochemical pathways in the body. One of these pathways includes the formation of Co Enzyme Q_{10}, which is an essential nutrient to sustain life. Co Enzyme Q_{10} is an essential nutrient in health that I will devote considerable attention to in a subsequent chapter in this book.

If I do use pharmacological agents, I now only select perhaps a fourth or a fifth of the dose. I personally use this program with much success and recommend it to my patients. With the exception of the *Optimum Health International Vitamins*, most of the ingredients to this program can be obtained at your supermarket or local health food store. The plan includes eating high-fiber/low-fat foods, using foods that heal and consuming vitamins, minerals, herbs and other nutritionals.

This simple nutritional strategy for cholesterol-lowering contains approximately 25 grams of fiber. Most individuals will probably consume an additional five to ten grams of fiber from the rest of their daily diet. This degree of fiber, in combination with psyllium seed and cascara will result in an increased frequency of bowel cleansing. Some individuals may also experience some temporary bloating and excessive gas. This program supports the National Cancer Institute's recommendation for at least five to nine fresh fruits and vegetables per day.

By following this program, individuals will be getting plenty of bioflavonoids, pectins and soluble fibers which will protect the body. The nutritional strategy will also inhibit constipation and bowel irregularity. Remember that this program includes no pharmacological drugs; it is perfectly *natural*. It will not only lower your cholesterol and lipids, but will also make you feel considerably better.

- Breakfast should include a serving of oat-bran, raisin bran, shredded wheat or bran flakes with fresh fruits such as blueberries, strawberries, raspberries, bananas, peaches, etc.
- Consume ½ clove of garlic, raw, or as a condiment in cooking, or take one Kyolic Tablet after meals only.
- Eat ½ grapefruit, including all white pulp
- Eat one pear daily. Eat one apple or one medium-sized carrot daily.
- Consume one teaspoon of Perfect 7 Psyllium/Herbal Combination 3 days a week.

INFORMATION ON SUPPLEMENTS

- The following supplements should be taken daily:

1. Take one flax seed oil capsule containing linolenic Acids, 1000 mg capsule after each meal. (See Section in "Fat, Fat and Fats" about this essential fatty acid).
2. Take one Optimum Health Multivitamin after each meal.
3. Take one Formula #1 Immuboost with bioflavonoid complex daily.
4. Take niacin, 250 to 500 mg, after your largest meals one to two times per day. Nicotinic acid (niacin) is the oldest lipid lowering agent and generally the most beneficial in terms of reducing bad cholesterol. It is also the most potent agent for raising levels of HDL's. Niacin is available in two preparations. One is quick-acting and the other slow-acting. It is the slow acting group used in large dosages which has caused some serious side effects to the liver. I would not recommend these long-acting preparations because of

the rare possibility of bad side effects. However, the short release formulation is popular and has been extensively studied over the past three decades. These studies show that niacin not only demonstrates a reduction in cholesterol; it also yields a significant reduction in long term mortality rates.

The unpopularity of niacin for both patients and physicians has been related to the unpleasant, hot skin sensations that patients may feel over the head and neck. I remember the first time I took niacin; I thought my skin was burning! My whole upper torso felt "on fire." It was a hot day in July when I took it, and I took off my shirt because the heat sensations were so intense. Fortunately, these skin sensations only last for a few minutes, and the reactions can be markedly reduced when taking the vitamin with aspirin or after a large meal. Some people even enjoy the sensations, particularly in colder weather. Nevertheless, it is very important for you to be aware of this minor yet unpleasant (for some people) reaction to niacin.

I usually recommend niacin in doses of 250 to 500 mg one to two times per day, depending upon patient tolerance. I do believe that the rapid-release niacin is not only more effective than the slow-release niacin, but also much safer. Niacin has a long safety record and is very inexpensive.

5. If you have high triglycerides in addition to high cholesterol, take an additional 200 mcg of chromium picolinate. Another fat fighter is chromium picolinate. In the diabetic literature, for example, dosages of up to 400 mcg of chromium picolinate have been shown to lower triglycerides. Triglycerides are fats carried in the blood and stored in the fatty areas of your body, like your waist, thigh, back of your arms, etc.

   There have been other studies demonstrating that chromium picolinate has been useful in transforming body fat to lean muscle mass, but I am not yet comfortable with this particular research. More studies are needed. The research on triglyceride lowering, however, is well substantiated.

6. For refractory cholesterol elevations that do not respond readily, 2-3 grams of L-Arginine can be taken at bedtime. L-Arginine is another nutritional support item that you could consider for refractory cholesterol elevations. Because of its membrane stabilizing properties, this amino acid has been gaining increasing popularity

as an "anti-aging" strategy. L-Arginine has been known to stimulate the endothelial cell releasing factor, which is a nitric oxide derivative that helps keep blood vessels open. Nitric oxide helps to prevent the many chain reactions that cause the hardening of blood vessels. In animal studies, L-Arginine has also been known to reduce cholesterol levels and retard plaque formation in blood vessels. L-Arginine has also been reported to increase the immune response, improve wound healing and retard tumor progression.

7. Consume one green tea beverage after lunch or dinner. Another phytonutrient with not only antioxidant activity but also antiplatelet and hypocholesterolemic activity is the customary green tea which is taken after almost every meal in Japan. Some researchers believe that the polyphenol activity in green tea protects you from coronary artery disease by its interaction with cholesterol. Perhaps this is one of the reasons that the Japanese have the lowest incidence of coronary heart disease in the world.

Green tea extracts contain various polyphenols and tannins which protect us against the harmful effects of free radicals. In addition, studies have demonstrated the polyphenol-rich green teas have been shown to reduce cholesterol by inhibiting the absorption of dietary cholesterol and promoting its excretion. Like the polyphenols derived from quercetin (See Chapter 8, "French Paradox"), the polyphenols of green tea are phythochemicals that I have placed in my antioxidant vitamins and mineral formulas.

8. Consider taking the phytonutrient guggul - an old yet very "new" cholesterol fighting agent. This resin, guggul, contains a complex mixture of phytonutrients called diterpenes and esters, as well as gluccosterones. Research in the mid 1960s clearly demonstrates that guggul significantly lowered cholesterol. There have been more than twenty clinical studies since the mid 1960s which clearly show that guggul not only can lower blood cholesterol and blood triglycerides; it also lowers LDL and raises HDL. Comprehensive pharmacological studies done on animals and humans have shown that cholesterol lowering of up to 30-40% has occurred by this safe and effective lipid lowering agent.

This powerful ancient Indian ayurvedic secret is now being utilized by manufacturers as a nutritional support system for cholesterol lowering. During the time I was writing this book, I worked with a manufacturer on a cholesterol support system which included guggullipid extract, niacin and chromium picolinate in a softgel base of borage seed oil, oat bran and ligans (flax).

In the future you will be seeing some new exciting and creative ways of lowering your cholesterol. All that is needed is an open mind without any bias or prejudice.

For additional information regarding cholesterol lowering support systems, or for information regarding the *Optimum Health International* formulas, you may call one of our nutritional counselors at 1-800-228-1507.

Seven

FAT, FAT AND FATS

German singer, Ernestine Schumann-Heink, struggled through the orchestra pit in a cramped Detroit concert hall, knocking over music racks with every step. "Sideways, madam," the conductor urged in alarm. "Sideways!"

"Mein Gott!" cried the singer in reply. "I haff no sideways!"

On another occasion, Enrico Caruso saw her seated in a restaurant with a very large steak on her plate. "Stina," he said, "surely you are not going to eat that alone?"

"Of course not alone," she laughed, "mit potatoes!"

Fat constitutes almost half of the total calorie consumption of Western cultures. As stated previously, it comes in various forms. Fats are the most calorie-dense food we eat. In addition to providing our bodies with considerable energy for our muscle needs, fat also provides insulation against cold and protects us from injury. In our food, fat improves the taste and frequently makes us feel full. Biochemically, fat is a chemical combination of carbon, hydrogen and oxygen atoms. Saturated fats contain single carbon chains with hydrogen atoms attached. Monounsaturated fats have fewer hydrogen atoms than saturated fats, and polyunsaturated fats have still fewer hydrogen atoms attached to the carbons. It is this hydrogenation (adding hydrogen atoms) that makes the oils more saturated. Hydrogenation also yields an oil with a more solid consistency at room temperature and a longer shelf life. So the more hydrogenated an oil, the more saturated it is, thus the more harmful it is.

There have been recent conflicting investigations regarding the trans isomers of naturally occurring cis-unsaturated fatty acids, produced when liquid vegetables are chemically hydrogenated to produce margarine and other solid-fat products. These compounds, found predominantly in margarines and vegetable shortenings used in baked goods, are created when the liquid oils are hydrogenated to make them more solid. Although some cardiologists have recommended margarine over butter because of its smaller proportion of saturated fats, several investigations have indicated that trans-fatty acids may raise levels of harmful LDL cholesterol and reduce the levels of the favorable HDL cholesterol - thus increasing the likelihood of coronary heart disease.

However, there is conflicting data on this issue. The February 4, 1995 issue of *The Lancet*, suggests that although there is no convincing evidence that trans-fatty acids are an important cause of coronary heart disease, it is possible that a high intake of these trans isomers may interact with other risk factors for coronary heart disease. My own recommendation is to avoid margarine and butter until further investigation clarifies this issue. If you must have a solid fat, my preference would be Land of the Lakes Whipped Butter in a container. And remember, less is more!

As you know from the analysis in the previous chapter, saturated fats usually come from animal products with the exception of coconut and palm oil, and their high intake has been linked to an increased cholesterol and thus a greater risk of heart disease. Unsaturated or polyunsaturated fats are liquid at room temperature and most come from plant sources. These compounds usually contain double bonds as opposed to a single bond found in saturated fatty acids (Table 6). Examples of polyunsaturated fats include sunflower oil, corn oil and grapeseed oil. Monounsaturated fats are composed of a fatty acid chain with only one double bond. An example here would be the oleic acid found in olive oil. Thus, if the fatty chain has more than one double bond it is called a polyunsaturated fat (PUFA). Recent research indicates that monounsaturated fats such as olive and canola oil are the least threatening to the cardiovascular system. However, we need to be very conscientious of the fact that all oils are 100 percent fat and, therefore, contain some saturated fat. Although olive oil and canola oil contain mostly unsaturated fats, they do contain small quantities of saturated fat and will raise cholesterol levels. Remember that one tablespoon of any oil contains 14 grams of total fat. I recommend that you keep the consumption of oils to a minimum, but if you need to choose an oil, it would be advisable to *use either olive oil or canola oil.* My own particular preference, possibly fostered by my Italian heritage, includes *cold pressed extra virgin olive oil.* I use this type of olive oil in my salads and in most of my cooking.

Representation of Chemical Bonds in
Saturated, Monounsaturated, Polyunsaturated Fats

SATURATED	MONOUNSATURATED	POLYUNSATURATED
H H H H H H	H H H H H H	H H H H H
-C̦-C̦-C̦-C̦-C̦-C̦-	-C̦-C̦-C̦-C̦=C̦-C̦-	-C̦=C̦-C̦=C̦-C̦-
H H H H H H	H H H H	H

Olive oil is an interesting entity in itself. Several years ago while doing research for a presentation in Brussels on the cultural and international aspects of heart disease, I learned that the island of Crete had an insignificant incidence of heart disease when compared to several other countries in Western Europe. In fact, the data indicated that not one person on the island of Crete died of a myocardial infarction (heart attack) over a 10 year period. However, the cholesterol for an average inhabitant of Crete is over 200. This presented somewhat of a paradox for me. The author indicated that it must have been the sunny climate and lack of stress that resulted in the lower incidence of heart disease. I felt that the lack of emotional stress and tremendous family comraderie and support was a major factor in the low incidence of heart disease. I have since realized, however, the residents of Crete consume generous quantities of olive oil. As olive oil has been shown to preserve good HDL and lower LDL perhaps these effects were significant despite the average cholesterols being over 200. (It is best to use extra virgin olive oil as it is cold-pressed and of the highest quality.)

There are many distinct advantages of monounsaturated fats over the polyunsaturated fats. When substituted for saturated fatty acids in the diet, olive oil and other MUFAs such as canola and almond oil lower LDL levels. They also do not appear, however, to reduce HDL. This is a favorable point of information. PUFAs will lower LDL when substituted for saturated fatty acids. However, large intakes of PUFAs are also associated with lowering of HDL. This is not favorable for the cardiovascular system. In addition, animal studies have also demonstrated that high intakes of

PUFAs may promote tumor development after pretreatment with chemical carcinogens. PUFAs also present a paradox. Although PUFAs are essential in cellular membrane function, they are easily oxidized, making the cells more vulnerable to harmful change. For example, the oxidation of these fatty acids in the retina of the eye may make the retina susceptible to degeneration.

For example, olive oil, (a MUFA) has been reported to have blood-thinning properties and contains antioxidants that may help protect cells. Although some of us prefer the taste of polyunsaturated fats, clinical research favors monounsaturated fats for optimal health. Canola oil is a MUFA that comes from rapeseed and it has a lighter taste than olive oil.

ESSENTIAL FATTY ACIDS

Canola oil contains small amounts of the essential fatty acids, linoleic and linolenic acids. As these acids cannot be manufactured by the body, they *must* be consumed in the diet. Linolenic acid, found in soybean and flax, is an Omega-3 fatty acid, similar to the fatty acids found in fish oils. Recent research has shown that an insufficient intake of these two fatty acids may predispose some individuals toward heart disease.

Researchers suggest that low levels of these fatty acids cause the body to produce an abnormal fatty acid called mead fatty acid, resulting in additional cholesterol production and, thus, hardening of the arteries. While most cardiologists recommend a low-fat diet as a preventive measure in reducing coronary heart disease, the link between low linolenic/linoleic fatty acid intake and coronary heart disease is real. Although it is wise to reduce our fat intake, it is best not to be exceedingly rigid in our over all approach to fats. Soybean products, seeds, flax oil, tofu, oatmeal, some nuts, as well as occasional fish, need to be consumed to keep the body supplied with adequate linolenic acid. Since many of the vegetable oils have considerable qualities of linoleic acid (Omega-6), deficiencies of linoleic acid are not common.

HAVE FUN READING LABELS

Keeping this data in mind, you ought to read labels carefully when you shop. But food labels sometimes don't tell us "the whole truth." For example, *some labels may state no cholesterol, but that does not necessarily mean it won't contain saturated fat, which when ingested will be trans-*

formed to cholesterol. Additionally, the word "hydrogenated fat" may be used as a euphemism for the highly saturated palm oil and coconut oil. So be aware and beware! *The best thing to do when reading labels is to look at the content of saturated fat, polyunsaturated fat and monounsaturated fat* (Table 7).

It is important to organize your shopping around low-fat, low-cholesterol concepts. Reading labels can also be fun. When reading labels, it is interesting to try to figure out the percentage of calories from fat. For example, if we are on a 2,000 calorie diet, the recommended fat intake is approximately 20 percent. Twenty percent of 2,000 is 400 calories. Four-hundred calories equals approximately 44 grams of fat. Thus, this should be our total fat intake for the day. (The American Heart Association Diet is more lenient with 30 percent calories from fat. I prefer less than 20 percent.) Of this total fat intake, only ten percent of the fat intake should come from saturated fat. This means that only four to five grams of fat should come from saturated fats.

In addition to organizing your menu around fats, it is also important to keep tabs on the fiber content. Remember that by increasing the fiber content and reducing the fat content, weight loss may be considerable (Table 8). When considering weight loss, you need to know your daily intake of fat. Remember we are not counting total calories but only the grams of fat (Table 9). In my own particular situation, I try to take in less than 20 grams of fat per day. Again, this is the equivalent of a one-quarter pound hamburger found in many of the fast food restaurants. Keeping the intake of grams of fat to a respectable level will not only reduce total body fat, but will also reduce caloric intake.

In our previous discussions we mentioned that excess calories are predominantly stored in the body as fat; you're familiar with this type of fat that is around the waistline, thighs and backs of our arms. Cardiologists refer to it as "triglycerides in the body," but in simple terms this is our body fat. Body fat can be determined by anthropometric measurements using calipers. Accumulation of body fat is a simple mechanism. We either eat too much or we exercise too little.

TABLE 7
COMMONLY USED FATS AND OILS

Type of Fat	Saturated	Monounsaturated	Polyunsaturated
Almond oil	1.3 (grams)	9.1 (grams)	3.6 (grams)
Beef fat	7.1	6.0	0.5
Butter	9.0	4.1	0.6
Canola oil	0.8	8.4	4.4
Chicken fat	4.2	6.4	3.0
Coconut oil	11.7	0.8	0.2
Corn oil	1.7	3.4	7.9
Cottonseed oil	3.6	2.6	6.9
Fresh Flax	1.3	2.2	10.5
Grapeseed oil	1.6	2.4	9.9
Lard	5.6	6.4	1.6
Margarine	2.0	5.0	4.0
Mayonnaise	2.0	3.0	7.0
Olive oil	1.9	9.8	1.2
Peanut oil	2.6	6.2	4.1
Pumpkinseed oil	1.2	4.8	8.0
Safflower oil	1.3	1.7	10.0
Sesame oil	1.8	6.4	5.7
Soy oil	2.0	3.1	7.8
Sunflower	1.4	2.8	8.7
Walnut oil	2.2	3.9	7.8

Avoid	Substitute	Substitute
Highest Saturated Fat	Highest Monounsaturated	Highest Poly w/Omega-3
Coconut oil	Olive	Flax
Butter	Almond	Fish Oil
Beef fat	Canola	
Lard		

TABLE 8

HIGH-FIBER/LOW-FAT FOOD

Food	Serving Size	Fiber	Fat (g)	Calories
Health Valley Chili	5 ounces	12.2	3	160
All Bran	⅓ cup	8.6	1	70
Multi-grain Pancake mix (Arrowhead Mills)	3 pancakes	8.0	2	290
Prunes	5 large	7.9	Trace	115
Oatmeal (Old Wessex Irish Style)	⅓ cup	7.0	2	110
Chickpeas	½ cup	6.2	Trace	115
40% Bran	¾ cup	6.0	1	95
Kidney Beans	½ cup	5.8	Trace	110
Pinto Beans	½ cup	5.3	Trace	115
Slit Peas	½ cup	5.1	Trace	115
Pear	1 pear	5.0	1	110
Raisins	½ cup	4.9	Trace	220
Broccoli	1 spear	4.5	Trace	55
Lima Beans	½ cup	4.4	Trace	105
Peas, green	½ cup	4.1	Trace	65

TABLE 9

MAXIMUM FAT INTAKE

Most of us are unaware of how many calories we should eat, much less how many grams of fat we should intake. The following chart is a helpful index regarding your daily caloric needs as well as the maximum total fat allowance. For the purposes of this chart, your caloric needs are determined by your activity. For example, if you are very active, multiply your weight in pounds by the number 16. If you are moderately active, multiply by 15. If you are inactive, multiply by 14, and if you are sedentary, multiply by 12. For someone like myself, weighing approximately 150 pounds and being moderately active, I would need 2,250 calories, of which my maximum fat intake would not exceed 50 grams. Being a cardiologist, however, I am aware of the hazards of fat intake and, therefore, probably eat less than 25 grams of fat per day, which is approximately ten percent of total daily calories from fat. For *Optimum Health,* if you can keep your fat intake to less than 20 percent per day, as well as increase the fiber intake, you will gradually lose weight. The following table offers examples of the maximum fat intake per day. To figure out your caloric intake, use the formula as suggested.

MAXIMUM TOTAL FAT INTAKE
MODERATELY ACTIVE
MALE & FEMALE

Ideal Body Weight	Calories	Fat (g) per/day
120 (lbs.)	1,800	40
130	1,950	43
140	2,100	47
150	2,250	50
160	2,400	53
170	2,550	57
180	2,700	60
190	2,850	63
200	3,000	67
210	3,150	70
220	3,300	73
230	3,450	77
240	3,600	80
250	3,750	83

SINK OR SWIM

In our passive exercise study of women at the New England Heart Center, we determined the amount of fat in several areas of the body. In our study, we concluded that exercise in combination with a high-fiber/low-fat diet actually reduced body fat. Significant reductions in body fat were noted, particularly in the suprailiac (waist) and triceps (back of upper arms) areas. Although fat does have its functions, most Americans have too much body fat. There is some disagreement, but it is safe to say that 15 to 20 percent of body fat for men and 20 to 25 percent body fat for women is considered the maximum range for a healthy person. One can be slightly out of this range and still be healthy, but it is my belief that less body fat is more acceptable. We should strive to keep our body fat to a minimum.

We also need to know that as we get older our body fat increases. This is why the older we get the easier it is to float in water. I remember when I was a collegiate wrestler I had less than 10 percent body fat. I was also taking scuba diving lessons at the time. During my certification for scuba diving, it was apparent to everyone in the class that I did not need lead weights to get me to the bottom. I indeed had negative buoyancy - I sank like a rock! Neither could I float as other people could. I really thought there was something wrong with me. I thought perhaps I had heavy bones or lead in my pants. What I really had was less body fat than every-one else, and since fat is lighter than muscle, the others floated. Being able to float is a direct response to having body fat. I was too dense to float! Thus, one consolation to getting older is being able to float in the ocean!

Through my training as a cardiologist, I have been able to keep my weight down, almost to my college wrestling level. This nutritional aware-ness has been a long-term process for me. Gradually, I have been able to reduce the saturated fat in my diet but only to a point where I still don't feel deprived. For example, most of my diet includes vegetables, grains and pastas. Although I used to be a terrific meat eater, I have reduced my intake of meat, only having red meat on rare occasions and poultry approximately one to two times a month. But there is also another reason why I avoid fat in the diet. I really believe our planet is in danger. Numerous chemicals and pollutants that affect the earth are being absorbed first in roots and vegetables and later in the animals that con-sume them. Just as PCBs and mercury are stored in fish fat cells, pesti-cides and other chemical pollutants are stored in animal fat cells. As you can see from the graph, pesticides and pollutants increase as the fat chain increases (Table 10). This is an area of intense investigation that you need to be aware of for your overall physical health.

Fighting cancer is another reason why we need to decrease the fat in our diet. There are several studies that show the casual relationship between fat intake and the occurrence of cancer. Population studies, as well as studies in animals, show convincing evidence that *an increase in the intake of total fat increases cancer, particularly of the breast and colon.* Researchers from the Harvard School of Public Health found that men with the lowest fat intake had half the rate of precancerous colon polyps as men with the highest fat intake. The Harvard study also demonstrated the impact of fiber, in that the high-fiber group (greater than 34 grams a day) had only one-third as many polyps as the group with the lowest fiber intake (less than 17 grams a day). In addition to cancer and cardiovascular disease, obesity, diabetes and gout are also associated with high-fat intake. If the weight of all these negative effects of fat consumption does not serve as a "noteworthy factor" to make some dietary changes, I don't know what would. Maimonides, in 1198, was indeed correct when he stated the simple fact, "Fat is bad."

TABLE 10_____

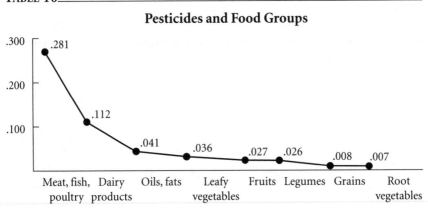

Pesticides and Food Groups

Meat, fish, poultry	Dairy products	Oils, fats	Leafy vegetables	Fruits	Legumes	Grains	Root vegetables
.281	.112	.041	.036	.027	.026	.008	.007

Source: *Runner's World*

Eight

THE GOOD, THE BAD AND THE UGLY—WATER, ALCOHOL AND CAFFEINE

Are you a drinker? I hope so.

The human body is mostly made up of water. Our blood, for all practical purposes, is similar to seawater. Water is involved in almost every body process, including digestion, absorption and excretion. Water helps maintain the proper body temperature and is essential for carrying waste material. Since water is continuously lost through excretion of urine, elimination, sweating and breathing, it is important to replenish the proper amount of water each day. Most researchers agree that drinking at least eight glasses of water a day is necessary for good health. And water is also germane to weight loss. Studies have shown that a decrease in water consumption will cause an increase in fat deposits, while an increase in water can actually reduce the amount of fat in the body.

The mechanism is simple. If the kidneys cannot function properly, due to dehydration, some of that responsibility has to be taken up by the liver. Since the liver metabolizes stored fat for energy, it cannot work at full capacity if the kidney is compromised. Therefore, the liver metabolizes less fat, and more fat then remains in the body, resulting in weight gain.

Water is an extremely important catalyst in weight loss. For example, in our hospital-based weight loss program, each participant had to drink large quantities of water continuously. If water was not consumed adequately, dehydration would occur and weakness and lethargy would result. The best way to give your body water is to replenish it. Since water is a major factor in fat metabolism, it makes sense for an overweight person to drink as much water as possible. The health implications of drinking plenty of water are numerous to say the least. In addition to helping rid the body of toxins, water can help relieve constipation as well. When the body gets too little water or too much salt, or if the patient is given too much diuretic, the body will take water from its internal sources. The colon is one such source. The result is constipation.

WATER TRICKS

Drinking enough water is not only essential to weight loss, but is also essential to good health. In medical school, I trained with one of the top kidney experts in the United States. He was one of the original investigators of kidney dialysis. When we used to make rounds in the hospital wards, *my professor would never pass a water fountain without drinking.* By watching him I learned a lot. He continuously drank water each day to give his kidneys the nurturing they needed. If that was good enough for a professor of nephrology, it was certainly good enough for me. I tried to remind myself as much as possible about the medical consequences of deficient water intake. In summary, *we need to drink at least eight eight-ounce glasses of water every day.* This is about two quarts of fluid. *During weight loss, we should drink at least one glass of water during each meal and a glass at least one hour prior to the meal.* As previously stated, too much salt depletes our natural stores of water. Excess sodium in the diet causes unnecessary fluid retention in the tissues, even edema (swelling), and depletion in other parts of the body such as the colon and upper gastrointestinal tract. In order to flush ourselves of excess salt, we need to drink more water.

Too much common table salt (sodium chloride) is harmful to our bodies in many ways. In higher concentrations it disturbs the mineral balance in the body. Too much salt in our diet can cause fluid buildup, thus creating an increase in pressure. This can lead to high blood pressure and possibly heart disease. The National Cholesterol Education Program (NCEP) recommends a sodium intake of less than three grams per day. Excessive salt intake has been incriminated in disease not only in urbanized societies but also in primitive societies as well. Natives in the Caribbean who cook their foods in seawater, for example, had much higher levels of blood pressure than those who cooked in fresh water. *In order to get rid of extra body salt we need to drink more water.* As water is forced through the kidneys, it takes away the excess sodium.

Unfortunately, salt does not only come from the salt shaker. Processed foods make up approximately 50 percent of the average American diet and these foods often contain a considerable amount of hidden sodium. Again, we need to read labels. For example, some of the commercially prepared soups contain almost a gram of sodium per can and a fast food hamburger may also contain at least one gram of sodium. A large kosher dill pickle contains greater than one gram of sodium. An over-consumption of processed foods with little dietary awareness leads us to be vulnerable to excess sodium in our diet. For example, we need to be aware that additional sodium is often added to bread products. Salt in this country is considered to be an excellent preservative.

Since sodium occurs naturally in most foods, as well as water, there is no danger of our body not getting enough. You really don't need any additional sodium chloride. Salt is not a food; salt has no nutritional value. The only time I would favor utilizing salt is in individuals who are losing a lot of sodium chloride through excessive work and perspiration. Elderly patients also suffering from low blood pressure who do not have any heart muscle disease may also be permitted to use salt. Under these circumstances the best way to get salt into the body would be in the form of natural fruits and vegetables. Celery and sea vegetables, for example, contain natural quantities of sodium chloride in its organic form.

LAST CALL FOR ALCOHOL

Alcohol is another source of empty calories, providing no vitamins, minerals or other essential nutriments. This is certainly one type of beverage that should not be utilized in anyone trying to undergo weight reduction. Alcohol just adds calories to the diet. It is really not a food, but rather a drug. Alcohol may be considered a poison. It causes metabolic damage to the body and depresses the immunological system. As a clinical cardiologist I can attest to the amount of heart disease that alcohol causes. I have seen hundreds of patients with no previous known history of heart disease come into my office with "heart muscle disease." The most common etiology of such heart muscle disease in the absence of other factors such as coronary artery disease, viral illnesses or valvular heart disease, is alcohol-induced cardiomyopathy.

Studies on alcohol are too numerous to count. But one particular study showed that at least two ounces of alcohol per day can cause deterioration of the heart muscle over a short period of time. This was seen in one study in which a group of volunteers drank two ounces of vodka per day and the control group drank water. At the end of the experiment, the ones who took alcohol had heart muscle deterioration on microscopic analysis.

In addition, alcohol can damage almost any organ in the body. The heart, the brain and the liver are perhaps the most vulnerable. Much of my medical internship and residency included treating alcoholics. The amount of disease entities common to alcoholics are incredible: Pneumonia, liver disease, arthritis, eating disorders, delirium, dementia and nerve and muscle diseases are common to the alcoholic. The emotional destruction that alcohol causes is almost as profound as the physical destruction.

Another important fact to consider about alcohol is its effects on sleep. Alcohol is probably the leading cause of insomnia. While alcohol does not induce ideal sleep, in some individuals it may cause the body to be anesthetized, seeming as though in a deep sleep. The sleep pattern, however, is not a good one. After ingesting alcohol and particularly after eating sweets, perhaps in a dessert after a nice dinner, many people have difficulty falling asleep because of the vasodilating effects of alcohol and the rapid heart rate that follows.

One of the more common things I see in my office is alcohol-induced cardiac arrhythmia. The patients come in with many different scenarios: skipped heartbeats, irregular heartbeats and rapid heartbeats. Many of these arrhythmias have their origins in alcohol. Other causes may be emotional distress, which is frequently compounded by the patient's use of alcohol as a remedy. Overall, my recommendation on hard alcohol is to try to avoid it.

Wine, on the other hand, has been used as a healing remedy for centuries. Written records dating back 4,000 years refer to the dietary and medicinal uses of wine. While it is not a good idea to drink it every day, wine contains polyphenols which are agents that kill viruses and bacteria. Polyphenols, like some vitamins, have antioxidant capabilities or the ability to tie up free oxygen radicals that cause destruction to cells. One particular polyphenol found in red wine is quercetin, a bioflavonoid known for its antioxidant and antihistamine properties, and touted as the main ingredient in the "French Paradox."

THE FRENCH PARADOX

The French Paradox is indeed a paradox! That is, the typical Frenchman has a high serum cholesterol, but a low incidence of coronary heart disease. In fact, in one major clinical study involving various cultures, France was second to Japan with the lowest incidence of heart disease in the world. If a typical Frenchman eats a lot of cheese, sauces, paté and other high fat foods, why should he have a lower incidence of coronary heart disease? The answer is the ingestion of red wine.

Many researchers believe it is the consumption of red wine that counteracts the French diet. But what is it about red wine that makes it so medicinal? Current studies indicate that specific compounds such as quercetin and tannins protect the body from harmful cholesterol. Tannins are found in the skin and seeds of grapes. They give wine a characteristic color. Red grapes contain considerably more tannin than white grapes. Quercetin, in addition to protecting the heart, has also been known to protect cells from abnormal behavior. For this reason, quercetin has been acclaimed as an anti-cancer agent, as well.

After the observations of the French Paradox were published in the medical literature, newer investigators tested the tannin-quercetin hypothesis. For example, experimental groups consumed red wine and other forms of alcohol, such as vodka or placebo, before ingesting a meal. It was clearly demonstrated that one to two glasses of red wine, and red wine only, before dinner can sustain antioxidant activity for up to four hours. Antioxidant activity protects and prevents the oxidation of cholesterol, leading to plaque build-up.

The Dutch, in a more recent follow-up study, showed similar findings of the French Paradox. They clearly demonstrated that older men, aged 65 to 85, showed a reduction in death rate in those that consumed greater proportions of onions, green apples and green tea (foods high in quercetin). Not only do flavonoids protect one against heart disease, but also have been shown as a class to develop a defense against cancer.

Some investigators have also suggested the use of an evaporated wine residue to be used as a salve remedy in treating cold sores and herpes simplex infections. The low alcohol content in wine may offer yet another advantage in healing. Recent investigations have supported the hypothesis that light alcohol consumption may actually reduce the risk of coronary heart disease, perhaps by favorably influencing HDL and blood clotting mechanisms. Wine, however, is alcohol and like caffeine it needs to be used in moderation.

Although one cannot recommend loosely for patients to consume liberal quantities of red wine to counteract the fat in their diet, the fact remains that the antioxidant and anti-cancer activity of red wine does exist.

A WORD TO THE WISE ABOUT CAFFEINE

Caffeinated beverages such as coffee were once highly utilized as drug therapy by physicians in Western Europe. In 1859, caffeine was administered as a respiratory treatment and written up in the medical journals as the "prescription of choice" for bronchial asthma. The pharmacological properties of caffeine are similar to the xanthines, a group of compounds that stimulates the central nervous system and the heart, as well as relaxes smooth muscles (especially the bronchial tubes) and empowers the brain. Caffeine also acts as a diuretic, resulting in increased blood flow to the kidney and allowing more water to be excreted. Drinking a cup of coffee and getting stuck in a traffic jam can have some undesirable consequences.

The average American citizen consumes approximately two to five cups of coffee a day, representing 200 to 300 mg of caffeine. Decaffeinated coffee does contain caffeine but in insignificant quantities. Caffeine is also found in chocolate, tea and cocoa. A cup of tea usually contains less than half the amount of caffeine as a cup of coffee (Table 11).

Excess caffeine intake has been noted in young children who drink colas. The symptoms of irritability, hyperactivity and insomnia are frequently due to excess quantities taken into the body. In my own clinical practice, I have seen scores of patients with problems related to caffeine intake. For example, I remember a case involving a young 25 year old male with a history of a psychiatric disorder. Since his psychiatrist prescribed tranquilizers to control his mood, he was referred to me for cardiological evaluation because of an exceedingly high heart rate, frequently greater than 120, and a blood pressure as high as 220/120.

An in-depth medical history on this individual, however, disclosed that he was drinking ten cups of coffee per day. He was also drinking considerable quantities of cola beverages. This individual suffered not from a "drug-induced" heartbeat problem, but from *caffeinism* - a condition where the heart rate and the blood pressure increase, and the patient feels very irritable and hyperactive.

TABLE 11

AVERAGE CAFFEINE CONTENT OF SELECTED ITEMS (mg)

BEVERAGES

Soft Drinks (12 oz serving)		Caffeine (mg)
Cherry cola, Slice		
(Diet or Regular)		48.0
Cola-Cola		
(Diet or Regular)		46.0
Cola (decaffeinated)		0.18
Mellow Yellow		53.0
Mountain Dew		54.0
Pepper type		37.0
Pepsi Cola, Diet		36.0
Pepsi Cola, Regular		38.0

Coffee	Serving Size	Caffeine (mg)
Brewed, Regular	6 oz.	103.0
Brewed, Decaf	6 oz.	3.0
Instant, Reg	1 rounded teaspoon	57.0
Instant, Decaf	1 rounded teaspoon	2.0

Tea Hot/Cold	Serving Size	Caffeine (mg)
Brewed Commercial	5 oz.	20-50
Brewed Imported	5 oz.	25-80
Instant	5 oz.	10-20
Iced Tea	12 oz.	70
Crystal light	8 oz.	11

Milk	Serving Size	Caffeine (mg)
Chocolate Flavor		
Dry Mix with milk	2-3 teaspoons	8
Chocolate Syrup		
in whole milk	2 tablespoons	6
Cocoa/Hot Chocolate		
with water	4 teaspoons	6

Table 11 *(concluded)*
AVERAGE CAFFEINE CONTENT OF SELECTED ITEMS (mg)

Candy

Chocolate	Serving Size	Caffeine (mg)
German Sweet (Bakers)	1 oz.	8
Semi-sweet (Bakers)	1 oz.	13
Milk-Chocolate (Cadbury)	1 oz.	15

Over-the Counter-Drugs	Caffeine (mg)
Anacin	32
Excedrin	65
No Doz	100

Patients will frequently complain of an erratic heartbeat, skipping of the heart and fluttering. Frequently, they will also have insomnia. The treatment of this condition is simple; one needs simply to reduce or eliminate all caffeine intake. I have counseled several patients with similar conditions of this type. Many patients have come to me with cardiac arrhythmias who simply were ingesting too much caffeine. Many other patients with cardiac-induced arrhythmias will aggravate their symptoms and arrhythmia frequencies if they do not eliminate caffeine.

As a diuretic, too much caffeine can wash out our body's vitamins and minerals. Too much caffeine has been incriminated as an agent in reducing the body's calcium, magnesium and potassium.

Caffeinated beverages, especially coffee, have also been known to enhance gastric acid secretion and aggravate ulcers. Every physician knows that if a patient is suffering from excess acid production or abdominal discomfort to instruct them to avoid caffeine, alcohol, nicotine and aspirin, as these are the four most common harmful chemical compounds that affect the gastrointestinal tract. Caffeine, like nicotine and alcohol, is considered a drug. Therefore, we must weigh the potential benefits versus the hazards. Some physicians believe coffee is harmful and should be avoided altogether. For the asymptomatic individual, limited quantities of caffeine (1-2 cups of coffee a day) may be acceptable. The benefit for some individuals may be increased mental mood, alertness and concentration. The trade-off, however, could be lethargy and fatigue as a result of the low blood sugar that may occur in the hour after consuming coffee. I know that during my days as an athlete and particularly during my days as a medical student, I relied on caffeine to keep me mentally alert and physically sharp over the short term. Coffee is definitely considered a "pick me up."

On the other hand, we can risk poisoning our bodies with too much caffeine. Please understand: caffeine is indeed a drug with considerable side effects. *I would recommend consuming no more than one to two cups of coffee per day and none after 3:00 p.m.* Decaffeinated beverages may be consumed in moderation.

In summary, caffeine, like alcohol, needs to be considered carefully. Although deprivation does not need to occur with these beverages, caution needs to be exercised when using them. Remember *the best beverage is water,* definitely a major player in the search for *Optimum Health* philosophy. Be aware, however, that many of our water supplies are contaminated with heavy metals, chlorine and environmental pollutants. If you don't use water filters, or obtain high quality bottled water, it is a good investment to have your water analyzed.

Nine

THE TRUTH ABOUT FREE RADICALS, VITAMINS AND ANTIOXIDANTS

I'd like to share a "Letter to the Editor" I wrote to my local newspaper in Connecticut, responding to an article about whether or not to take vitamins.

As a physician, father, cook and recent author who has thoroughly researched the medical literature, I can tell you that although there is no substitute for a balanced diet, the fact remains: vitamin and mineral deficiencies do exist in our population. Nowadays, many of our soils have become "worn out;" water has become polluted, industrial toxicities fill the atmosphere, automobile emissions pollute the environment, heavy metal toxicities are springing up everywhere and nuclear waste dumps are poisoning the depths of the earth. These toxins create an undesirable metabolic stress on the body. One way of protecting our bodies is by binding free radicals with antioxidants.

For example, if excessive fat is consumed *after* we have just eaten in our favorite fast food restaurant, or if excessive radiation is taken in when we are at the beach on a bright, sunny day, or if toxic fumes are inhaled (driving in traffic on a hot humid day), or if heavy metals are ingested (lead in our drinking water), the body, in trying to protect itself, becomes involved in a biochemical war between the invading toxins and our immune system. The by-products of these biochemical reactions may result in toxic wastes accumulating in the body, thereby causing hormonal changes which may lead to symptoms of allergy, palpitations, nausea and shortness of breath, to mention a few. Such events over the short and long-term may lead to biological changes, diseases and aging. This is where vitamins and minerals come in.

Although eating fresh fruits and vegetables on a daily basis would help, it is a known fact that transport and storage cause some produce to lose valuable vitamin content. Take, for example, the comment in the article about eating a fresh orange over vitamins. The question is, how fresh is fresh? And is the orange laced with toxic chemical agents and pesticides? We also need to be aware that many vitamins and minerals are not particularly consumed in the diet. Take Co Enzyme Q_{10}, for example, a vital nutrient, especially for the cardiovascular population. Q_{10} is found in abundance in beef heart muscle, pork, mackerel and sardines. But who eats that particular diet? And what about the population on antibiotics, oral contraceptives, corticosteroids, alcohol and excessive caffeine?

All of the above entities frequently deplete the vitamins and minerals in our body. What about the patient who has undergone coronary artery bypass surgery and has been placed on a heart-lung machine? It is a known fact that once the blood is circulated through a heart-lung machine, the vitamin, mineral, and co enzyme factors of the blood are destroyed. I could go on and on about why we need vitamin and mineral supplementation in today's world. Certainly the Japanese do not have a problem with this. Since Co Q_{10} went on sale in April of 1974, approximately six million Japanese take it every year. If I were writing the article on "To Be or Not To Be Taking Vitamins," I, as a clinical cardiologist, a modified vegetarian who eats very little meat and consumes considerable quantities of grains, fresh fruits, vegetables and herbs, would continue TO *BE* taking vitamin and mineral supplements and, in addition, continue recommending them to my family and patients.

As a lay person and particularly as a young doctor, I never held vitamins or minerals in high esteem. After all, I always felt I ate well, and why should I supplement my body when I consumed grains, fresh fruits and vegetables? Being a doctor, I thought I *knew* what was beneficial. But again, my patients became my best teachers. Frequently, I needed to prescribe drugs for various conditions. But I, like many other doctors, had some pharmacological failures. While sometimes I had to ask myself if my patients were really taking the medications, more often I knew that they had accepted my advice and followed instructions.

It was only after careful scrutiny and much investigation that I discovered many of my patients were not really *absorbing* the medications. I knew that because of diminished hydrochloric acid in their stomachs, some people cannot absorb medicine. Could the same thing happen with foods? If so, how would we know? Through becoming ill? It became increasingly clear to me that not all the agents we put into our bodies will be absorbed. Even if we were to absorb all the nutrients we eat, is this enough to optimally sustain our bodies in today's environment?

Over the last few years as I continued to read and practice preventive medicine, I gradually began to believe more and more in the healing powers of vitamins, minerals and natural healthy foods. There are subtle changes that may occur in the body which frequently are missed by the individual. In my particular case, I had psoriasis on my elbows and knees for years. After taking vitamin and mineral preparations that I personally developed, within one year, many of my psoriatic symptoms cleared up. Although I still continue to get occasional flare-ups, my skin, in general, is much healthier in these localized areas. It was only by trial and error that I learned I was not receiving all the nutrients I thought I was getting. Again, I was eating well. Although there are no clinical studies to prove such effects, in my case this was highly significant. It goes to show that even if we are not sick, we may unknowingly be in a state of less than perfect health.

ASK FOR HIGH-GRADE FUEL

I like to think of the body as a Porsche with a finely tuned engine requiring a high-performance fuel to operate. When the fuel is of an inferior grade, the engine may spurt and sputter. When the engine has no fuel, it stops. The human body reacts in a similar fashion. We need food and nourishment in order to keep our engine going. However, if we do not give ourselves the proper nutrients, if we consume insufficient nutrients, or perhaps even poor-grade nutrients, our bodies will not function in a smooth and timely manner.

This reasoning can also be applied to the many vitamin and mineral formulas that are presently on the market. Some formulas have high-grade nutrients, while others contain inferior-grade nutrients, as well as inferior delivery systems.

The problem with most of us is that we believe we are getting all the vital nutrients we need from our diet. But is this true? Overcooking foods or microwaving them may alter the biochemical makeup of vitamins and enzymes. This is particularly true in the elderly, who frequently cannot get out to purchase fresh fruits and vegetables, and who use microwaving as their preferred way of cooking. Microwaving can seriously impair B vitamins. Recently, it has been discovered that there are now large deficiencies of B vitamins, especially in the elderly population. I am very skeptical of these small magnetic ovens. I personally don't have a microwave in my house.

Habits like microwaving, in a sense, are similar to using a low-grade fuel. Freshness can also be fleeting. Frequently, fresh produce will lose much of its vitamin value because of storage, shipping, and handling. Asparagus, for example, loses up to two-thirds of its vitamin C after just two days of being at room temperature.

Although the vitamins and minerals found in natural whole foods will give us some protection against illness, I *do* believe that *supplementation enhances our health*. It is a little known fact that *certain vitamin and mineral supplements can significantly protect individuals against the increasing dangers of radiation and chemical pollutants*. As a clinical cardiologist, I have seen numerous articles on the beneficial effects of beta carotene and vitamins C and E, as well as selenium. These nutrients are frequently referred to as antioxidants, which protect our bodies from the formation of free radicals sometimes associated with the diseases of modern man.

FREE RADICALS AND DISEASE

While we cannot readily see what is happening in the body, common examples of oxidation (free radical damage) occur - like the browning of a freshly cut apple or the rusting of metal. Such oxidation can be the result of the normal body's metabolism or the result of external sources, such as radiation, air pollution and alcohol or heavy metal intoxication, to name a few.

Free radicals are highly reactive molecules produced during such oxidative normal metabolism. Interfering with enzymatic reactions, they do their damage by attacking the cells in the body. By having unpaired electrons, they collide like unguided missiles, causing disruption of cells, membranes and even DNA itself. The body, in trying to protect itself, becomes involved in a biochemical war between the invading toxins and the immune system. During such biochemical battles, toxic wastes of combat accumulate in the body, producing an enormous metabolic stress.

Our industrialized and over-polluted environment also creates a continuous attack on our bodies, adversely affecting us in numerous ways. For example, heavy metals, such as iron, lead and cadmium are increasingly present in our drinking water. Where I live in Manchester, Connecticut, our water has been tested and found to have too much lead. In addition to harmful metals, increasing radiation from the technology of industry and our old friend, the Sun, conveyed through a receding ozone layer, places an enormous stress on the body.

Other man-made risk factors like auto emissions, cigarette smoke, pollutants in the air we breathe, and electromagnetic contamination incidiously poisons our bodies. Flying at 30,000 feet in an airplane, for example, or worse yet, sitting near a jet engine on the plane, creates a fire storm of free radicals in our bodies. Free radicals are also generated by walking past our refrigerators, watching TV up close, sitting down at a computer and probably cooking with microwaves. These electromagnetic waves are invisible forces of electricity that continually zap us! The increasing use of fats in our diet also causes relentless biochemical reactions that are toxic to the body.

Unfortunately, free radicals can be produced by the body itself. This results from the oxidation of food, especially fats. As oxygen is utilized in the burning of fat (oxidation), and if the fat is rancid, an alarming number of free radicals are produced. Consider all the free radicals you have in your refrigerator, like the leftovers sitting in a sea of fat. Or consider the margarine that has turned a funny color, or the leftover butter that's soft, warm and rancid. And remember the mayonnaise that is half-full? The surface, by being infiltrated with the air, may turn color, producing a rancid situation. These little things, totally unknown to us, provide the raw materials for causing dire reactions in the body.

Another unknown entity is the radiation that is emitted from the ground. There is considerable investigation into the impact of radon on the formation of free radicals, which seems to be a major factor in the development of lung cancer. Radon is found deep in the earth in rocks. Over time, the toxic effects of radon in our homes can infiltrate our bodies. For example, I have a patient with lung cancer who never smoked, but his home was contaminated with radon. Since radon gas is radioactive, he is currently involved in a state-wide study to determine the degree of the relationship between radon and lung cancer. Environmental toxicities that can produce free radicals are all around us.

While the effects of free radicals on health and disease are not completely understood, they are believed, over time, to cause biological changes resulting in aging or an acceleration of a variety of chronic diseases, such as heart disease, cancer and cataracts. For example, in cancer, free radicals may disrupt DNA, and in heart disease, the oxidation of LDL is now believed to be the focal cardinal reaction in atherosclerosis. Macular degeneration, cataracts, arthritis and premature aging (dementia) may also be free radical-mediated. Although more research is needed to establish causality between free radicals and disease, multiple studies have shown the benefits of an antioxidant defense system.

ANTIOXIDANTS

Antioxidants act like "friendly guardians" or "bodyguards" that neutralize free radicals. Sacrificing themselves in chemical reactions by donating electrons, they act like "Pac-men," engulfing free radicals before they can do their damage to the body. Antioxidants protect DNA, cellular membranes and even various enzyme systems involved in the metabolism of fats, carbohydrates and lipids. Thus, the integrity of every cell in the body depends on the balance of free radicals and antioxidants.

Biological antioxidants can be single nutrients such as beta carotene, vitamin E, vitamin C or selenium, to mention a few. Or, they can be elaborate antioxidant enzyme systems (such as glutathione peroxidase or superoxide dismutase). Although antioxidant enzyme systems are thought to be genetically predetermined, the concentration of antioxidant vitamins and minerals is directly related to the intake of diet and supplements.

This free radical/antioxidant theory appeals to me as a doctor. Many of us not only eat high-fat diets that can form free radicals, but also are exposed to harmful metals, chemicals, drugs, toxins, pesticides and the various forms of electromagnetic contamination and radiation that I have discussed. I am especially concerned about radiation.

As a clinical cardiologist, I frequently encounter radiation. Performing cardiac catheterizations and inserting pacemakers requires working with x-ray devices which produce radiation. The patient gets a small dose, and so does the doctor. Since radiation accumulates over time, many small doses add up and can certainly be disruptive to the body. In my particular case, I stopped performing cardiac catheterizations because of hemorrhages found in my corneas that I believe were related to radiation.

HEALING POWER OF VITAMINS - MY EYES

Radiation is a factor in the formation of cataracts. Since eye diseases run in my family, I took a personal interest in nurturing my eyes. I researched much literature about the healing properties of vitamins, minerals and antioxidants for the eye.

I found one study indicating that a vegetable diet rich in vitamin A supported healing in the eyes. In this same study, women who took vitamin C supplements also had a significant reduction in the development of cataracts. In this study of over 50,000 female nurses, those who took the highest quantities of vitamin A, and others who used vitamin C supplements, over a long period of time, had a 40% reduction in cataracts. Since cataracts are the most common sign in the aging process, this study was *eye-opening* to me!

Antioxidants and antioxidant-rich vegetables help to prevent the oxidation of protein in the lens which leads to the formation of cataracts. In the women's heart study, 50,828 nurses showed that a high vitamin A carotenoid diet of carrots and spinach could protect the eyes. These findings were later validated in the JAMA November 9, 1994, article entitled, "Dietary Carotenoids, Vitamins A, C and E, and Advanced Age-Related Macular Degeneration."

Age-related macular degeneration is the leading cause of blindness over the age of 65. The macula is the most sensitive point of the retina for vision. Previous observational studies and animal experiments have demonstrated antioxidant benefits to the retina. The outer retina is rich in poly-unsaturated fatty acids and is susceptible to free radical attack and oxidation. Antioxidants and other nutritionals help maintain the cellular membranes of the blood vessels that supply the vulnerable macular region of the retina.

Lutein and zeaxanthin are dominant pigments found in the retina that filter out the harmful blue light which accelerates the oxidation process. Lutein is found in spinach, collard greens, apricots, corn seeds, red peppers and peaches. As the carotenoids lutein and zeaxanthin are significantly decreased in advanced AMD, it makes sense to incorporate this nutritional healing to protect our precious eyesight. I personally try to eat spinach, apricots and other sources of these excellent carotenoids almost every day. In addition, I take my multi-vitamin mineral supplement containing beta carotene, vitamin C, vitamin E and zinc, all of which have been shown to be protective for the eye.

As a result of this self-healing endeavor for my eyes, I continued my incessant investigation in other areas of health and healing, using vitamins, minerals, antioxidants and other nutritionals.

My investigations continue to include computer searches and extensive reading. Although I eat a very healthy diet of fruits and vegetables, I still take vitamin and mineral supplementation. Since we are all exposed to radiation and chemical pollutants in our environment that may be destructive to many vitamins and essential fatty acids, it is a good idea to try to protect ourselves with these added nutrients.

Many of us consume fats, particularly fried foods, and most of us have eaten in fast-food restaurants where fats and oils are cooked at high temperatures. Remembering that the waste products of oxidized fats are toxic, it makes sense to supplement our diets with vitamins and minerals. Vitamins C, E, beta carotene, Q_{10} and others offer an antioxidant defense against free radical invasion. It is this critical ingredient in winning the body's unrelenting biochemical war with our diet that is so essential in halting tissue deterioration.

But how much vitamin and mineral supplementation is enough? We need to be aware that the recommended daily allowance (RDA) was instituted *approximately 50 years ago* by the U.S. Food and Nutrition Board to determine the daily amount of vitamins and nutrients necessary to prevent illness directly due to vitamin deficiencies such as scurvy, beriberi, etc,. The RDA's, however, are considered to be only *minimal* doses that ward off such conditions, and these diseases are rare today. It has become apparent that larger doses of vitamins, but not megadoses, may provide more protection for the body. What I mean is *the RDA may not be enough, given today's electromagnetic, over-radiated and chemically-polluted environment.* We need to consider a larger dose than the RDA recommendation to provide an optimal daily allowance that is health-enhancing.

WHAT DOES RDA MEAN?

In the 1940s, the federal government developed the RDA (Recommended Daily Allowance) for nutrition. These recommended daily allowances are published by the Food and Nutritional Board of the National Academy of Sciences National Research Council. In the following chart, the US RDA's are listed. The chart represents the bare minimal essential nutrients that the average person needs.

VITAMINS	Children Under 4 Years Old		Adult & Children 4 Years Old & Older	
Vitamin A	2500	I.U.	5000	I.U.
Vitamin D	400	I.U.	400	I.U.
Vitamin E	10	I.U.	30	I.U.
Vitamin C	40	mg	60	mg
Folic Acid	0.2	mg	0.4	mg
Vitamin B-1	0.7	mg	1.5	mg
Vitamin B-2	0.8	mg	1.7	mg
Vitamin B-6	0.7	mg	2.0	mg
Vitamin B-12	3	mcg	6	mcg
Niacin (B-3)	9	mg	20	mg
Pantothenic Acid (B-5)	5	mg	10	mg
MINERALS				
Calcium	800	mg	1000	mg
Phosphorus	800	mg	1000	mg
Iodine	70	mcg	150	mcg
Iron	10	mg	18	mg
Magnesium	200	mg	400	mg
Copper	1	mg	2	mg
Zinc	6	mg	15	mg

When considering nutritional supplementation, remember that *taking vitamins and minerals in their proper balance is important.* For example, high doses of isolated B vitamins may cause depletion of other B vitamins, and too much of the mineral zinc may cause anemia. It was observed in the *Journal of the American Medical Association* that large numbers of elderly patients may be ingesting too much zinc. Consequently, a careful history about zinc ingestion is necessary when evaluating elderly patients for anemia. We also need to be aware that some vitamin supplements, particularly vitamins A and D, can cause serious illnesses if taken in excess dosages. *The key here again is moderation.* The following list points out some potential dangers from excessive supplementation.

HAZARDS OF VITAMINS/MINERALS MEGADOSE/OVERDOSE.

1. Vitamin A – A fat-soluble vitamin and is stored in the body. Do not consume in excess. Vitamin A greater than 50,000 units per day may cause weight loss, skin difficulties, bone pain, bleeding, etc.

2. Vitamin D – Another fat-soluble vitamin. When taken in greater than 3,000 units per day, may cause kidney impairment, weight loss and thirst.

3. Vitamin E/Coumadin – Rare occurrences of bleeding may occur. Use caution if you are taking more than 200 I.U.s of vitamin E per day in the presence of Coumadin (a blood thinner). Check with your physician before taking a higher dose of vitamin E.

4. Vitamin C – Caution needs to be used in patients on hemodialysis or with chronic renal failure. Approximately two percent of the population may have an iron overload state which indicates that the body may have too much iron. If you are taking more than a 1000 mg of vitamin C per day, I recommend having your iron level evaluated by your physician. Vitamin C will enhance the absorption of iron and act as a pro-oxidant in the presence of iron overload.

5. Iron/Copper – Are potent oxidants. Do not take them unless recommended by your physician.

6. Calcium – Avoid in renal failure.

7. Zinc – Greater than 100 mg per day may cause immunosuppression which may make people more susceptible to infections. However, in dosages less than 50 mg daily, zinc will help to stimulate your immunity.

8. Selenium – Greater than 300-400 mg per day may cause anemia, poor appetite and liver cirrhosis.

9. Beta carotene – Use with caution in the presence of alcoholic liver disease.

10. Vitamin B-6 – Greater than 300 mgs daily may cause liver and neurologic toxicity.

Later in this chapter, I will give you specific recommendations concerning nutritional vitamin and mineral supplementation. I do prefer using beta carotene over vitamin A, and unless your physician is treating you for osteoporosis, I would not use more than 400 I.U.s per day of vitamin D. Although I recommend Co Enzyme Q_{10} to most everyone in my practice, caution should be utilized in nursing mothers. I would also not administer Co Q_{10} to small children, as they have healthy livers and their bodies should contain abundant sources of it.

Now that I have told you about the downside of excessive vitamins and minerals, I want to discuss with you the many advantages of antioxidants, vitamins, minerals and targeted nutritionals. Unfortunately, the medical profession in general has not been very supportive of targeted nutritional supplementation. There has been much negativity and personal bias on this subject. I know this is true, because I was biased against vitamins back in the late 70s. And why has this been true for so many health professionals?

Over the years, few doctors were trained or knowledgeable in the field of nutrition, and until recently, only a few professionals believed that supplemental vitamins would be beneficial. There were very few scientific studies demonstrating health benefits in humans as compared to placebo. It was believed that a balanced diet would supply all the vitamins and nutrients needed to prevent the various vitamin deficiency diseases such as scurvy, beriberi and rickets, that we rarely see today.

Such was the thinking of the 1980s. However, the 1990s began to show us that anitoxidants, minerals and nutrients, in significant doses, can help prevent other diseases.

In the past couple of years, there has been an explosion in medical literature about vitamin and mineral supplementation. You cannot pick up a medical journal today without seeing a reference to vitamins, minerals or antioxidants. Numerous well-controlled scientific studies have shown impressive prevention benefits, especially for the antioxidant vitamins and minerals (beta carotene, C, E, Co Enzyme Q_{10}, selenium and others). Consider the following facts for prevention of heart disease, cancer and cataracts:

1. The Harvard Physician's Study showed a 44 percent reduction in heart attacks and a 49 percent reduction in strokes for the group given 50 mg of beta carotene every other day. Similar findings in heart disease and strokes were also shown in a large study involving 87,250 nurses over a period of eight years. These studies also have shown decreasing trends in the development of cancer.

2. In a California study, a vitamin C intake of greater than 300-500 mg per day suggested increases in life expectancy due to a decrease in heart attacks and various forms of cancer.

3. High vitamin diets reduce cataract risk. In a study of over 50,000 female nurses, those with the highest intake of vitamin A and C had a 39 percent lower risk of cataract formation.

4. Vitamin E has been shown to play a major role in the prevention of atherosclerosis in both men and (especially in) women. As presented recently in the *New England Journal of Medicine*, an approximate 26-41 percent reduction in heart attacks occurred after a two year period in participants taking 100–400 I.U. of vitamin E per day.

5. In a Chinese study of 29,000 participants, the ingestion of beta carotene, vitamin E and selenium showed a 13 percent reduction in esophageal and gastric cancer, and a nine percent reduction in deaths as compared to the population not taking supplements.

6. Vitamin E supplements promoted regression in coronary artery disease in men following coronary bypass surgery.

7. Beta carotene studies have demonstrated a decrease in tumor size in patients with oral leukoplakia (precancerous mouth legions).

9. There is strong population evidence that high dietary intake of vitamin C offers protection against non-hormone-dependent cancers of the esophagus, larynx, oral cavity, pancreas, stomach, rectum, breast, cervix and lungs.

10. Positive health benefits have also been demonstrated for numerous other vitamins and minerals. Hundreds of articles have appeared in several medical journals over the past year on these topics, demonstrating some positive health benefits. There are many large population studies and clinical trials presently underway that will yield further information concerning vitamins, minerals and antioxidants.

Although vitamin and mineral supplements are no substitute for a proper diet, they are a beneficial, nontoxic and easy way to promote *Optimum Health*. Unfortunately, even the rare individual who eats a balanced diet (nine percent of Americans) consisting of five to nine fresh fruits and vegetables a day does not get the larger amounts of these minerals demonstrated to be effective in scientific studies.

Therefore, supplemental vitamins and minerals are the easiest way to make up this deficit. The problem here is that most vitamins and minerals are unregulated as to potency and absorption. The *Center for Science in the Public Interest* in Washington, DC, found tremendous variability in potency when 50 vitamin preparations were analyzed. Furthermore, many vitamin preparations are hard to absorb and much of the product goes in and goes out with many of the nutrients not being absorbed into the blood stream. Choosing the right vitamin and mineral formula is a complex yet crucial task!

A FAMOUS-BUT-FLAWED STUDY

Choosing the right vitamin and mineral formula is not only difficult for the general population, but also for investigators performing major clinical studies. For example, you probably have heard of the famous Finnish Trial. In *The New England Journal of Medicine*, 1994, the authors indicated that beta carotene supplements may cause lung cancer. The disclosure of this study hit the media like an explosion. The results were portrayed all over the televisions and newspapers of America. This study got more press than any other study in the history of medicine. The question is, why?

The results of this study appeared just before the passing of the famous Hatch-Richardson Freedom of Acts Bill regarding the purchase of vitamin and mineral supplements. The study population in the Finnish Trial included approximately 29,000 male smokers in Finland. Most of these individuals had been smoking for 30 years. Since the average fat content of the Finnish diet was at about 38 percent total calories, most participants had high cholesterol levels. In addition, many of the participants drank considerable quantities of alcohol.

Although this study had serious flaws and limitations from the beginning, the question remains, "Why would researchers choose a population with such serious risk factors for heart disease and cancer, and try to resurrect them at the 11th hour with antioxidant supplements?" (The supplements were also of low quality and low dosage).

The trial showed the following results: the men taking vitamin E had fewer lung cancers, but the results were not significant statistically. The men taking beta carotene had 18 percent more lung cancers which was statistically significant. The men taking vitamin E had 34 percent fewer prostate cancers and 15 percent fewer colo-rectal cancers. The men taking beta carotene had slightly more cases of cancer (other than lung cancer), but that result was not statistically significant.

The researchers could not find a reason why these smoking men taking beta carotene were observed to have more cancers. My own personal interpretation of this study includes a major concern involving the choice of the vitamins and minerals. I previously told you that a China study showed a reduction in cancer. The supplements used in the China study were manufactured in the USA. These vitamin supplements did not contain quinoline yellow (yellow dye #10), consistent with good manufacturing practices. Since quinoline yellow is not FDA certified for use in this country in food additives, it was not used in the China supplements. However, all formulations in the Finnish study were colored with quinoline yellow, a water-soluble powder that may be used in coloring cosmetics and drugs. They were not manufactured in the USA under GMP regulations.

Since the Finnish study is at variance with all other clinical studies and had such unexpected results, the question about the impact of quinoline yellow remains. Certainly, vitamin E and beta carotene are not considered drugs nor cosmetics. Laced with quinoline yellow, could the experimental agents become ineffective, lose potency or possibly become harmful? And no one has looked at the biochemical interactions of yellow dye #10 and beta carotene in animal studies.

If we consider real science, we need to look at the impact quinoline yellow has on these food nutrients. Certainly, the American FDA has an opinion on quinoline yellow since it is not certified for use in the United States. Nevertheless, the Finnish study has had a tremendous negative impact on people in this country. People seem to forget that it is at variance with over 200 published population studies showing a lower risk of cancer and cardiovascular disease in populations consuming dietary antioxidants, vitamins C, E and beta carotene. People forget that even the authors of the article were skeptical of the results. They indicated, "An adverse affect of beta carotene seems unlikely, in spite of all of its statistical significance, therefore, this finding may be due to chance."

My reason for discussing this flawed study with you is to raise your awareness about the advantages and possible limitations of not only supplements, but also of the studies that evaluate them. As this study was doomed to fail from the beginning because of poor quality ingredients, toxins and poor design, we must certainly question its results. In the next section, I will discuss some of the vitamins and minerals that are necessary in the proper functioning of our body.

VITAMINS

Vitamins are a group of organic compounds that regulate the metabolism of carbohydrates, proteins and fats. Vitamins are considered micronutrients and act as a catalyst for chemical reactions in the body. Frequently, a vitamin will be described as a co enzyme because it works with enzymes in assisting biochemical functions. Since vitamins cannot be produced by the body, we rely on getting them through the diet and/or in vitamin and mineral supplements.

Some vitamins may be fat-soluble, such as A, D, E and K, and do not need to be replenished on a daily basis, as the body can store them in the adipose tissue. The water-soluble vitamins, however, such as the Bs and vitamin C, must be ingested on a daily basis, as they cannot be stored in the body.

Vitamin A

Vitamin A is essential to prevent night blindness and the formation of cataracts. It is also important in the development of healthy bones, skin, hair and mucous membranes. It enhances immunity and is important in epithelial tissue (skin and mucous membranes) maintenance and repair. As an antioxidant, vitamin A helps protect against the adverse effects of radiation and chemical pollutants. Although high doses of vitamin A can be utilized for infections and conditions of physical or emotional stress, supplements of vitamin A should not be taken in high dosages for a long period of time, as it is a fat-soluble vitamin and can be stored in the body. There have been cases on record where megadose therapy resulted in hypervitaminosis A, causing liver damage, skin rash and brain dysfunction.

Beta-Carotene

Pro-vitamin A, or beta carotene, is a precursor of vitamin A and is converted into vitamin A by the body. *Beta carotene is a yellowish compound contained in carrot juice, canteloupe, watercress and other fruits and vegetables, especially those with yellow, orange or dark green hues.* Unlike vitamin A, beta carotene has been shown to have few toxic side effects. Except for the tendency to turn the skin a slight yellow-orange color when used to an extreme, the only other caution should be when treating medically uncontrolled diabetic and hypothyroid individuals, as they have difficulty metabolizing beta carotene.

Beta carotene has become the focus of much research. In a recent study by Harvard medical experts, it has been claimed in supplement form to contribute to the prevention of cancer as well as coronary artery disease.

In large population studies, people eating foods high in beta carotene also had fewer heart attacks than those taking in less beta carotene. Both vitamin A and beta carotene are extremely important to the immune mechanisms of the body and may help to fight the common cold and other flu-like illnesses. Beta carotene also has been reported to protect the lung from increased ozone and smog in polluted city environments and is helpful in combating the toxic effects of automobile emissions.

The RDA for vitamin A or beta carotene is 3,000 I.U.s for children and 5,000 I.U.s for adults. We usually get plenty of vitamin A in the diet. *Foods that contain considerable quantities of vitamin A include carrots, beets, cantaloupe, broccoli, Swiss chard, dandelion greens, garlic, kale, parsley, red peppers, sweet potatoes, spinach, yellow squash, turnip greens and watercress.* For an animal source of vitamin A, I recommend *fish liver oils, particularly cod liver oil, as I do not recommend eating calves liver or other organ meats.* Although I'm sure vitamin supplements would be preferable, one tablespoon of cod liver oil contains 11,000 units of pre-formed vitamin A. Similarly, three and one-half ounces of carrots offer approximately 11,500 units of vitamin A. It is also important to note that antibiotics, cholesterol-lowering agents, some laxatives, various antacids, and excessive quantities of alcohol or caffeine may interfere with vitamin A absorption.

Vitamin B complex with vitamin B-1 (Thiamine)

My first exposure to a patient with vitamin B-1 deficiency occurred during my internship. A man in his mid-fifties was presented to the Albany Medical Center Hospital with congestive heart failure. He reminded me of "Popeye." His arms and legs were very swollen and he was suffering from chronic heart failure. This man was an alcoholic. Although he responded to the usual treatment for heart failure at the time, i.e. diuretics and Digoxin (a heart-strengthening medicine), he did not appear to improve significantly until he received vitamin B-1. Thiamine enhances circulation and is needed for the normal functioning of the heart muscle and smooth muscle of the gastrointestinal tract. It is also an important constituent for the central nervous system. Vitamin B1 is administered to many patients with alcoholism as it protects the brain. If not taken in the diet, deficiencies may occur. *Excellent sources of vitamin B-1 include brown rice, whole grains, green vegetables, peas, wheat germ, soybeans, dried beans, green vegetables, Brussels sprouts, oatmeal, prunes, raisins and sunflower seeds, to mention a few.*

Vitamin B-2 (Riboflavin)

Riboflavin is necessary for antibody production, cell respiration and metabolism of fats, carbohydrates and proteins. Signs of riboflavin deficiency include cracks and sores at the corner of the mouth. It also has been suggested by researchers that riboflavin may alleviate allergic conjunctivitis, a common problem for hayfever sufferers. Riboflavin is also beneficial for the skin, nails and hair. It may be helpful in controlling dandruff. High dose riboflavin (100 mg), when taken with other B vitamins in combination with magnesium, has been known to prevent and reduce the discomfort of migraine headaches. *Sources of riboflavin include leafy green vegetables, whole grains, spinach, poultry, fish, meat, asparagus, broccoli, Brussels sprouts, currants and sea vegetables.* It is also important to know that oral contraceptives may increase the need for riboflavin, and this is one particular vitamin that is easily destroyed by overcooking and the use of alcohol. Incidentally, riboflavin is responsible for the bright yellow urine you may have noticed following the ingestion of a multi-vitamin.

Vitamin B-3 (Niacin)

Niacin is an important vitamin for circulation, energy production and functioning of the nervous system. In large doses, it is helpful in lowering cholesterol. I already told you something about my personal experience with niacin. I took niacin in the powdered form, only to realize that instead of following the instruction of teaspoons, I took tablespoons. I immediately developed a "niacin flush" accompanied by the tingling of the skin associated with a hot flash.

I really thought I was having an allergic reaction. I immediately went back to one of my textbooks on vitamins and found that this sensation, to my surprise, is welcomed by many people who experience it. Some people even use niacin as a sexual stimulant for enhancing sexual pleasure. Some of my patients found this out by accident and now take dosages up to 500 mg at bedtime. Deficiencies in niacin may cause abnormalities in the central nervous system. *Excellent sources of niacin include meat products, broccoli, grains, dried beans, potatoes, tomatoes and nuts.*

Vitamin B-5 (Pantothenic acid)

Pantothenic acid, also referred to as vitamin B-5, is known as the "anti-stress vitamin" because of its crucial role in energy metabolism. Under situations of severe emotional and physical stress, it is not uncommon for some individuals to need an additional 500 mg of pantothenic acid per day. Although the human requirement for pantothenic acid is not known, ten mg is considered sufficient. However, more of the vitamin is required after injury, stress or during antibiotic therapy. Although symptoms of pantothenic acid deficiency are rare, considerable amounts of the vitamin are lost in the processing, canning and cooking of foods, especially in acidic or alkaline solutions.

The brain contains the highest concentration of pantothenic acid in the body, therefore, a deficiency of pantothenic acid, like all the B vitamins, would include symptoms such as easy fatigue, depression and insomnia. The alcoholic is one individual who may be particularly prone to a B vitamin deficiency, especially if foods high in B-5 are not consumed. *Excellent sources of pantothenic acid would include whole grains, meat, cabbage, cauliflower, beans, eggs, saltwater fish and poultry.*

Vitamin B-6 (Pyridoxine)

Vitamin B-6 is an important vitamin in the regulation and formation of blood cells. It is required for the synthesis of nucleic acids. Some investigators reported that vitamin B-6 helped some individuals recall dreams. It also has been used to calm the effects of premenstrual syndrome and is helpful in the treatment of allergies and asthma. In weight loss, B-6 has been reported to be a useful nutrient as well. The use of 200 mg of B-6 on a daily basis has also been helpful to some of my patients with carpal-tunnel syndrome. Since vitamin B-6 has absolutely no toxicity at this dosage, it may be a suitable alternative to surgery, particularly since people may respond to dosages as low as 40 to 100 mg per day.

Oral contraceptives may increase the need for vitamin B-6. An urologist may prescribe vitamin B-6, as it is useful in preventing calcium oxalate gravel in the urinary tract. In short, vitamin B-6 is an important co enzyme in the metabolism of amino acids that can affect our mental and physical health. Most foods contain small amounts of vitamin B-6. *The best sources include green vegetables, brewers' yeast, carrots, fish, meat, peas, sunflower seeds, avocados and green peppers.*

Vitamin B-12 (Cyanocobalamin)

Vitamin B-12 is necessary for the formation of blood cells and actually prevents anemia. It is also necessary in the maintenance of a healthy nervous system. A prolonged absence of vitamin B-12 may cause pernicious anemia. This is a type of anemia that may cause weakness, lethargy and damage to the nervous system. I remember one of my elderly patients who had an absorption problem with vitamin B-12. When he came to my office with angina, he almost underwent coronary artery bypass surgery because of his severe coronary disease. We discovered, however, that his angina possibly could have been provoked by a low blood count resulting from a vitamin B-12 deficiency. After he received vitamin B-12 injections, he felt considerably better with less symptoms of angina. He now visits his family physician on a monthly basis to obtain B-12 shots which completely corrected the problem. He has been with this particular treatment for approximately ten years and, at the age of 84, still has a good quality of life. *Sources of vitamin B-12 include all animal foods, cheese, eggs, milk, tofu and sea vegetables. Since B-12 is not found in most vegetables, vegetarians need to be cautious and supplement B-12 in their diet.*

Folic Acid

Over the past couple of years, this B vitamin has received tremendous attention in the medical literature. The public health service has recently recommended that 400 mcg be available to every childbearing women in the United States. Even our FDA has agreed to this health claim. Folic acid has been shown to have a positive impact on reducing the amount of birth defects of the spinal cord and central nervous system. Spina bifida, as is it is commonly called, is a horrible congenital neural tube defect which not only causes despair and anguish for families, but is also economically devastating to care for. Folic acid will prevent spina bifida up to 70 percent of the time.

Unfortunately, when a young woman gets pregnant, if there are suboptimum levels of folic acid in her blood, the likelihood of congenital birth defects is higher. Since folic has also been shown to decrease the incidence of cervical cancer in women, it is not unreasonable to recommend this vitamin to large segments of the female population. But what about males? Do they need folic acid, too?

The most exciting research in the cardiovascular literature over the last few years has involved, you guessed it, folic acid. Why has folic acid become so fashionable? Coronary artery disease, peripheral vascular disease and vascular disease in the brain may now be considered diseases of aging. If the body has low levels of folate, vitamin B-6 or vitamin B-12, the likelihood of premature aging in our circulation occurs. But why? And why should we have low levels of folate, vitamin B-6 or B-12? I previously told you that microwaving and over-processing of foods and poor dietary habits deletes these essential ingredients. However, there is another major demon lurking in disguise - red meat.

Red meat contains the amino acid, methionine. In order for methionine to be properly metabolized, the body needs sufficient quantities of folic acid and other B vitamins. If these vitamins are lacking, methionine can not be broken down properly, and the dangerous amino acid, homocysteine, arises. Homocysteine is extremely toxic to the walls of blood vessels and capillaries, causing cellular and membrane inflammation. The blood vessels become vulnerable to toxic LDL cholesterol. This chronic process results in plaque deposition within the blood vessel wall, thus causing artheroschlerosis. This can also occur in young people. In recent studies, including the Health Physician Study at Harvard and the Framingham Study in Boston, it has been demonstrated that high levels of homocysteine in the body cause premature vascular disease, including stroke and heart attack.

The antidote to all of this is folic acid and, to a lesser degree, vitamin B-6 and vitamin B-12. Although it is wise to eat less red meat, it is perhaps wiser to take a vitamin B supplement containing all of this protection. Since this data is very new and has only been in the medical literature during the last few years, perhaps three quarters of the physicians in this country, including cardiologists, haven't had a chance to assimilate this. One problem in our society today is the poor eating habits of young adults and teens who don't consume foods rich in folic acid. My recommendation is to give B vitamins to everyone, including young children.

Other B Vitamins

Other B complex vitamins include biotin, choline, inositol and para-aminobenzoic acid (PABA). These vitamins are found in many of the foods mentioned in vitamins B-12, with the exception of PABA, which is found in *molasses, liver and kidney*, as well as whole grains. Para-aminobenzoic acid is an antioxidant which may protect against sunburn and various skin cancers. Since most preparations of B vitamins include a multi-B complex and are water-soluble, it is only necessary to take these in small doses on a daily basis, as the excess amount is excreted.

Generally, there are no known toxicities if the B vitamins are taken in small amounts. In large amounts, however, one has to utilize caution, particularly with the long-acting preparation of vitamin B-3, which can be injurious to the liver. There are no known side effects for vitamin B-5, pantothenic acid. It is also important to note that alcohol and caffeine, as well as birth control pills and estrogen replacements, can have a negative impact on B vitamins. Caffeine and alcohol, for example, may affect the elimination of B vitamins; oral contraceptives or estrogens may result in a functional deficiency of the B vitamins. This is related to complex hormonal pathways in which relative B-6 and B-12 deficiencies may occur. Thus, in patients on estrogen, it is reasonable to meet the body's increased need for B-2, B-6 and B-12 with additional nutritional supplements.

Vitamin C

Vitamin C has been the subject of considerable controversy over the last few years, particularly when Linus Pauling first publicized it as the "cure for the common cold." Numerous research studies have indicated that vitamin C improves the immune system. In the animal model, for example, vitamin C has been shown to protect against lethal doses of radiation. Perhaps the most famous and noteworthy effect of vitamin C is preventing the disease of scurvy. Scurvy is an illness in which subcutaneous bleeding occurs, along with a loss of appetite, tender joints and a low grade anemia, accompanied by slow wound healing. Centuries ago, sailing ships used to carry limes in order to prevent scurvy. Recently, there was a case of scurvy at a major university center. A young male who was vitamin C deficient had been eating out of cans for six months. He presented himself to the doctor with bleeding and funny "corkscrew" type hair. This modern case of scurvy was caused from eating only processed foods, with no fresh citrus. Vitamin C was the antidote.

Vitamin C is a powerful antioxidant that is necessary for tissue growth and repair, particularly in the gums. Vitamin C also plays a crucial role in the absorption of iron, which is necessary for the formation of red blood cells, thereby preventing anemia. Doctors frequently will administer vitamin C in combination with iron, for example, to increase the iron assimilation in the body. Vitamin C creates a favorable acidic pH in the stomach so that iron-bound compounds can be absorbed. Vitamin C is also an essential constituent in the metabolism of amino acids, particularly tyrosine and phenylalanine.

During psychological and emotional stress, vitamin C may become depleted from the adrenal glands. Dietary supplementation with foods rich in vitamin C or vitamin supplements may help prevent the body's negative reaction to prolonged stress. Some clinical studies have also demonstrated a reduction in serum cholesterol with vitamin C supplementation. Since the body cannot manufacture its own vitamin C, it must be obtained through the diet or in nutritional supplements. Since most vitamin C is water-soluble and can be excreted in the urine, it needs to be taken on a daily basis.

Although the evidence linking vitamin C to cardiovascular disease is gaining increasing popularity, it is well known that many groups at an increased risk for heart disease also have lower vitamin C levels. If one scrutinizes the literature, the groups at risk for heart disease, such as men, the elderly, diabetics and hypertensives, have lower vitamin C plasma levels. In addition to these population groups, smokers are especially deficient in vitamin C and should seriously consider taking vitamin C as a supplement.

In other clinical studies, vitamin C has been shown to decrease platelet aggregation, similar to the Omega-3 fish oils.

Another interesting function of vitamin C is that it raises the body's level of glutathione. In a double-blind study performed at the University of Arizona, experimental subjects placed on 500 mg of vitamin C showed glutathione levels were increased by 50 percent. Glutathione is a powerful antioxidant in itself and is perhaps one of the body's most potent free radical scavengers. Thus, vitamin C may help maintain glutathione levels and improve overall antioxidant status.

Common sources of vitamin C include green leafy vegetables, bell peppers, broccoli, squash, cabbage, strawberries, lemons, kale, grapefruit, oranges, currants, parsley, onions, green peas, radishes, rosehips, spinach, Swiss chard, tomatoes, turnip greens and Brussels sprouts.

Once again, it is important for us to remember that oral contraceptives and corticosteroids may reduce the levels of vitamin C in the body. Alcohol is also an antagonist to vitamin C. Although symptoms of a toxicity are rare with high intakes of vitamin C, kidney stones could occur if vitamin C is taken in large doses and not accompanied by adequate hydration. In doses greater than 5,000 mg a day, some side effects may occur. Excess urination, diarrhea or skin rashes may be experienced as some tolerable side effects.

Vitamin D

Vitamin D is the bone vitamin. A deficiency of vitamin D may impair the growth and development of bone structures. This is commonly seen in the pathologic entity called rickets in children and osteomalacia in adults. In addition to bone, the maintenance of healthy teeth is enhanced by vitamin D. *The principle source of vitamin D comes from the sun's ultraviolet rays.* A deficiency of vitamin D could result from lack of exposure to the sun, especially if the natural vitamin is not taken in the diet. Nursing home inhabitants, for example, who do not wish to go out into the sun are susceptible to vitamin D deficiency.

This is an important consideration since vitamin D is not self-activated and requires conversion by the liver, in either its natural or supplement form. Regular sunshine, perhaps as little as one-half hour per day, is all that is necessary to activate the vitamin D metabolism in the body. It is also important to note that in the elderly, vitamin D can help in the overall treatment of osteoporosis, an illness resulting from gradual loss of bone, predominantly in the spine and hips, that affects approximately 50-60 percent of all women over the age of 50. When treating osteoporosis, it is important to know the overall health of the patient. Many of these individuals may have kidney and liver disease and are frequently diabetic. Thus, vitamin and mineral supplementation is critical in this population.

As vitamin D is a fat-soluble vitamin which is stored in the body, it may be toxic if taken in megadoses. This can be particularly serious in children or in individuals with kidney disease. Some drugs, such as steroid hormones, interfere with the action of vitamin D in the intestines; others, such as cholesterol-lowering drugs, may also interfere with the absorption of vitamin D. *The dietary sources of vitamin D include fish oils and saltwater fish, especially fatty fish like halibut, salmon, mackerel and bluefish. It is also found in abundance in eggs, liver, milk, sweet potatoes and sunflower seeds.*

Vitamin E

Vitamin E is gaining more and more popularity with cardiologists. An article concerning vitamin E and its inverse relationship to angina was published in the prestigious medical journal, *Lancet.* Vitamin C and beta carotene were also cited as being beneficial in treating angina. Although the mechanism for vitamin E and its protective effects on the heart is not well established, recent research indicates that vitamin E is an important antioxidant that may help protect unsaturated fatty acids from breaking down and causing the formation of free radicals. Vitamin E may help lower the deleterious influence of LDL on cellular membranes, thus preventing the oxidation of LDL - the cardinal step in artherosclerosis. In addition, it has been reported to aid against the long-term effects of aging and may be used as an adjunct in cancer treatments.

Over the last two to three years, vitamin E has been the subject of careful scrutiny. There have been multiple studies regarding cancer and cardiovascular disease. Perhaps the most noteworthy studies included the Nurses Health Study of 87,000 women. There was a 41 percent reduction in risk of heart disease among women who took vitamin E supplements for more than two years. There was also a significant improvement in risks, with supplements as low as 100 I.U., and slightly more improvement at the 200 I.U. level.

In a follow-up study involving almost 40,000 men, similar findings were found. However, the vitamin E intake for men showing the lowest risk was at 400 I.U.s. Thus, men may need higher supplementation than women.

In a study regarding coronary artery angioplasty, researchers in Atlanta demonstrated a favorable trend in those patients taking vitamin E over placebo for recurrent restenosis (recurrent narrowing of the balloon-inflated vessel). Since the restenosis rate for angioplasty is high, I am working with some major medical centers to assess the efficacy of multi-mineral combinations versus placebo in preventing closure of the vessels following balloon dilation.

Perhaps the most exciting news about vitamin E came out of a June 1995 research paper in the *Journal of the American Medical Association.* This landmark study should raise the eyebrow of any reputable cardiologist who has had a negative bias about the crucial preventive aspects of vitamin E. In this study of 156 men, aged 40-59 with a previous history of coronary artery bypass surgery, those subjects given supplementary vitamin E intake greater than 100 I.U.s per day had less coronary artery progression than did subjects on placebo or those given less than 100 I.U.s per day. The data was also confirmed by cardiac catheterization, a procedure that takes pictures of the coronary vessels that wrap around the heart. This is indeed a landmark study, for the results indicate a positive association between supplemental vitamin E intake and reduction in coronary artery disease.

Previous studies also demonstrated that the higher the plasma vitamin E level in the blood, the less the occurrence of heart disease symptoms such as angina and even heart disease death. Multiple population studies have also demonstrated that countries who take in higher vitamin E in their diet have less incidence of coronary artery disease. The study further strengthens the positive impact of vitamin E supplements on the regression of coronary artery disease. Once again, the mechanism of vitamin E is probably related to its antioxidant effect against preventing the harmful oxidative effect on low density lipoprotein (LDL). Although most cardiologists I know take vitamin E, I am sure this information will persuade even the most resistant cardiologists and other physicians to consider vitamin E supplements.

The favorable effects of vitamin E on the immune system were also demonstrated in an animal study using lethal doses of radiation. In one particular study, two groups of mice were radiated. One was given vitamin E and the other was not. The mice who were radiated but not given vitamin E succumbed to the radiation. The experimental group given the vitamin, however, had an increase in survival, thus showing the protective effects of vitamin E against radiation and on the overall immune response. Vitamin E has been shown to be effective against many common pollutants in the environment, such as nitroamines (carcinogens found in many processed meats), chlorine, mercury and carbon monoxide. The once thought of "sex vitamin" is now standing on its own as an effective healing agent, not only for its merits in cancer and cardiovascular disease, but also in its effectiveness as an antipollutant vitamin. When combined with beta carotene and vitamin C , vitamin E is extremely helpful in neutralizing the deleterious effects of industrial pollutants and toxic heavy metals.

Vitamin E has also been reported to be effective in thinning the blood, eliminating leg cramps and aiding in the prevention of cataracts, as well as decreasing the breast tenderness and swelling experienced in the PMS syndrome. *The best sources of vitamin E include vegetable oils such as wheat germ oil and peanut oil. Green leafy vegetables, nuts, seeds, dry beans, brown rice and whole wheat are other good sources of vitamin E.* Vitamin E is found in fats, oils and margarines. Therefore, if you consume a low-fat diet, you may not get the RDA of vitamin E.

As a supplement, approximately 200 to 400 units of vitamin E per day is suggested to enhance the body's health and immunity. Although not all the mechanisms of vitamin E are clear, medical research has revealed yet another secret of the role of vitamin E in health. It has recently been discovered that vitamin E's role may be important in increasing the production of Co Enzyme Q_{10}.

Co Enzyme Q_{10}

I'd like to share with you a letter I sent to the editor of the *Journal of the American Medical Association* about the use of Co Enzyme Q_{10} in congestive heart failure:

> Targeted nutritional supplementation with fat-soluble and water-soluble minerals is important adjuvant therapy in patients with congestive heart failure. As a clinical cardiologist who works on a day-to-day basis with many patients, both from the physiological and psychological point of view, I fully support the inclusion of psychological and nutritional approaches in the overall care of the patient. In addition to what was mentioned in the article, I would recommend the addition of Co Enzyme Q_{10} to patients with diminished left ventricular function.
>
> I have had the opportunity to treat hundreds of patients with Co Enzyme Q_{10}, and for a significant number, there has not only been a significant improvement in left ventricular function, but also in quality of life. I have even had heart transplant patients refuse transplantation following the use of Co Enzyme Q_{10}. Although these are anecdotal cases, there have been at least 50 major articles published in the last ten years in reputable journals on the use of Co Q_{10} in cardiac-related diseases, especially congestive heart failure and idiopathic dilated cardiomyopathy.
>
> The contractive ability of the heart depends on the functional capacity of myocardial cells to expand and contract. Congestive heart failure often involves insufficient myocardial contractive forces. Literally, heart failure is an energy-starved heart. The cardiologist cannot focus only on fluid retention, but also on the biochemistry of "pulsation." It is important to consider the molecular and cellular components of the heart.
>
> When it comes to the heart, cardiologists need to think bioenergetically. This is where Co Enzyme Q_{10} comes in. Although Co Q_{10} has major therapeutic mechanisms in reperfusion injury, it has also been demonstrated to scavenge free radicals produced by lipid peroxidation, stabilize cellular membranes and prevent depletion of metabolites necessary for the resynthesis of ATP in mitochondria. As the oxygen-based production of energy takes place in the mitochondria, it is not unusual that the ubiquinone concentration of myocardial cells is approximately ten time greater than brain or colon cells. Cardiac muscle is one of the few tissues in the body to be continuously aerobic, thus requiring ATP

support. Co Q_{10} enhances ATP/ADP production in mitochondria, thus helping to drive the "machinery" of the cell.

As side effects of Co Q_{10} are rare, I suggest this as another nutritional additive to the treatment of congestive heart failure, cardiomyopathy and in those patients with abnormal systolic and diastolic dysfunction. Certainly, one set of researchers in Naples, Italy, has concluded that the treatment of every 1000 cases of congestive heart failure patients with Co Q_{10} for one year could reduce hospitalizations by 20 percent. In this era of cost containment, this is indeed remarkable.

Stephen Sinatra, MD, FACC

One of the most exciting and intriguing insights that I learned in researching this book was the personal discovery of the health benefits of Q_{10}. Actually, I first learned about Q_{10} several years ago in an article that appeared in the *Annals of Thoracic Surgery* in February of 1982. In this particular study, a control group and an experimental group were designed to investigate the impact of Q_{10} on cardiovascular heart function in patients placed on the heart-lung machine during open heart surgery. The article concluded that patients given Q_{10} prior to open heart surgery actually had an improvement in their heart function. It also reported that the preoperative administration of this vitamin-like substance could favorably increase one's tolerance to the low oxygen state that occurs during open heart surgery. Thus, Q_{10} increased cardiac output and overall heart efficiency.

Although this study was highly provocative, my openness to such vitamin and mineral therapy at that time, to say the least, was nonexistent. As a well-trained traditional cardiologist, I saw no need for such nutritional supplementation, particularly since drugs such as Digitalis, diuretics and other myocardial stimulants were considered highly useful. It took several years of experience, growth and humility to teach me that vitamins and other natural remedies can be a useful adjunct to traditional medical therapies.

Congestive heart failure is a term that cardiologists refer to as a weakening of the heart muscle. When the heart muscle becomes so weak that it cannot pump the blood effectively to the organs of the body, patients may develop swelling of the ankles, lack of appetite, fatigue and shortness of breath on activity. Sometimes, the pumping ability of the heart is so impaired that the blood, instead of being pumped out of the heart, backs up into the lungs. At this time patients will complain of shortness of breath during activities and sometimes while at rest, especially when lying down. Congestive heart failure is a failing heart or an energy-starved heart. For all practical purposes, the tiny myocardial cells are so exhausted that they cannot sustain sufficient intrinsic cellular energy, thus they cannot contract and effectively create a pumping mechanism for the blood to be circulated around the body. Congestive heart failure is indeed the most frustrating and challenging dilemma of my profession.

Over the last 20 years I have seen hundreds of patients with congestive heart failure. For some, the diagnosis is obvious; that is, if a large heart attack destroys a considerable quantity of heart muscle, the contracting action of the heart is so impaired that the remaining viable myocardial cells eventually become exhausted and worn out in sustaining the circulatory pumping action of the heart.

A long-standing history of high blood pressure can also impair myocardial function. Valvular disease, frequently induced by childhood rheumatic fever as well as viral illnesses and toxins such as chronic alcohol abuse, can likewise impair the functioning of the heart muscle.

As a clinical cardiologist, I can also attest to numerous cases of unexplained heart failure. These are individuals who have "cardiomyopathy" of an unknown nature; that is, in these individuals, there was no known cause of heart muscle weakening. There was no history of diabetes, heart attack, high blood pressure, alcohol abuse, rheumatic fever or severe viral illnesses. Some patients just develop weakening of the heart from no apparent cause. Some of the cardiomyopathies have also been found to be due to a nutritional origin. Vitamin deficiencies such as beriberi, thiamine deficiency and the rare postpartum cardiomyopathy of pregnancy may be related to nutritional deficiencies that have been known to cause congestive heart failure.

Although some patients with cardiomyopathy improve, the majority of these individuals deteriorate. For the cardiologist, the treatment of heart failure is similar to the oncologist treating a life-threatening cancer. Although we can find drugs to help control symptoms, there is really no known cure for cardiomyopathy. Like some form of incurable cancer, there is frequently a deterioration that ultimately ends in death. One of the most heartbreaking weeks of my practice occurred approximately four years ago. During that one week period, I lost five male patients from congestive heart failure. Many of these patients were also my "friends" for several years.

NEW HOPE

My rediscovery of Q_{10} in the preparation of this manuscript has now given me an exciting charge of optimism that may offer an improvement in quality of life and hope in the treatment of these patients! It is true that in February of 1982, a very favorable article was reported in a major cardiology journal. But most of my colleagues and I probably did not really appreciate the true meaning of this article.

Then, one of my colleagues in endocrinology, Dr. Lester Kritzer, questioned me about the healing properties of the co enzyme. He gave me a book entitled *The Miracle Nutrient Co Enzyme Q_{10}* by Emile G. Bliznakof, M.D. and Gerald L. Hunt. After reading the exciting contents of the book, and particularly after looking at the bibliography, I began to inquire about Q_{10}. I went to the library and requested major articles that were listed in the cardiology literature. As I read some of these articles, I became excited and also intrigued.

Surprisingly, another timely and fortuitous event happened. One of the most reknowned cardiologists in the world was speaking at our hospital as I was reviewing the literature on Q_{10}. As the Director of Medical Education, I had invited Dr. William Frishman, a Professor of Medicine at Albert Einstein College of Medicine, to address our medical staff on high blood pressure in the geriatric population. As we were chatting a few minutes prior to his discussion, he inquired about what I was doing with my life. He knew of my training as a psychotherapist with a special interest in the emotional aspects of heart disease. I shared with him my development of this book on nutritional and emotional healing. I then directed him to my inquiries about Co Enzyme Q_{10}. His energy changed and his eyes lit up. Not only did he know about Q_{10}, but he had published a major article in the respected journal, *Medical Clinics of North America*, on cardiovascular pharmacology in January 1988.

I almost fell off my chair! He proceeded to tell me that Q_{10}, in his clinical studies, was considered therapeutic not only in congestive heart failure, but cardiac arrhythmia, and high blood pressure as well! My interest was now overwhelming. I became so excited about this fortuitous discovery that I was determined to learn all I could about the nutrient. I proceeded to request our Pharmacy Department to place it on formulary and, furthermore, to disseminate information to the medical staff about its use.

WHY HAVEN'T YOU HEARD ABOUT Q_{10}?

So why has the discovery of Q_{10} not made more of an impact on physicians? The answer can probably be traced to two reasons. First of all, Q_{10} was not identified until 1940. It was not until the mid 1960s that it was first demonstrated to be of use in the treatment of cardiovascular disease. Thus, it is a very recent discovery in the medical world. Clinicians in general are not very open to the healing properties of natural vitamins, herbs and co enzymes. Admittedly, I, too, was not very interested in Q_{10} after my first exposure to it 14 years ago. But after becoming a bioenergetic analyst over the last 12 years and studying the impact energy has on the organism, I came to realize the profound importance of the energetic principle, especially at the cellular level. This appreciation left me with an unquenchable thirst for the subsequent investigation of Q_{10}.

So enough of all this. *What is Q_{10}?* Co Enzyme Q_{10} is a vitamin-like substance that is similar in structure to vitamin K. Like vitamin E, it is a powerful antioxidant. In humans, Q_{10} is found in high concentrations in various organs, particularly the heart which has its highest concentration. In cells, the highest concentration of Q_{10} is found primarily in the mitochondria or so-called powerhouses that supply energy to the cell.

The function of Q_{10} is to stabilize cell membranes and act as an antioxidant and free radical scavenger by preventing the depletion of products necessary for the production of adenosine triphosphate (ATP). ATP is used in almost every energy transaction in the body. Thus, Q_{10} enhances the production of cellular energy by stimulating the formation of ATP at the mitochondrial level. Q_{10} is critical for the production of energy and healthy functioning of the cell.

Since Q_{10} is necessary for the optimal functioning of the cell, can a deficiency of Q_{10} impair such energy production? The answer to that question is *yes*. An intriguing speculation can therefore be raised. Can cardiovascular malfunction such as congestive heart failure be caused by a deficiency of Q_{10}? The answer to that question is also *yes*.

The father of Q_{10} research, Dr. Carl Folklers, demonstrated that patients with cardiovascular disease are deficient in Q_{10}. He found that levels of Q_{10} in cardiac patients are lower than in age-matched controls. Moreover, through autopsy and biopsy studies on both diseased and healthy human hearts, Folklers has also determined that once internal levels of Q_{10} drop below 25 percent of normal, disease may develop. If levels drop below 75 percent, serious pathology and even death may occur. Although more research needs to be done, Folklers predicts that Q_{10}

therapy will one day be an accepted international treatment for congestive heart failure. I personally use Q_{10} in every one of my patients with congestive heart failure if they are willing to take it. Recently, I have been using much higher dosages, even giving some very ill patients 300 mg per day.

Japanese and more recent USA studies have shown the favorable impact of supplementing Q_{10} to individuals with congestive heart failure. By increasing the level of intrinsic cellular energy, Q_{10} has a direct and beneficial effect on the energy-depleted muscle cells of the failing heart. Since Q_{10} protects critical cellular components from low oxygen states, the administration of Q_{10} enhances the energy production in a cell and an organ that is literally starving for energy. Since it has been demonstrated that Q_{10} declines with advancing age, perhaps idiopathic cardiomyopathy may be related to a deficiency of cellular and mitochondrial Q_{10}.

For some unexplained reason, the body's ability to extract Q_{10} from natural food sources declines with the aging of the organs, the liver being the most significant. Thus, supplemental Q_{10} may be a significant healing remedy in selected populations - especially the elderly. In experimental animal studies, those animals administered Q_{10} showed their heart cells were protected from the damaging effects of oxygen deficiency. Multiple clinical studies also show that Q_{10} protects individuals from the chest pain or discomfort that doctors frequently refer to as angina pectoris. For example, exercise studies in patients with angina pectoris have shown a longer duration of exercise time in patients treated with Co Enzyme Q_{10}.

The protective effects for angina probably come from Q_{10}'s increased resynthesis of ATP, which increases energy production and oxygen delivery. The utility of Co Enzyme Q_{10} in the treatment of angina pectoris and congestive heart failure has been demonstrated in multiple double-blind and placebo-controlled studies. The cardiovascular literature has also demonstrated a reduction in blood pressure as well. Apparently, some hypertensive patients may be deficient in Co Q_{10}. In one placebo-controlled double-blind study, patients given Q_{10} demonstrated a reduction in both systolic and diastolic blood pressures over matched controls. I have been using more and more Q_{10} as a natural approach to lowering blood pressure, and with favorable results.

OTHER BENEFITS

We have spoken about the myocardial protective effects of Co Enzyme Q_{10} during open heart surgery. In addition, Co Q_{10} has also been found to be an anti-arrhythmic agent. This has been demonstrated in both animal and human studies. Q_{10} has also been used in treating other disorders. For example, some forms of muscular dystrophy have been known to respond to Q_{10} therapy. In addition, Q_{10} has been used in the treatment of periodontal disease and has recently been used in bolstering the effects of the immune system and thus has been utilized in the treatment of immunodeficiency diseases. The use of Q_{10} in the AIDS syndrome has been under investigation with preliminary research showing a positive impact.

Weight reduction is yet another useful attribute of Q_{10}. In my counseling of patients about weight loss, it became apparent that some patients actually did adhere to a diet, but could not lose weight. Perhaps these patients did not burn calories, possibly as a result of a lower metabolism. In one European study, obese patients were found to be deficient in Q_{10}. As in congestive heart failure, this raises more intriguing speculation. Could Q_{10} be a helpful adjunct in diet therapy? Although this may appear to be speculative, the use of Q_{10} in selective individuals with a presumed low metabolism may appear to be quite useful. An anecdotal case comes to mind. Mary, a woman in her fifties, came to our weight reducing program out of frustration because she had tried several programs before. She had a tremendous inability to lose weight. Although her resistance was apparent both on psychological and physical levels, her conscious drive perpetuated her persistent struggle for weight loss. Unexpectedly, after two weeks on our high-fiber, low-fat program, Mary lost no weight. At that point I sensed her tremendous despair. She was really trying.

After carefully going over her program, it was apparent that she was "staying on the diet". At this point, I suggested some dietary supplements that would enhance her metabolism. I placed her on a formula of Q_{10}, vitamin B-6, zinc, chromium picolinate and my multi-vitamin and mineral complex. She was told to take these supplements after every meal. She persisted in her high-fiber, low-fat regimen and, to her surprise, lost five pounds in the following week. According to the group leader who counseled Mary, this was the first time in several years that she lost the weight. Perhaps, as others, she may have had a low metabolism and, in addition, perhaps a subtle deficiency in selected vitamin and mineral nutrients. At the end of this chapter, various formulas for vitamin and mineral supplementation will be addressed.

Clinical research has also revealed the use of Co Enzyme Q_{10} has multiple beneficial effects in brain disorders, aging, and in situations of allergy. For example, Q_{10} has the ability to counteract histamine and may have considerable utility in the treatment of asthma. Q_{10} has also been used as a favorable agent for tumor regression in breast cancer.

The usual dose of Q_{10} may range from 30 mg, one to three times a day, to up to 200-350 mg as pharmacological doses for the treatment of congestive heart failure, angina and hypertension. The highest dosages are required for treating congestive heart failures. In clinical studies where 150 mg has been used, no significant side effects have occurred. In a large study of over 5000 patients taking a dose of 30 mg, abdominal discomfort was reported in 20 patients and loss of appetite in 12. Since Q_{10} is neither a protein nor a foreign substance, only very rare side effects can be anticipated.

The best sources of Q_{10} are usually found in red meat such as beef and pork. Other good sources of Q_{10} would include mackerel, salmon, sardines, eggs, wheat germ, spinach and broccoli. Since the highest concentrations of Q_{10} are found in red meats, particularly organ meats, this usually may create an undesirable deficiency, particularly for the cardiac patient who is discouraged from eating red meats, organs (liver) and eggs. Therefore, *supplements are probably necessary*, especially in the elderly and for those on vegetarian-type diets.

I personally take between 30 and 60 milligrams of Co Enzyme Q_{10} per day. I take the vitamin for several reasons. First of all, as a physician, I encounter many individuals with flu-like illnesses. As a cardiologist, I am frequently faced with stressful events such as radiation and life threatening situations. I take Q_{10} to bolster my immunity. I also believe that, like vitamin E, Q_{10} will prevent the oxidation of LDL. I usually do not eat many foods that contain Q_{10} with the exception of broccoli and salmon, so I take it for preventive reasons. My own personal experience with Q_{10} has been extremely favorable, to say the least. My allergies have improved, particularly allergic conjunctivitis. I have even placed small amounts of Co Enzyme Q_{10} in my Multi-Vitamin Antioxidant formulas. In addition, Co Q10 is a major ingredient in one of my Immu-Boost Formulas for enhancing immunity.

My experience with my patients has also been extremely rewarding. To this date, I have well over 1000 patients on Q_{10} therapy. I also have recommended Co Enzyme Q_{10} for several patients with cardiac arrhythmias who were reluctant to take standard anti-arrhythmic drugs because of persistent side effects. One patient who suffered from a "panic disorder" was continuously plagued by cardiac irregularities. It was not uncommon for him to go to the emergency room on several occasions because of an irregular heart beat. After adding Q_{10} therapy, vitamins and herbs, his admissions have ceased. For scores of patients with congestive heart failure, the addition of Q_{10} had a considerable impact on their quality of life. Many other patients with high blood pressure were able to lower their pharmacological drugs with the addition of Co Q_{10}. Some were even able to discontinue all of their hypertension medications while being treated with Co Q_{10}.

Thus, in the cardiovascular patient, Q_{10} may serve as a valuable adjunct in therapy, with minimal risk of any side effects. In addition to the treatment of heart disease, Q_{10} may have beneficial effects in cancer and obesity, as well as the immunodeficiency diseases. It is also interesting to note that Q_{10} has been officially approved by the ministry of health in Japan and is on formulary in all Japanese hospitals. Since there is overwhelming medical evidence supporting the the use of Q_{10} and negligible, if any, risk, it is my recommendation that this nutrient be utilized in treating many of the common degenerative, nutritional and infectious diseases of our day.

So, where can you get Q_{10}? And how much does it cost? In my own experience of soliciting many health food stores, I was able to find Q_{10} in perhaps two-thirds of the stores I visited. In grocery stores where vitamins are sold, I have yet to find one grocery store or chain that included Q_{10} in their product line. Manufacturers will sell Q_{10} in its pure form or use it in combination with a multi-vitamin and mineral combination. When Q_{10} is purchased in capsules, make sure that it is a yellow color, especially since Q_{10} in its pure form is yellow in color. In the very near future, Q_{10} will be available in a softgel. The bioavailability will be significantly improved with this type of delivery system. In my own antioxidant line of nutrients, I have switched to a softgel preparation of Q_{10}, which is now red.

The price of Q_{10} varies from one health food store to another. The usual cost for 50 capsules is approximately $15 - $20. In our health food store in Manchester, Connecticut, we are offering fifty 30 mg softgel Q_{10}'s for $15.95. When purchasing Q_{10}, make sure there's an expiration date and a lot number on the bottle, as Q_{10} can become ineffective if the expiration date has expired. Do not purchase Q_{10} from anyone if no expiration date is on the bottle.

Although there have been several hundred articles in the medical literature on Q_{10}, one needs to keep in mind that the FDA has not studied Q_{10} and, therefore, it is not considered a drug. If the FDA investigates

Q_{10}, it could possibly be taken off the market and regulated under the auspices of the FDA. If such is the case, the cost of this nutrient could go considerably higher, particularly if a doctor's prescription is necessary and if the "vitamin" is only sold at pharmacies. It is my hope that this will not happen since this could place an unnecessary economic burden on those wishing to take this vitamin on a daily basis.

Ten

MINERALS, BOTANICALS AND ENZYMES

L ike vitamins, minerals perform many functions in the body essential to health, particularly at the cellular level. They are important components of bone and blood, maintaining healthy nerve and organ function. Minerals are inorganic substances that come from rock formations deep in the earth. After the breakdown of rocks by erosion, minerals are then passed from the rocks to the soil and then to plants and the rest of the food chain. *If you eat whole foods and simply wash the vegetable skins, as opposed to peeling them, the absorption of minerals will be greater.*

It is important to note that once minerals are absorbed, they may be in competition with each other. For example, excessive zinc can deplete the body of copper, while high calcium levels may affect magnesium and manganese absorption. We also need to consider that people on high-fiber diets containing phytate, a binding agent, may risk mineral deficiency when their mineral intake is low or borderline low. High-fiber intake may increase transit in the intestines, resulting in a decrease in mineral absorption. Thus, high-fiber diets and/or vegetarian diets may require additional mineral supplementation. When taking mineral supplements, it is important to take a multimineral supplement rather than individual minerals, unless recommended by your physician.

A full discussion of minerals is beyond the scope of this book. As with vitamins, I will try to emphasize the overall importance of several of the major minerals and their usefulness in some of the common medical syndromes that doctors frequently see, such as high blood pressure, osteoporosis and chronic fatigue syndrome.

CALCIUM

Calcium is an important mineral and is necessary for good bone and tooth development. It is also a major mineral in cardiac electrical conduction and in the transmission of impulses through the nerves. Calcium is also necessary for muscle contraction and blood clotting.

Calcium deficiencies may cause muscle cramps, cardiac arrhythmia, brittle nails, tooth decay and numbness in the arms and legs. The most critical period for adequate calcium intake is in childhood when the skeleton is developing. The recommended daily requirement for children is 800 to 1,200 mg per day (Table 12). It is also crucial for women to take the RDA minimum since they are at risk of developing osteoporosis, particularly in the postmenopausal state. Recently, the RDA of calcium has been increased to approximately 1500 mg for postmenopausal women.

Calcium taken in the diet slows aging bone loss. Recent evidence indicates that providing calcium supplements to postmenopausal women allows for slower bone loss both with or without accompanying hormone replacement. Whatever age, women and men should aim to meet the recommended dietary allowance for calcium.

The absorption of calcium is variable. Usually only 20-30 percent of the calcium taken in through our diet is absorbed into the blood. Caffeine may limit its absorption, as may refined foods or foods grown in calcium-deficient soil.

The best sources of calcium include dairy products, seafood, green leafy vegetables (except lettuce), asparagus, broccoli, cabbage, molasses and sea vegetables (Table 12). *Sea vegetables are among the richest sources of calcium and magnesium in the world.* One ounce of wakame seaweed, for example, has approximately the same amount of calcium as eight ounces of milk. *Other wonderful sources of calcium include figs, dates, parsley, prunes and sesame seeds.* Utilizing sesame seeds as an accent in our foods is extremely healthful. Sesame can be used when marinating fish or chicken, as well as in salads or on a bowl of rice. One cup of sesame seeds has as much calcium as three cups of milk.

Cheeses also provide tremendous sources of calcium, but they are also a major source of fat. Cream cheese, for example, provides significant quantities of calcium, but also has approximately 11 grams of fat per one ounce serving.

TABLE 12

RECOMMENDED DAILY DIETARY ALLOWANCES FOR CALCIUM

Age or Condition	Calcium
1-10 years	800 mg
11-24 years	1,200 mg
25-50 years	800 mg
51 years and older	800 mg
Pregnancy	1,200 mg
Lactating (first year)	1,200 mg
Post menopausal women (1994)	1,500 mg

1989 Food and Nutrition Board, National Academy of Science/National Research Council

Similarly, ice cream provides abundant calcium, but also has considerable fat. Some gourmet ice creams, for example, may contain as much as 34 grams of fat per serving with 150 mg of calcium. *Low-fat frozen yogurts*, on the other hand, contain very little fat and the same amount of calcium. *Skim milk and very low-fat milk products are excellent sources of calcium that do not contain the excessive fat.* Here again, awareness is necessary. All milk, regardless of whether we are discussing whole milk, two-percent, one-percent, or even skim milk for that matter, provides about 300 mg of calcium per cup.

When taking calcium supplements, it is important to remember to take them throughout the day and before bedtime. Too much calcium, however, can be harmful. A prolonged, excessive (well above FDA) intake of calcium and vitamin D has been shown to cause hypercalcemia, which can affect one's blood pressure as well as kidney function. It is also important to note that excessive calcium may impair the absorption of zinc and manganese. Calcium supplements should be utilized with caution in anyone with kidney disease or advanced diabetes.

ZINC

Zinc, an essential trace mineral, has many functions. It is most important in supporting the prostate gland and the growth of reproductive organs. Patients with diets low in zinc have been found to have an increase in acne and prostatitis. Low levels of the mineral have also been found in prostate cancer.

TABLE 13
RECOMMENDED FOODS HIGH IN CALCIUM

Cereals	*Nuts and Seeds*
Oatmeal (Quaker Instant)	Sesame seeds
Cheese	Soybeans
Feta	*Vegetables*
**Ricotta, Part skim	Asparagus
Fruits	Broccoli
	Cabbage
**Figs	**Daikon
Dates	Turtle beans
Prunes	Collards
Milk/Yogurt	**Kale
	Kelp
**Skim milk	Parsley
**Low-fat yogurt	Wakame
**Skim yogurt	**Tofu
One-percent milk	White beans

** Foods Highest in Calcium

Zinc is equally important to the immune system, particularly in the healing of wounds. Necessary for the absorption and maintenance of vitamin E and the B-complex vitamins, zinc is now noted to be essential in the wound healing of diabetics. Zinc plays a key role in helping the body eliminate toxic heavy metals such as aluminum, lead and excess copper.

Zinc is found in abundance in fish, meats, poultry and whole grains. Alcohol consumption, diuretics, excess calcium or diarrhea may lower zinc levels. Since alcohol is known to interfere with the absorption and metabolism of zinc, zinc deficiencies are commonly found in alcoholics. Diuretic users and those with eating disorders are also at risk for a zinc deficiency.

Recently it has been shown that a deficiency in zinc may be related to excess fat storage, contributing to weight gain. Zinc is therefore an important mineral to consider in weight reduction as it relates to glucose metabolism. In a state of zinc deficiency, sugars may be only partially metabolized, thus leading to an increased availability for fat production and storage. In a pediatric study of overweight children having low levels of zinc, weight loss was retarded until zinc was supplemented in the diet. *Therefore, zinc may be important to investigate in individuals who remain resistant to weight loss after a thorough medical examination and modification of lifestyle and nutritional habits.*

MAGNESIUM

Magnesium is the cardinal mineral for the heart. Along with potassium (which we will discuss next), it is extremely important in myocardial function. Magnesium is involved in over 300 enzymatic reactions in the body. In the last few years medical trials have demonstrated that a magnesium deficiency is highly correlated with multiple medical illnesses. Low magnesium is one of the most underdiagnosed serum electrolyte abnormalities in clinical practice today. It is found in several medical conditions: insulin dependent diabetes, heart failure, Crohn's disease and alcoholism.

Magnesium deficiency is frequently seen in other electrolyte abnormalities such as low potassium, sodium and calcium situations. It is also found in individuals on diuretics, as well as in those taking commonly prescribed medicines for gastro-intestinal distress. In the athlete, magnesium stores may be severely depleted as a result of long-term physical training.

But why has the magnesium story only surfaced in the last few years? Over the last 30 years, researchers have demonstrated that a deficiency of magnesium can lead to atherosclerosis in animals. Other clinical studies demonstrated that people who consumed hard water, that is, water high in magnesium and calcium, had a lower risk of heart attack. It appears from these clinical studies that magnesium is protective for the heart. In the 1990s, magnesium has become an extremely popular adjunct in the management of acute heart attack.

Magnesium deficiency can result in a host of cardiological disorders including life-threatening arrhythmias, heart muscle disease, and potentially fatal heart attacks (Table 14). *As a cardiologist, I cannot overemphasize the importance of magnesium.* Cardiologists are well aware that magnesium deficiency is a leading cause of cardiac arrhythmia when potassium depletion fails to respond to usual therapies. It is well known, for example, that low magnesium states will significantly exacerbate the pro-arrhythmic effect of low serum potassium, especially in patients taking an excess of Digitalis preparations (Digoxin, Lanoxin). Usually, potassium and magnesium depletion are commonly present in heart patients, and treatment involves administering both agents.

TABLE 14

POTENTIAL CARDIOVASCULAR CONSEQUENCES OF
MAGNESIUM DEFICIENCY

- [a] Cardiac arrhythmias (Abnormal rhythm)
- [a] Coronary atherosclerosis
- [a] Cardiomyopathy (Failure of the heart muscle)
- [a] Coronary vasospasm (Chest pain)
- [a] Heart attack
- [a] Sudden death

In a study performed on human nutrition in France, the link between magnesium, free radical damage and LDL cholesterol was established. This animal study showed that magnesium deficiency was linked to an increased association of free radical damage to LDL cholesterol, implicating an association to hardening of the arteries.

As many Americans consume less than the RDA recommendation for magnesium, increasing magnesium-rich foods and/or supplements may help reduce the risk of marginal deficiency and cardiovascular complications.

Recently, the medical literature has also cited low red blood cell magnesium levels as a potential cause of the chronic fatigue syndrome.

Chronic fatigue syndrome is characterized by the presence of fatigue for more than six months, impairment of memory and concentration, and a variety of symptoms such as muscle aches, muscle tenderness, joint pain, headaches and depression. Although the specific cause remains unknown, a generalized immune deficiency seems to be a major factor. Viral illnesses, for example, have also been known to cause chronic fatigue. Usually the treatment of such a condition includes rest, alleviation of stress and vitamin and nutritional therapy.

In one particular study, one group of chronic fatigue syndrome patients was treated with magnesium while another group received placebos. The magnesium-treated patients reported heightened energy levels when compared with controls. Red cell magnesium levels were normalized in all the treated patients, compared with only one control subject. Thus, magnesium has a potential role in the treatment of chronic fatigue syndrome.

In another recent magnesium study, supplementation was proven to be an effective treatment for premenstrual syndrome. In this double-

TABLE 15_____
CAUSES OF MAGNESIUM DEFICIENCY

1. Excessive Urinary Loss
    Diuretics
    Alcohol abuse
    Diabetic ketoacidosis
    Antibiotics
    Postobstructive diuresis
    Hypercalcemia
    Syndrome of inappropriate antidiuretic hormone secretion
2. Decrease in Intestinal Absorption
    Prolonged gastrointestinal suction
    Surgical resection of bowel
    Diarrheal states
    Various bowel diseases
    H-2 receptor antagonist therapy (Tagamet or Zantac)
3. Decreased Intake
    Alcohol abuse
    Parenteral alimentation IV therapy inadequate in
    magnesium
    Protein-caloric malnutrition
    Starvation

blind placebo-controlled study, both pain and mood change were positively affected by oral magnesium preparations.

Magnesium serves as a co enzyme for approximately 80 percent of the enzymes in the body and is the fourth most abundant element in the human body. Researchers believe that magnesium levels may be decreased as a result of stress, anxiety or low physical activity. A major factor that contributes to magnesium deficiency, however, is a reduction in available dietary magnesium. There is also a low concentration of magnesium in our water and soil. The overprocessing of foods also appears to enhance the deficiency of magnesium in the diet. In addition, there are numerous medical conditions that produce a net loss of magnesium from the body (Table 15).

In the absence of renal disease, magnesium supplements may be taken without fear of adverse reactions. Magnesium chloride is a good choice in that it is well absorbed. *The best sources of magnesium in the diet are sea vegetables, sesame seeds, green leafy vegetables, fish, meat, seafood, brown rice, soybean products, whole grains, bananas, apricots, nuts and seeds* (Table 16).

Magnesium also has one other vital protective function in the body. *It helps to counteract aluminum toxicity*, which is gaining attention in both the medical and lay literature. A few years ago in England, industrial contamination of the water supply with aluminum caused a small outbreak of central nervous system cases similar to Alzheimer's disease. *Newsweek*, 1991, published an article on Alzheimer's disease mentioning its casual relationship to aluminum. More recently, there has been further evidence suggesting that there is a connection between aluminum toxicity in the environment and the development of lesions in the brain that cause Alzheimer's disease. Like many of the other environmental toxins, the accumulation of aluminum may go on for years, eventually taking its toll on the body.

Aluminum is a toxic metal; unfortunately, it is still being used in drugs, food (particularly junk food), food additives and packaging, as well as pots and pans. Aluminum is also the major component used in our cans. It is found in antacids, foil, deodorants, bleached white flour, and even in our water. Aluminum has no known benefit to the human body. In addition to the possible connection with Alzheimer's disease, aluminum may cause other central nervous system disturbances as well as enhance the process of osteoporosis.

It makes sense to avoid aluminum as much as possible, particularly since the environment is so overwhelmed by it. My recommendation would be to *exchange any aluminum cookware for stainless steel, iron or glass*. I recommend avoiding canned foods. When possible, substitute with jarred, frozen or fresh products. (Also avoid drinks in aluminum cans when plastic or glass containers are available.)

Read labels to avoid compounds containing aluminum. *Eat a diet high in fiber and foods that inhibit aluminum absorption, including almonds, spinach and rhubarb*. The B vitamins, particularly B-6, are also recommended. In addition to a high-fiber diet, magnesium, calcium, vitamin C and zinc are helpful nutrients in counteracting aluminum toxicity.

POTASSIUM

Potassium is a mineral that truly concerns physicians. The effects of either low potassium or high potassium can be life threatening. Drugs for the

TABLE 16
RECOMMENDED FOODS HIGH IN MAGNESIUM

Cereal and Grains	Vegetables
All Bran	Adzuki beans
Brown rice	Black beans
	Navy beans
Fish	**Kelp
All seafood	Spinach
	Wakame
Fruits	**Tofu
**Figs, dried	White beans

Nuts and Seeds

**Pumpkin seeds
Sesame seeds
Soybean nuts
Sunflower seeds

**Foods Highest in Magnesium

treatment of high blood pressure or congestive heart failure may interfere with potassium absorption and excretion. Since potassium is necessary for the healthy functioning of nerves, cells and membranes, it is an important electrolyte to monitor. Low potassium is a major cause of cardiac arrhythmia. Although potassium supplementation is usually not necessary, individuals on diuretics, laxatives, or who have excessive diarrhea, may require extra potassium. Caution should be taken, however, in those individuals with renal insufficiency, as additional potassium in the diet may not be excreted by the kidney. You should be able to get all the potassium you need from your diet. *The highest levels of potassium are found in sea vegetables, fruits, vegetables, fish, lean meat, poultry, garlic, raisins, bananas, apricots and whole grains* (Table 17). Coffee and alcohol may deplete potassium in the body. Alcohol can deplete the body's magnesium levels as well. When consuming such beverages, it is important to maintain a proper potassium intake.

TABLE 17

FOODS HIGH IN POTASSIUM

Cereals

All Bran
Bran Buds
Raisin Bran

Dates

**Figs
Nectarines
**Prunes, dried
**Raisins

Fruits

Apricots
Bananas
Cantaloupe
Bamboo shoots

Fish

Anchovies
Bass, fresh water
Bluefish
Catfish
Clams
Crab, Blue
Flounder/Sole
Haddock
Halibut
Lobster
Mackerel
Mussels
Perch
Salmon
Snapper
Swordfish
Trout
Tuna

Meats/Poultry

Rib eye
Beef round eye
Goose without skin

Milk/Yogurt

Skim milk
Low-fat yogurt
Skim yogurt

Nuts and Seeds

**Soybean nuts

Vegetables

**Avocado
Beet greens
Chard, Swiss
Chickpeas
French beans
Garlic
Potato with skin
Squash, Acorn
Sweet potato

Beans

**Adzuki beans
Black beans
Kidney beans
Lentils
**Lima beans
Navy beans
Pinto beans
Natto (soybean prod.)
Nori
Turtle beans

**White beanas   ** Foods Highest in Potassium

Potassium, calcium and magnesium deficiencies have all been incriminated in blood pressure elevation. In my natural approach to blood pressure control, adequate supplementation of these minerals is crucial. (See Table 17A)

TABLE 17A
NATURAL BLOOD PRESSURE LOWERING PROGRAM

This program is a natural, non-pharmacological approach to lowering blood pressure. It includes increasing calcium and magnesium intake, decreasing sodium and adding Co Enzyme Q_{10} to your daily regimen. If you would like to try this program, consider my following suggestions.

1. Reduce all salt intake and be careful of processed foods. Read labels! Be aware of food additives and food enhancers, particularly monosodium glutamate. Avoid canned vegetables, canned soups, diet soft drinks, preservatives, meat tenderizers, soy sauce, etc. If you are overweight, watch the amount of fats and calories that you consume. Try to lose weight if you can.
2. Do not take nonsteroidals such as Motrin, Advil, Nuprin, etc.
3. Consume a high-fiber diet. Eat at least five to nine servings of fresh fruits and vegetables per day. Drink 8 glasses of clean, filtered, bottled water per day.
4. Avoid cheeses, meats and dairy products, as well as all processed meats (including bacon and sausage).
5. Maintain a regular exercise/walking program.
6. Avoid Nutrasweet and any antihistamines.
7. Take 250 to 500 mg of a magnesium supplement per day.
8. Take a daily antioxidant, multivitamin/mineral formula that contains no iron, copper, oils, preservatives, fillers or animal products.
9. Take 30 mg of Co Enzyme Q_{10} after each meal.
10. Consume as much parsley and garlic as possible. Use fennel and rosemary as well as other important herbs. Increase intake of calcium-containing foods such as kale, white navy beans, raisins, figs and lima beans.

SELENIUM

Selenium is considered a cardiologist's mineral because it protects the heart. Selenium is an active antioxidant scavenger of free radicals. It is important to the immune system and has been regarded as an agent in the protection from cancer. For example, the Orient has considerable quantities of selenium in its soils, making the Asian diet rich in the mineral. Not surprisingly, cancer and heart disease occur considerably less in the Oriental cultures than in the West. Studies have corroborated that *people who eat selenium, whether in food or in supplement form, develop less cancers, particularly of the breast, colon, and prostate.*

In the United States, there is an inverse relationship between breast cancer and selenium content in the soil. For example, Ohio tends to have the highest incidence of breast cancer and the lowest amounts of selenium in their soils. Conversely, the Dakotas have the highest soil concentrations of selenium and a lower incidence of breast cancer.

A selenium-rich diet has been proven in animal studies to reduce skin tumors when these animals were exposed to overwhelming ultraviolet light. The results seem to indicate that increasing selenium may significantly reduce the risk for developing UV induced skin cancer.

When combined with vitamin E or Co Enzyme Q_{10}, selenium's efficacy is much greater, making it a very powerful antioxidant. This type of synergism was reported in a small study of heart attack patients. Those patients receiving a combination of selenium and Co Enzyme Q_{10} had a better index of survival one year following their heart attack. The data was gathered from 61 patients during the year following their heart attacks. Six patients (20 percent) of the control group died of repeat heart attacks, while only one patient (three percent) died from the group taking the selenium/Q_{10} combination. Although this was only a small sample, it does suggest the cardiovascular protective possibilities of Q_{10} and selenium.

Selenium also protects against environmental pollutants such as lead and cadmium and is a major antagonist against the toxic effects of mercury, which is prevalent in dental fillings, cosmetics, pesticides and in saltwater fish, particularly tuna. *Prominent sources of selenium include fish, sea vegetables, whole grains, wheat germ, garlic, onions, chicken, brown rice and broccoli.* There are no known side effects at levels less than 300 mcg per day. The recommended daily maintenance dose of selenium is approximately 50-200 micrograms.

IRON

Iron, in simple terms, is essential for the production of hemoglobin, which is found in red blood cells. Since iron is the mineral most prevalent in blood, a lack of it causes anemia. Deficiencies in iron include anemic symptoms such as fatigue, pallor and dizziness. Other symptoms of iron deficiency include brittle hair, hair loss and ridging of the nails.

Several factors influence the amount of iron absorbed in the diet. A degree of hydrochloric acid (natural stomach acidity) must be present in the stomach in order for iron to be absorbed. Vitamin C can also increase iron absorption by as much as 30 percent. Iron absorption can be decreased by antacids, aspirin, caffeine and some food preservatives.

The most common cause of iron deficiency results from bleeding, either through the gastrointestinal tract or through excessive menstrual bleeding. Iron deficiency is more likely to occur in rapidly growing teenagers as well as menstruating women. Iron supplementation is recommended in pregnancy as well as in cases of chronic blood loss. The RDA for iron is approximately ten-18 mg per day. Since we can obtain much of the iron needed from our diet and environment, it is not recommended for healthy men to take iron supplements. Young women, however, could take iron on a daily basis, especially when pregnant.

Iron overload can go unnoticed and may be quite insidious in its onset. Since iron is stored in the body, excessive iron taken over a considerable period of time can cause problems, particularly in the liver, heart and pancreas. Individuals who drink considerable quantities of iron in their drinking water in addition to taking iron supplements may develop headaches, shortness of breath and easy fatiguability - symptoms of iron overload. Iron cookware is yet another source where one can obtain additional amounts of iron from the environment. In the previous analysis, I discussed with you the cautious use of excess vitamin C in situations of iron overload. If your serum iron and other iron indices are elevated, you need to be cautious about ingesting iron and vitamin C in your body. It is best to see your physician if you are in doubt about the iron stores in your body.

The best sources of iron include sea vegetables, green leafy vegetables, whole grains, lean meats, eggs, poultry, dates, prunes, beans, lentils, parsley, peaches, raisins, rice, dried fruits, molasses and sesame seeds.

TABLE 18

FOODS HIGH IN IRON

Cereals and Grains	*Fruits*
Oatmeal	**Figs, dried
Bran Buds	Peaches
Bran Flakes	Prunes, dried
Product 19	Dates
Brown rice	Raisins

Fish	*Nuts and Seeds*
Clams	Sesame seeds
Oysters	Pumpkin seeds, dried

Vegetables	*Miscellaneous*
Artichokes	Eggs
Chickpeas	Prune juice (best
Great Northern beans	bet for Iron)
Kidney beans	
Lentils	
Lima beans	
Navy beans	
Spinach	
Tofu	
Turtle beans	

**White beans
**Foods Highest in Iron

IODINE

Iodine is especially important in the healthy functioning of the thyroid gland. It calms the body and relieves nervous tension. Although it is only needed in trace amounts, iodine deficiencies can occur, particularly if drinking water is chlorinated. If too little iodine is taken into the diet, it affects the mental and nervous systems. Some of the possible side effects are the inability to think clearly, irritability and difficulty sleeping. Iodine deficiency may also result from soils that are not laden with iodine. *The best sources of iodine include sea vegetables, saltwater fish, Swiss chard, watercress, turnip greens, mushrooms, bananas, cabbage and onions.*

MINERALS AND YOU

There are many important minerals that the body utilizes in normal functioning. Many of these are trace elements that are extremely useful in preserving the health and everyday maintenance of the body, referred to by doctors as "homeostasis." At the time I was writing my book, *Lose to Win*, I had the opportunity to visit a chemical laboratory where vitamin and mineral supplements were produced. I learned from the chemists on staff that the FDA would occasionally inspect the laboratory for quality control.

After going on a tour through the factory and seeing firsthand the process of making vitamins and minerals, I was quite impressed by the complexity of the formulas and delivery systems. However, many of these vitamin and mineral formulas contained questionably large amounts of metals like iron and copper.

Although some vitamin manufacturers do not place iron in their formulas because of its pro-oxidant properties, many multi-vitamin and mineral preparations do include, in my opinion, excess quantities of iron. Naturally, if iron supplementation is required for iron deficiency anemia or in menstruating young women, then it could be taken without any undue side effects. However, since iron is stored in the body and accumulates over time, it is one mineral that should not be consumed unless prescribed by a physician. In my opinion, men who don't have any evidence of chronic blood loss should not take any iron unless it is clearly demonstrated that they are iron deficient.

Copper is another oxidant that should be limited to small quantities. The RDA for copper is two mg. Although copper is needed to make red blood cells, we tend to get all the copper we need from our drinking water, as it usually journeys through the copper pipes in our schools, homes and work places. Frequently, multi-vitamin and mineral preparations will include copper in their formulas. Although I am not recommending that you stay away from such formulas, keep in mind that an over-consumption of copper, like iron, could exist. Therefore, I recommend you choose vitamin and mineral formulas that are devoid of these metals or contain much less than the RDA requirements.

Many physicians have come to me, knowing that I have a strong interest in nutritional healing, and have asked what vitamin and mineral formulas I recommend. Since I developed formulas with absolutely no toxicity and no iron or copper, I advocate them without any reservations. Consequently, thousands of health professionals use my supplements across the country.

I developed the *Optimum Health Formula* personally, in consultation with a panel of experts, including pharmacists, chemists and other physicians with expertise in this field. Our aim was to create an all inclusive formula with sufficient potency and absorbability to provide optimum levels of all nutrients worth supplementing. We wanted to eliminate guess work, inadequate self-dosing and the need for most other supplements. And we wanted to do so at a significantly reduced cost.

Most vitamin preparations can be criticized due to one or more of these three major drawbacks:

1. Potency varies up to 29 fold (2900 percent) from label strength, according to the Center for Science in the Public Interest, a consumer testing organization based in Washington, DC.
2. Bioavailability and absorption are rarely greater than 50% and frequently much less.
3. Formulations may not be current, may be incomplete, may have inadequate potency and/or potentially harmful ingredients.

The *Optimum Health Formula* has the following special features: (See formula on Table 19)

1. Full potency guaranteed and prepared by a manufacturing facility that observes the GMP (Good Manufacturers Procedures) of the pharmaceutical industries which follow FDA regulations.
2. Excellent bioavailability. A unique vegetable cellulose-activated base from natural sources offers a quick release of nutrients, and a Krebs cycle complex utilizes chelation for enhanced mineral absorbability.
3. Formulation. This is the most complete and effective nutrient preparation on the market.
   a. Antioxidant rich. All natural beta carotene, vitamin C and vitamin E.
   b. Full spectrum of effective minerals, including selenium, vanadium, chromium picolinate and zinc in a seawater base.
   c. Several lipotropic factors which support fat, glucose and cholesterol metabolism in a base of herbs.
   d. Complete vitamin B Complex to help neutralize homocysteine.
   e. Co Enzyme Q10, glutathione and quercetin, three outstanding nutritionals are included.

You will note that the fat-soluble vitamins, i.e. A, D and E, are not represented in very large doses. Here again, since these vitamins are taken on a daily basis and are stored in the body, high doses of these nutrients are not recommended. I presently take three to six captabs per day. This depends upon my energy needs, stress level and susceptibility to infection. For my patients with cancer, heart disease, arthritis and infections, I recommend a similar dosage schedule. For my healthy patients who consume a good diet of five to nine fresh fruits and vegetables daily, I recommend one tablet after each meal.

If you are interested in weight loss, additional supplementation may be required. In addition to the *Optimum Health Formula*, I use additional chromium picolinate, L-Carnitine and Co Q_{10}. Recently, Hydroxycitric Acid is another newcomer to the list of supplements that may be helpful in weight loss.

Coming from an exotic Indian fruit, Hydroxycitric Acid (HCA) not only helps to suppress the appetite, but also prevents some carbohydrates from being turned into fat. An advantage of using HCA is that it does not involve the central nervous system. Therefore, side effects such as irregular heartbeat, elevated blood pressure and excessive nervous stimulation do not occur. HCA avoids these problems because it acts locally at the level of carbohydrate metabolism. HCA has been tested for its safety in animals as well as humans. However, if you are pregnant or nursing, I would not use HCA.

You need to keep in mind that such supplements only serve as additional therapy to a well-balanced, nutritious, high-fiber, low-fat program. Many of these vitamins and nutritional supplements can be purchased in health food stores. In addition to vitamins, minerals and nutritionals, my comfort level with herbs has been increasing over the last few years.

BOTANICALS

For centuries, herbs have been used medicinally. Chinese cultures have long believed that certain plants support good health and prolong life. Present day Europeans use many herbal remedies to cure illnesses such as the common cold. Unfortunately, American medicine has a different approach to herbs. Most physicians in this country have been trained in American medical schools where the traditional herbal therapies of European and Oriental societies are simply not taught.

For example, the only medicinal herbs I learned about in medical school were the Digitalis, which comes from the flowering foxglove plant, and the Rauwolfia for high blood pressure, which comes from Asian plants. Most other medicinal herbs were not given any credibility, despite the fact that several common pharmaceuticals originated from plants and barks. Herbs were belittled and even scorned. Nevertheless, as my comfort level with botanicals grew, I decided to use them in many of my vitamin and mineral formulas. The following is a short synopsis of some of the herbs I frequently prescribe in my cardiological practice.

GINGER

Since my youngest son is often plagued with motion sickness, I tried countless cures for nausea. Eventually, I found ginger to be the most effective remedy. This discovery also helped my patients. Many of them suffer nausea and vomiting as a result of heart attacks, coronary artery bypass surgery or medications.

The phytotherapy that I use is simple ginger root, which has been used in Chinese medicine for thousands of years.

I have used ginger tea in coronary care units, my office and my home. Creating a tea infusion is, perhaps, the oldest form of preparing herbal remedies. The recipe for ginger tea is quite simple. I tell my patients to buy ginger root in any supermarket. If you take about a one-inch segment off the root and slice it into fine thin pieces, you can boil it as a tea. Let it stand for approximately one-half hour, add some honey and freshly squeezed lemon, and you will be amazed how your nausea, indigestion and even vomiting will cease after a few cups of the tea.

In addition to its use for digestive disorders, ginger has long been touted as an immune stimulant. It also yields excellent circulatory benefits by thinning the blood, relieves symptoms of PMS and may have a favorable impact on cholesterol as well. Ginger also hastens the delivery of cayenne.

CAYENNE (CAPSICUM)

Cayenne, or capsicum, comes from the fruit of the red pepper plant. Cayenne is cultivated all over the world. My first exposure to cayenne was the medicinal use for preventing the oxidation of harmful LDL cholesterol. For this reason I added capsicum to my *Optimum Health Vitamin and Mineral Formula.*

In addition to having a favorable impact on cholesterol, capsicum will also increase one's energy and has proven quite effective in arthritic situations. In both my cholesterol lowering programs and my natural healing for arthritis, I included cayenne as a phytonutrient. This botanical also contains valuable vitamins and minerals, such as vitamin C, beta carotene and sulphur.

I use cayenne externally as an effective pain killer. For years, I have seen patients in my office with herpes zoster, a painful viral neuromuscular affliction which causes terrible discomfort. Although some of the traditional medicines have assuaged the pain in these individuals, the external use of cayenne has been extremely helpful. Patients may report irritation and pain at the application of capsicum, but prolonged exposure deadens the nerves to pain and provides significant relief. Therefore, I always tell my patients that capsicum will at first stimulate and then inhibit the flow of pain from the skin and membranes.

It is important to note that taking cayenne internally (40,000 heat units) may cause irritation of the stomach. After a hot spicy bowl of chili, for example, it is a common experience to suffer abdominal irritation. This reaction is most likely due to the cayenne. The remedy for such an occurrence, either from food or from capsule form, is to eat bread or other starches.

GOTU KOLA

Gotu kola is a quick-acting, anti-fatigue medicinal plant popular in Pakistan, India and Ceylon. In Ceylon, it is considered a brain food and is reported to stimulate the memory. I once sat on a plane next to an anesthesiologist from India. He saw me reading material concerning gotu kola and told me that this plant is often used as a tea in his home country for enhancing memory and rejuvenating energy. Remember that gotu kola contains no caffeine.

Studies have also demonstrated that gotu kola is effective in treating inflammation and in stimulating the immune system. Gotu kola contains saponins which inhibit the growth of harmful bacteria. Consequently, gotu kola has been a focal remedy of ancient Ayurvedic Indian Medicine and today is held in high esteem by herbalist physicians all over the world.

GINSENG

I have become more and more impressed with another medicinal herb that contains saponins, the well known ginseng. The medicinal uses of ginseng have included bolstering immunity, increasing energy, reducing stress and even enhancing sexual desires. Ginseng comes in a variety of forms. Some of the preparations stimulate the body, while others may have a calming effect. Ginseng has been used in Asia by millions of people for over thousands of years. Ginseng is also cultivated in this country and has even been exported to China. American ginseng is considered more "Yin" and is used for reducing energy in the respiratory and digestive systems; Asian ginseng is "Yang," used for increasing energy and raising heat in the circulatory system.

Ginseng is thought to function as an "adaptogen," a substance which improves both physical and mental performance. It has been used as a general body tonic to alleviate physical and mental exhaustion. Chinese folklore indicates that it also helps to restore sexual vitality in middle-aged men.

This perennial root-like herb not only contains multiple saponins but also ginsenosides. Its chemical constituents have been known to stimulate immune functions, leading to improved resistance to infections. Panax ginseng is rightfully its given name, originating from the word *panacea* which comes from the Greek words *pan* and *akos*, referring to "cure all."

WILD YAM EXTRACT

Another agent with the potential to enhance sexual libido and psychological well being is wild yam extract, or dioscorea villosa. Wild yam extract is a precursor for DHEA, or dehydroepiandrosterone - the "mother" steroid of the body. The use of DHEA has been gaining increasing popularity recently, and I am following this trend with great interest.

Recent studies have demonstrated that low DHEA levels in younger men may be an indicator of myocardial risk. Current evidence in the cardiological literature has demonstrated increased heart attacks in men with low DHEA levels. These results suggest that higher levels of DHEA may offer protection against heart disease. Although it requires a medical research license to prescribe DHEA in this country, wild yam extract is an available form of DHEA that can be purchased without a prescription.

Wild yam extract may be found in most health food stores. Usually, 500 mg of wild yam extract is the equivalent of 5 mg of DHEA.

The medicinal properties of wild yams have dated back since antiquity. Natives in New Guinea, for example, praised the growing of wild yams. Prestige and authority were given to tribesmen who were able to grow the largest yams. The tribesmen practiced visualization to increase the size of their own yams and even used magic to cause rival tribesmen's yams to shrivel! Thus, the wild yam has historically been held in high regard by more "primitive cultures," long ago capturing the hearts of these native tribesmen.

HAWTHORNE BERRY

Hawthorne berry is another herb that I have come to use considerably in my cardiological practice. This botanical carries on many activities for vasodilatory action, which increase blood flow. In addition, hawthorne may significantly decrease free fatty acids. European research shows the berry to be an anti-cholesterol agent. I personally have used it many times in the treatment of cardiac arrhythmia, particularly atrial fibrillation, with much success.

Hawthorne berries can be taken as a tea, as a tincture or in tablet form. This herb is beneficial in improving the health of the heart, as it may have a toning action on the heart that compensates for age-related cardiac degeneration. I have even used hawthorne in combination with Digitalis for regulating rapid heart beats. In Germany, hawthorne is probably one of the most sought after medicinal preparations (next to the ginkgo biloba). I have yet to see any toxicities with its use.

THE GINKGO

In Western Europe the ginkgo is perhaps the most popular medication on the market, with doctors writing millions of prescriptions annually. The ginkgo tree is an ancient tree whose leaves have been used for medicinal purposes for the last 5,000 years. European studies demonstrate that the ginkgo has not only improved memory but has also enhanced mental alertness. I use it to help my patients with memory loss, depression and ringing in their ears. The flavonoids in ginkgo consist of a complex mixture of ginkgoloids and ginkgo flavonoids. Ginkgo also contains quercetin.

The mechanism of action behind ginkgo biloba is that it increases blood flow in deprived areas, particularly the inner ear and the macula. If it indeed improves circulation in these areas, it may have an effect on macular degeneration. In addition to its favorable effects on free radical damage and inhibition of blood clotting, ginkgo may have some utility in assuaging Alzheimer's disease, although there have been no clear-cut studies demonstrating this effect. No toxicity from ginkgo has been reported, even after prolonged treatments.

ECHINACEA EXTRACT

Echinacea extract is another herb I frequently recommend. Echinacea is one of the many cone flowers, a group of native American wildflowers which comes from the sunflower family. There are several species. Used widely by American Indians for a host of ailments, echinacea has the reputation for healing venomous bites from both spiders and snakes. When combined with goldenseal, echinacea has been very effective in stimulating the immune response. Both of these herbs can build up the number of T-lymphocytes in the body, thus bolstering one's immunity. I use it on myself and on my children for infections and flu-like illnesses.

I have found echinacea, goldenseal, garlic and other botanicals quite helpful in enhancing immunity. Echinacea is the perfect choice for colds and flu because it assists the body in the production of white blood cells and interferon, two substances capable of increasing the body's defenses to infection. European studies have demonstrated that up to 900 mg of echinacea has significantly relieved cold and flu-like symptoms. A combination of the botanicals also relieves inflammation. Although Prednisone and other corticosteroids effectively reduce the inflammation following coronary artery bypass surgery, they also can cause considerable side effects when used for several weeks. To avoid these side effects, I prefer to treat chest cavity inflammation with a combination of the botanical agents and a low dose of Prednisone.

Echinacea is most potent when taken for measurable periods of time. Because its immune-enhancing effect may be diminished after prolonged use, echinacea should not be used on a daily basis. It is important to give the body a "rest period" for perhaps several weeks if recurrent infections occur. For more progressive systemic diseases, such as tuberculosis, and for autoimmune diseases, such as lupus, severe rheumatoid arthritis and multiple sclerosis, echinacea should probably not be used.

ASTRAGALUS

Astragalus is another ancient Chinese herb which is frequently combined with ginseng to strengthen the natural defenses of the body. Astragalus has shown particular efficacy in stimulating the immune system, and also shows some vasodilatory cardiovascular effect. The anti-inflammatory actions of astragalus come from the alteration of the body's mast cells. Perhaps astragalus inhibits the interaction between allergens by preventing the breakdown of mast cells, thus preventing the release of histamines. Quercetin works in much the same way. Consequently, these two herbs could help relieve hayfever and other allergic conditions.

In China, astragalus has also been used in the treatment of cancer. Because of its potent activation of macrophages and T cells in the immune system, astragalus enhances the natural defense functions by stimulating the responsiveness of T-cell lymphocytes. I have personally used astragalus as a healing remedy for my seasonal hayfever. I have even included it in one of my Immuboost Formulas.

CHAMOMILE, MYRRH GUM AND FENUGREEK

Three other botanicals I use in my vitamin and mineral formulas are chamomile, myrrh gum and fenugreek.

Chamomile is heralded in Europe as a cure-all. Its gentle actions are safe for use by both children and adults. It has calming, anti-spasmodic and even anti-inflammatory effects. In my own household, when one of us has trouble sleeping, we drink a cup of chamomile tea. It may also be used for indigestion and headache, or in a steam inhalation for sinusitis. Chamomile's blossoms contain the chemical chamazulenes, which carries anti-inflammatory action. Chamomile has also been used topically, having enjoyed extensive use in facial and hair-care preparations. Compresses of chamomile have brought relief in a variety of irritating skin conditions such as eczema, sunburn and even diaper rash.

Myrrh gum, prized as a valuable herb since Biblical days, was presented as a gift by one of the wise men to the Christ child. It contains volatile oils which are ideally suited for promoting easier breathing during congestive colds and for clearing out mucous-clogged passages. Long noted for its antiseptic and healing properties, myrrh gum was used in ancient Greece for the treatment of wounds. It has also been used in oral preparations to tone the gums and to prevent tooth decay. Mixed with witch hazel, a tincture of myrrh may be applied to cold sores. It has even been mixed with water for an antiseptic douche.

Fenugreek seed is an herb that may affect cholesterol, similar to the way pectin does. European cultures use this as an important remedy to diabetes. Traditionally, fenucreek has been widely used, especially in the Middle East, to expel excess mucous from the respiratory and digestive systems.

There is a large volume of literature written on the medicinal properties of plants and herbs in many reputable texts. My purpose in this short section is to raise your awareness about how to use botanicals as an alternative or an adjunctive path in health and healing. I will discuss the healing properties of two other botanicals, onions and garlic, in Chapter Thirteen, *Nutritional Healing*.

Two other treatments which I also want you to become aware of are enzyme replacement therapy and the friendly bacteria, lactobacilli.

ENZYME REPLACEMENT THERAPY

A simple and easy approach to *Optimum Health* includes exercise, targeted nutritional supplementation and a well-balanced diet. Recently, however, physicians have recognized the need for enzyme replacement therapy. For even though there is truth in the saying, "You are what you eat," even truer is the statement,"You are what you absorb."

Let me explain. For cells to absorb and distribute nutrients to the body, food must first be properly digested. Unfortunately, many compounds in food may be undigestible by the body's endogenous enzyme system. Sugars contained in beans or other cruciferous vegetables may not be totally broken down. Complex sugars such as raffinose, stachose and verbacosce may be undigestible by the body's own enzyme system. These complex sugars pass down into the large intestine where they are then acted upon by the non-friendly bacteria, E coli.

The metabolic by-products of this functional maldigestion/malabsorption are the well-known gases, carbon dioxide, hydrogen and methane. Even if we eat small quantities of these complex oligosaccharides, it may produce considerable waste gases. This may cause cramping, discomfort and flatulence. It is no wonder then that beans, Brussels sprouts, broccoli, cabbage, cauliflower, etc. are avoided by some individuals. We all know what we can and cannot eat. We have an intuitive sense of which foods may give us excess gas, bloating or flatulence.

Fortunately, modern day technology has developed enzyme systems which are able to convert the offending large sugars into more simple, digestible sugars such as galactose, fructose and glucose. Laboratory tests have shown that various enzymes containing aspergillus can convert the large undigestible sugars into smaller sugars, creating better absorption and digestion. Thus, enzyme replacement therapy is gaining popularity for the breakdown of complex carbohydrates and proteins. Such compounds are marketed as Carbozyme and Digezyme for carbohydrates and Aminozyme (Aminogen) for proteins.

It is extremely important to have nutrients absorbed and not lost in the GI tract. For example, if there were a considerable amount of undigested or unabsorbed food in the colon, bacteria would multiply rapidly. In addition to producing noxious gases, the build up of toxic metabolites in the colon could even prove to be carcinogenic. It is therefore quite important to have sufficient digestive enzyme capability so that nutrients are absorbed in the small intestine before they arrive in the colon. Fecal material should be made up of water, bile salts, undigested food fiber and dead bacterial waste. It should not be composed of undigested or unassimilated food.

In addition to inefficient enzyme systems, there are many conditions that disturb the delicate workings of the gastrointestinal tract. Individuals complaining of long standing constipation, diarrhea or irritable bowel, or those with real pancreatic disease, gall bladder disease or inflammatory bowel conditions (with and without diverticulosis or hemorrhoids) may have disturbed gastrointestinal function. In addition, there are other factors that contribute to the maldigestion/malabsorption syndrome, including antibiotics, use of birth control pills, corticosteroids, processed foods and continuous overuse of the same foods. One way to enhance the health of the gastrointestinal tract is by supplementing it with friendly bacteria.

OUR BACTERIAL BUDDIES

Regular use of friendly bacteria such as lactobacilli and bifidobacteria will not only improve digestive health, but will also protect against fungal and bacterial infections. These bacteria will also improve the immune system.

Increasing our lactic bacteria is one important step toward *Optimum Health*. Lactic bacteria are single cell organisms which may occur singularly, in pairs or in short chains. These organisms have the ability to transform sugar into lactic acid. They play a significant role in the production of fermented milk, yogurt and some cheeses. When the sugar in milk (lactose) is broken down and converted to lactic acid by bacteria, the production of lactic bacteria in the intestine increases. Lactic bacteria can be increased through the fermentation of yogurt. Sourdough bread and sauerkraut are other foods that can increase lactic bacteria in the intestine. These food sources will increase the friendly bacteria in our GI tract. Freeze-dried supplements containing lactobacillus, acidophillus and bifidobacteria could also be taken.

Preparations containing lactase, which can be purchased in health food stores, may also enhance the digestion of milk and other lactose products. An increase in friendly bacteria not only promotes the production of B vitamins and amino acids, but also improves the immune function in the body. Friendly bacteria enhances the action of calcium, making it more available for absorption and use by the body. It is important to be aware that increasing the friendly bacteria in our body can have a broad impact in positively affecting our health.

TABLE 19

OPTIMUM HEALTH FORMULA

Contains Scientifically Balanced Composition of Vitamins, Minerals and Nutrients

SIX CAPTABS DAILY PROVIDE:

Vitamins:	%US	RDA
Vitamin A (Beta Carotene)	25,000 IU	500
Vitamin D (Cholecalciferol)	400 IU	100
Vitamin E (d-Alpha Tocopherol Succinate)	400 IU	1332
Vitamin C ("Esterified") (Abscorbic Acid)	600 mg	996
Vitamin B-1 (Thiamine Mononitrate)	40 mg	2666
Vitamin B-2 (Riboflavin)	40 mg	2353
Niacin (Niacinamide)	40 mg	200
Vitamin B-6 (Pyridoxine Hydrochloride)	40 mg	2000
Vitamin B-12 (Cyanocobalamin)	40 mcg	666
Biotin	0.3 mg	100
Pantothenic Acid (Calcium Pantothenate)	50 mg	500
Folic Acid	0.8 mg	200

Minerals:

Calcium (Calcium Phosphate Oxide)	250 mg	25
Phosphorus (Calcium Phosphate)	195 mg	20
Magnesium (Oxide)	280 mg	70
Manganese (Gluconate)	2 mg	**
Iodine (Kelp)	150 mcg	100
Selenium (L-Selenomethionine)	200 mcg	**
Zinc (Gluconate)	30 mg	200
Chromium (Picolinate)	100 mcg	**
Potassium (Citrate)	99 mg	**
Boron (Citrate - Aspartate)	1 mg	**
Vanadium (Vanadyl Sulfate)	5 mg	**
Molybdenum (Sodium Molybdate)	150 mcg	**
Trace Minerals (Sea Water)	60 mg	**

Lipotropic Factors:

Choline (Bitartrate)	100 mg
Inositol	100 mg
Taurine	30 mg
Methionine	30 mg
Betaine HCL	30 mg
L-Carnitine	25 mg
Pyridoxine 5 Phosphate	1 mg

Enzymes:

Papain (Papaya)	50 mg
Bromelain (Pineapple)	50 mg
Acidophilus (Lactobacillus Bulgaricus Bifidus)	5 mg
Aloe Vera	2.5 mg

Nutritionals:

Co Enzyme Q_{10}	25 mg
L-Lysine	20 mg
L-Glutathione	15 mg
Silicon (Vegetable Silica)	180 mcg
Quercetin	20 mg

Antioxidant Base: lemon, bioflavonoids, rutin, hesperidin
Herbal Base: papain, sarsaparilla, hawthorne berries, capsicum, gotu kola, hyssop, myrrh gum, peppermint, green pepper, ginger, fennel, fenugreek and chamomile.

Eleven

WOMEN AND CHILDREN FIRST

O ff the coast of Newfoundland on a cold and dark night, the phrase, "Women and children first," echoed throughout the icy, frigid air. The unthinkable was happening: The Titanic was sinking. While most of the men went down with the ship, many women and children were saved. This was a time for placing the lives of women and children above all others. However, in 1995, women and children are not first when it comes to prioritizing nutritional and metabolic needs.

Children are the most vulnerable to nutritional deficiencies, especially during their most active growth period. More and more children are consuming processed foods containing large quantities of additives, preservatives and sweeteners. In addition, the fast-food industry has created eating habits in children that are consistently high in fats and low in nutrients. Studies show that school children, particularly young children, may be prone to low nutritional levels, even less than the RDA.

In March of 1995, the *American Health Foundation* (a private New York organization) reported some alarming findings about children in grades two through six. In this questionnaire-based study distributed to 3,112 children, the findings revealed that American adults are doing a poor job of educating their youngsters about healthy ways of living. Of the children polled:

- 24% had eaten no fruit and 25% had eaten no vegetables the previous day.
- 15% said they thought cheese was a good source of fiber.
- 48% said they thought apple juice (which contains no fat) has more fat than whole milk.
- 36% said watermelon has more fat than American cheese.

This study confirms that bad habits, as well as good ones, start early. Awareness in education is certainly key, not only for adults, but also for their children.

There is growing concern that children may be deficient in vitamins B, C and E, as well as iron, calcium and zinc. In a report by *The Journal of the American Diabetic Association*, children exhibited serious deficiencies in folate as well as vitamin B-6. Allergies, lack of motivation, fatigue, skin problems and lack of academic interest may also be related to vitamin and mineral deficiencies. The National Cancer Institute recommends at least five to nine servings of fresh fruits and vegetables per day. On any given day, however, 40 percent of Americans do not even get *one* serving!

IRON, A DOUBLE-EDGED SWORD

As shown in *The American Health Foundation* study, this practice of neglecting nutrients particularly pertains to children. It is no secret that most children would rather go to bed without supper than eat their spinach.

Physicians and researchers have suggested that a multiple vitamin is good "insurance" as a supplement for growing children's physiological functions. Zinc, for example, is needed during growth and sexual development. Folic acid is crucial during the neonatal stages of development, as well as throughout adolescence. Iron is also needed. It is estimated that iron deficiencies affect about five percent of five to eight year olds, approximately two and one-half percent of adolescents and as much as 25 percent of pregnant teenagers. Iron deficiencies exist in young female athletes as well. To correct the problem, an increase in the absorption of iron is usually facilitated by including foods high in vitamin C with all meals. Drinking orange or tomato juice or even taking an iron supplement is also helpful.

Because of their growing bodies' needs, children should receive an ample supply of iron. Standard children's vitamin and mineral supplements often include small doses of it. Caution should be exercised in dispensing iron, however, for there have been several pediatric deaths due to iron overdoses in children. These deaths result from an over-ingestion of the mineral, which causes fatal shock to young, vulnerable children.

A typical overdose scenario involves a child tampering with his or her mother's vitamins which contain abundant sources of iron. Since only a few tablets could prove fatal to a very young child, it is absolutely essential that mothers keep any iron supplements away from children, as well as adult multivitamin/mineral preparations containing iron. I suspect that in the future there will be a warning from the FDA indicating that the ingestion of too much of the mineral can be harmful to young children.

Despite these concerns, parents can safely give their children vitamin and mineral supplements, providing that the iron is not more than the RDA. In addition to supplements, parents can certainly administer natural sources of iron in forms of foods and juices like prune juice and organic raisins.

One way to improve poor diets or "junk diets" is to utilize targeted nutritional supplements. For young children, I am a strong believer in multivitamin and mineral preparations, preferably chewable, without artificial colors, preservatives or oils. Since young children do not consume many fresh fruits and vegetables, vitamin preparations using natural food sources, such as alfalfa, chlorella, green barley, carrot juice, spinach and kale are preferred. A varied diet, consisting of a balanced supply of proteins, carbohydrates and essential fatty acids, combined with a minimum of sugar, fast and processed foods, will help provide the substrate for supporting a healthy metabolic lifestyle for a growing child.

Many parents are unaware of the harmful eating habits of their children. For example, school lunches, which contain a high concentration of surplus cheeses, processed meats and other dairy products, perpetuate a processed and junk food lifestyle. One major junk food that children consume daily is cola beverages, which contain phosphoric acid. Drinking too many carbonated beverages can literally remove calcium from the bone. If children drink these beverages while declining their intake of milk, they may be at serious risk for bone fractures. In a recent study of adolescent boys and girls, there was a strong association between cola beverage consumption and bone fractures, particularly in females. This gives further evidence that many junk foods out on the market really are "junk."

In response to this, many of my patients have asked me if their children need vitamin and mineral supplements, or even herbs for that matter. I have no problem recommending ginger, garlic and echinacea to children; nor do I have any reservations about giving children natural vitamin and mineral supplements. It is important to be aware that growing children may be deficient in B vitamins, iron, calcium, vitamin E, zinc and even vitamin C. Consequently, in addition to a healthy diet consisting of fresh fruits and vegetables, it makes good sense to consider targeted nutritional supplementation for every growing child. Children, like their mothers, have special needs and vulnerabilities that must be addressed.

WOMEN AND HEART DISEASE: SPECIAL RISKS AND SPECIAL NEEDS

I worry about the fact that most women do not get the kind of care they need for the prevention and treatment of heart disease. It is an established fact that in many large scale clinical trials, women have been under-represented. Data on the incidence and course of heart disease has been obtained from large cohorts of men, and then applied to women. Why? Because heart disease has not been thought to be a major health factor for women.

The facts, however, reveal that cardiovascular disease is the leading killer among American women. Although most women fear breast cancer as the number one threat to life, death from heart disease occurs a staggering five times more than cancer of the breast.

It is estimated that 50 percent of all American women will die of a cardiovascular disease, such as a stroke or a heart attack. Despite this high incidence of heart disease, data seems to indicate that misdiagnosis, under-diagnosis and lack of effective treatment are major problems affecting women today. Recent research reveals that women are different than men not only in terms of risk assessment, but also in treatment interventions. Most cardiologists continue to treat women less effectively and aggressively than they treat men, sometimes leading to catastrophic results. Because heart disease is considered a male-oriented phenomenon, physicians have sometimes failed to diagnose coronary disease in females.

For example, if a 45-year old woman comes into the Emergency Room with chest pain, and a 45-year old man comes in with similar complaints, most physicians would probably admit the male and explain to the female that her symptoms are likely due to stress and anxiety. It is a fact that most physicians are trained to view cardiovascular disease as a low probability in women. And yet, in the peri-menopausal and postmenopausal population, nothing is farther from the truth: the number of coronary events quadruples as women approach middle age.

Studies also indicate that women who are hospitalized for coronary artery disease undergo fewer diagnostic and therapeutic procedures than do men, and have a higher complication rate as well. When going through coronary artery bypass grafting, women may already be at a disadvantage due to a delay in diagnosis - the operative mortality for women following coronary artery bypass surgery is almost twice that of men. Post-operatively, women also have higher incidences of congestive heart failure, less symptomatic relief and greater psychosocial impairment.

Because of the small size of their coronary vessels, women have also been shown to have more complications with coronary artery angioplasty. This is only one of many clinical differences between men and women. If the same evaluation and diagnostic criteria are applied to women as to men, there may be greater risk of late or misdiagnosis.

In preventive cardiology, risk factor modifications also differ according to gender. Consider the following.

1. Risks from diabetes are higher for women than they are for men
2. Risks from being overweight are higher for women than for men.
3. Women have a higher risk than men if they have high triglycerides (fat storage).
4. Women have a higher risk than men if they have a lower HDL (good cholesterol).

Clinical research has shown that the incidence of diabetes and its complications is much higher in women. This increases the risk for heart disease to five to seven times in diabetic women, compared to only two to three times in diabetic men. This simple fact alone should raise the eyebrow of any reputable cardiologist evaluating suspected heart disease in diabetic women.

ONLY YOU CAN PREVENT HEART DISEASE

How can women prevent the onset of heart disease? For all women, proper heartsense includes reducing the risk of diabetes by increasing physical activity and maintaining an ideal body weight. Recent studies report that being a mere 20 pounds overweight correlates with a two-fold risk of heart disease in women. Thus, seemingly benign overweight status in women carries more serious implications for cardiovascular disease. It is absolutely essential for women to understand the potentially dangerous combination of risk factors that render them vulnerable to heart disease: mild to serious overweight status, low HDL and high triglycerides (fat storage).

High triglyceride levels appear to be a more significant risk factor in women than in men. Among diabetics, as triglyceride levels rise, cardio-vascular risks increase approximately three-fold in men, while an alarming two hundred-fold increase occurs in women. The interpretation of other cholesterol fractions also requires gender specific consideration.

Cholesterol levels have been a major issue of interest among cardiologists in treating and preventing cardiovascular disease. Much of the research has focused on a high LDL (low density lipoprotein) as a major risk factor in coronary artery disease. LDL is the "bad" cholesterol because of its tendency to become oxidized in your blood. Oxidized LDL is injurious to tiny blood vessels. According to the "response to injury" hypothesis, the oxidized LDL results in plaque formation and a decreased diameter of blood vessels which may lead to symptoms of heart disease or, ultimately, a heart attack. From research based on male patients, a high LDL has been proclaimed to be a powerful risk factor for heart disease. In women, however, it appears that a low HDL (high density lipoprotein) is a much stronger risk factor. HDL, or good cholesterol as it is commonly called, functions as the scavenger lipoprotein that helps prevent LDL from doing its damage.

It is important for your physician to know these differences concerning HDL and LDL in women. Why? Because the cholesterol-lowering strategies of many of the pharmacologic therapeutic agents on the market have different interactions and certainly different implications in women. Heartsense strategies in women should focus not only on lowering LDL, but also on enhancing other means of raising HDL, such as exercising and maintaining an ideal body weight. Another important risk reducing strategy to consider is Hormonal Replacement Therapy.

Hormonal Replacement Therapy (HRT) has become a highly controversial and important topic for women in the 1990s. For the first time in history, large numbers of women are living into their eighties and nineties. This means that for many, one third to one half of their lifetime will be spent without functioning ovaries and the hormones they produce. To take or not to take HRT may be one of the most important health care choices that women face. Long-term preventive benefits against osteo-porosis and coronary heart disease must be weighed against present qual-ity of life and the potentially increased risk of uterine and breast cancer. Although there is much we are still learning, the data we already have can be overwhelming, leaving many women confused and unsettled.

Even the physicians who care for these women often have mixed feel-ings about recommending HRT for the peri- and post-menopausal years (usually 40-85). The decision is complicated even further by the inescapable fact that each woman is an individual. There is no standard algorithm to apply when it comes to HRT. Before embarking on a course of HRT, a woman and her physician must consider her personal and fam-ily medical histories, her lifestyle, short and long-term risks and benefit profiles, as well as expectations regarding her quality of life.

Let's explore the pluses and minuses of this hotly debated treatment option.

One of the primary uses of HRT is to ease the physical and mental discomfort, sometimes extreme, of menopause. Most physicians are aware of the more common symptoms - hot flashes, night sweats and chills, insomnia, mood swings and irregular bleeding. As a cardiologist, I see many women with the less often recognized "hot flash equivalents" - palpitations, dizziness and unusual sensations in the hands and arms, such as tingling and numbness. All of these hot flash-like symptoms are manifestations of vasomotor instability and are triggered by declining estrogen levels.

Such symptoms are not only uncomfortable; they can also be alarm-ing. At times, the anxiety these women experience from believing some-thing is wrong with their heart is more incapacitating than the physical discomfort itself. I have even met some women who said that their menopausal symptoms had actually taken control of their lives. They felt exhausted, depressed, miserable, disconnected and out of control. Fortunately, hormonal replacement such as estrogen (ERT) works quite well to alleviate these problems, and most women can tolerate the hor-mone. The more common side effects, such as headache and breast ten-derness, usually disappear within three months. And there is certainly room for adjustment in medication, brand, dosage and dosing regimen. For women who are truly uncomfortable when suffering during menopause, quality of life itself is a valid reason to start HRT.

Be Careful When You Sneeze!

But what if your quality of life is not so bad? Are there other advantages to HRT? Definitely. Estrogen helps to maintain the integrity of the skin, hair and nails, and the cellular lining of the vagina and urethra. Of greater significance is the protective effect it has on the integrity of the structure of women's bones. Osteoporosis is a great crippler. While some bone loss is a normal part of aging, it is estimated that 25-35 percent of all post-menopausal women will develop severe skeletal problems. Approximately 93 percent of all women who do not take estrogen will have a fracture of the hip, spine, pelvis or forearm by age 85. Patients of mine have even suffered fractures from opening a window, lifting a baby, sneezing and being startled by a phone call.

When weighing the risks and benefits of taking estrogen, keep this in mind - more women die each year from complications of fractures brought on by osteoporosis than die from cancer of the breast and uterus combined. Estrogen replacement has clearly been shown to delay the onset of age-related bone loss and, in combination with calcium, is critical in the prevention and treatment of osteoporosis.

The National Institute of Health has recommended 1000-1500 mg of calcium per day for postmenopausal women, especially for those over the age of 65. Unfortunately, calcium intake of less than 600 mg per day is common for both men and women after the fifth decade of life. A related concern is inadequate levels of vitamin D. Necessary for the development of bone, vitamin D may be low in the older populations due to dietary restrictions or loss of mobility which keeps them confined indoors and away from exposure to sunlight.

In addition to these nutrients, remember the value of exercise. Besides contributing to overall well-being and cardiovascular fitness, weight-bearing exercise joins with calcium and estrogen replacement to form the optimum trinity for bone preservation.

My primary interest in recommending HRT centers on its cardio-protective functions. Estrogen produces favorable alterations in the cholesterol risk profile. By raising favorable HDL levels and lowering unfavorable LDL levels, estrogen decreases the probability that cholesterol plaques will be deposited in the blood vessels. Moreover, estrogen's dilating effect on the blood vessels permits optimum blood flow. It stimulates the release of endothelial cell releasing factor, which helps prevent the accumulation of harmful LDL within the vessels. There is also some evidence to show that the cardio-protective effect of estrogen may be related to better utilization of insulin, as well as improvement of the balance between blood coagulation and blood thinning. All these actions of estrogen may improve blood flow and reduce the potential of myocardial insufficiency. Finally, HRT is known to promote some beneficial antioxidant activity as well. Despite these advantages, a woman and her physician must balance the cardiovascular benefits of HRT with its potential risks.

Previously, I stated that most women fear dying of breast cancer despite the fact that cardiovascular disease is still the leading cause of death in women. If a woman has a positive family history of heart disease, or at least two or more of the risk factors, then it is extremely important to consider estrogen replacement therapy. The odds of developing breast cancer as opposed to cardiovascular disease were discussed in a study in the gynecological literature in 1986 and 1994.

In a hypothetical cohort of 10,000 women assumed to be at least 50 years of age, health outcomes were plotted to age 75. The risk ratios for mortality, as well as health and disease, were examined in the use of estrogen replacement therapy based on the studies reported in the literature. The data looks something like this. If you are approximately 50 years old and if you are taking estrogen replacement therapy for 25 years, there would be a decrease in fatal coronary heart disease events by 48 percent and a decrease in deaths from hip fracture by 49 percent. The downside includes increased deaths from breast cancer by 21 percent and increased deaths from uterine cancer by 207 percent (estrogen use only - not taken with progesterone).

What this means in real numbers, is that over a course of 25 years of estrogen replacement therapy per 10,000 women, approximately 574 deaths would be prevented. In a previous study, it was crudely estimated that approximately 5,250 women per 100,000 would be saved by this treatment. Thus, in these hypothetical, population-based evaluations, it appears that the health benefits of estrogen replacement therapy in the post-menopausal years exceeds the health risks.

Despite the clear and well documented benefits of HRT, an aura of fear and suspicion surrounding its use continues to linger in the minds of many women and the clinicians who care for them. The biggest and most actively debated source of this distrust is rooted in the fear of cancer of the breast and uterus. With respect to breast cancer, the research findings have been, at times, contradictory. Also, studies showing an increased incidence of the disease often involved higher dosages or types of estrogen not used in the United States.

However, a recent review in *The New England Journal of Medicine*, June 1995, indicates that there is an increased risk of breast cancer associated with long-term hormone replacement therapy (HRT). In this study, women over 55 years of age had a significant increase in the risk of breast cancer and death if they took HRT for five years or more. The results of this study suggest that approximately 300 women per 100,000, ages 55 and above, will develop breast cancer without any hormone use. For women on HRT for five years or more, the incidence of breast cancer doubles to slightly more than 600 cases per year. (A major weakness in this study is its failure to take into consideration how many women on HRT would have been saved from heart disease.)

In contrast, a small July 1995 JAMA study reported no increased risk of breast cancer associated with short or long term HRT (estrogen - progestin). What conclusions can we make from all of this? It is important to weigh the trade-off between risks and benefits, especially among older women who take hormonal therapy. I recommend every woman and her physician weigh the potential risks of breast cancer against the substantial reduction in cardiovascular disease.

Cancer of the uterine lining has also been an issue of concern with ERT. Estrogen promotes the growth of the uterine lining, the endometrium. If the growth continues unabated, it causes a condition called endometrial hyperplasia (overgrowth), which in some instances may be a precancerous development. To prevent this, physicians usually prescribe a form of progesterone to be used in combination with estrogen, for a woman with an intact uterus. The progesterone may be used for part of each month or at lower doses on a daily basis. Taking it this way virtually eliminates the risk of endometrial cancer. For those women who cannot tolerate progesterone, ERT may be used alone; the patient must then be followed up with regular endometrial biopsies. An endometrial biopsy includes taking a small piece of tissue from the lining of the uterus and analyzing it under a microscope for the investigation of any abnormal cells.

One other problem with taking HRT may be fibroid tumors. These are benign tumors arising from the uterine muscle. The growth of fibroids may be stimulated by taking estrogen. As in estrogen dependent cancer, ERT stimulates the growth of these benign tumors but does not cause them. Also, the commonly used dosages of estrogen may be sufficiently low as to have no effect whatsoever on fibroid growth.

It appears that HRT confers a number of life enhancing health benefits with relatively little increased risk for the vast majority of women. But what about women who are not suitable candidates for HRT, cannot tolerate its side effects or who choose not to take it? What options are available to them? Fortunately, a woman may choose from a number of dietary modifications, vitamin and mineral supplements and herbal preparations to support her passage through menopause and preserve the health of her postmenopausal years.

ALTERNATIVES TO HRT

Phytoestrogens are compounds found naturally in a variety of plants. They are especially plentiful in soybeans and soy based products. These phytonutrients have manifested different degrees of estrogenic activity. Thus, in women who are reluctant to take pharmaceutically prepared estrogens, phytoestrogens could be an alternative therapeutic agent. They are even good for the heart. Population studies conducted in China and Japan have shown that people who consume large quantities of phytoesterogen-containing plants (soy products) have a low occurrence of heart attack. Soy products such as miso, tofu and soy milk are typical of the traditional Japanese diet. Menopausal symptoms are usually uncommon among Japanese women. Bioflavonoids, found in citrus fruits, especially the pulp and white of the rind, also have estrogenic properties, and for some women, are helpful in controlling hot flashes, anxiety and mood swings.

Certain dietary restrictions may be beneficial to women undergoing the transition of menopause. These guidelines may also help younger women who struggle with premenstrual syndrome. Foods high in fat, refined sugars and chemical additives can cause disruptive fluctuations in hormonal levels. For example, the often-craved chocolate can increase breast tenderness and possibly intensify mood swings. Eating large amounts of "nightshades" - potatoes, tomatoes, eggplant or peppers - may heighten women's symptoms. Excessive use of caffeine, sugar or alcohol can increase anxiety, irritability, insomnia, mood swings and vasomotor instability (which causes more hot flashes, palpitations, numbness and tingling sensations). Furthermore, these substances deplete the body of B vitamins and minerals, especially calcium. Vitamin C and B vitamins are also important supplements for menopausal women, especially for treating irritability and fatigue.

Women on HRT should also be taking extra B vitamins, as HRT may negatively affect a woman's nutritional status. As with oral contraceptives, women who take HRT may have a relative deficiency of B vitamins and thus an additional need for folic acid, vitamin B-12 and vitamin B-6. Salt and water retention and weight gain have also been reported by women taking estrogen. And some women may experience headaches, abdominal cramping, diarrhea or even nausea while taking estrogen replacement therapy.

In addition to these problems, calcium requirements may increase as well. Generally, because iron levels are higher in postmenopausal women than in younger women, most women in this age group do not need to supplement iron. To alleviate the hot flashes , anxiety and irritability that accompany menopause, some women may use vitamin E as an estrogen substitute. Vitamin E may be taken orally or applied directly to the vaginal tissue. It is also used to reduce the size of breast cysts and, when combined with magnesium and vitamin B-6 , may ease premenstrual tension.

MENOPAUSE AND OPTIONS

It is a very common practice for women in mid-life to cut back their fat intake as a way of controlling weight gain. However, menopause is not the time to reduce the intake of essential fatty acids. These linoleic and linolenic acids are extremely useful in preventing dryness of hair, skin and vaginal tissues. Evening primrose oil and black current oil are useful in regulating the body's natural prostaglandins. Prostaglandins can have a positive effect on the hormonal shifts that occur during both menopause and the premenstrual syndrome. These oils have been useful in alleviating many of the mental and physical effects that accompany these hormonal changes. They can be taken in supplemental form or can be found in seeds, wheat germ, fish and soy products.

In addition to vitamins, minerals and other nutrients, a number of herbs are extremely useful in managing specific symptoms of menopause. For example, hot flashes may be cooled by blue and black cohosh, wild yam root and dong quai.

Dong quai is a favorite Chinese Herb for women, long prescribed by traditional Chinese and Indian herbalists in balancing the vital energy of the body. In the West, dong quai is primarily used to relieve menstrual cramps of the premenstrual syndrome and to regulate hormonal imbalances in the menopausal woman. Dong quai works by dilating the blood vessels and reducing spasms and cramping. Dong quai's vital estrogen compounds mimic natural estrogen in the body; this probably explains its effectiveness in relieving both menopausal symptoms and the cramping of PMS. In the post-menopausal woman, dong quai may alleviate vaginal dryness as well. Dong quai can be taken by women entering menopause or before menstruation. It should be avoided during pregnancy and has been known to cause sun sensitivity.

Fatigue, another major symptom of the climacteric, may be lifted by ginseng, ginger and cayenne pepper. Anxiety, irritability and insomnia may be stilled by valerian root, chamomile, hops and passionflower. Passionflower is gentle enough to treat overly nervous children and can be used for the elderly suffering from sleep disorders as well. To soothe the anxiety and irritability of both menopause and PMS, try a nice combination of chamomile tea with a few concentrated drops of passionflower. Other effective nutrients in treating the menopausal syndrome include alfalfa and licorice root. Specific dietary modifications, exercise and even mental imagery can also be of great assistance to women who experience hormonal symptoms from PMS or menopause.

Menopause and PMS are both situations of hormonal imbalances. In PMS, there is an imbalance with excessive estrogen and low progesterone. Although the increasingly popular sarsaparilla is mainly used for flavoring beverages, it has also been employed as a tonic or diuretic. In PMS, sarsaparilla may enhance the natural production of progesterone. Since both PMS and menopause are related to hormonal imbalances, acupuncture, yoga and other therapies focusing on the body's energy centers have also proved effective in assuaging the physical and mental symptoms that occur from these hormonal swings.

As I have discussed, today's menopausal women have an abundance of options. Begin by selecting a physician who will work as your partner. Then read, experiment and talk to other women. Do whatever is necessary during this important transitional time to maximize your health and well-being for all the years to come.

PREVENTIVE HEALTH FOR WOMEN

If you are a woman reading this chapter, you are probably wondering about an easy self-help program for *Optimum Health*. The approach is really quite simple. First of all, *don't smoke*. In addition to causing heart disease and cancer, smoking is a participating demon in the syndrome of bone loss or osteoporosis. Smoking also pollutes the blood with heavy metals and chemicals, raising havoc with the immune system. It contributes to many unwanted symptoms - ranging from the common cold and bronchitis to cardiac irregularities and even rare instances of sudden cardiac death.

In the previous analysis I told you how risk factor profiles for heart disease differ greatly between men and women. For women, the major risk factors include diabetes, being overweight (by as little as 20 pounds), low HDL and high triglycerides. If, however, a woman has high blood pressure or smokes, the risk goes considerably higher, and in the post-menopausal situation, the risk becomes higher still. Thus, it makes heart-sense for women to become more proactive in reducing their risk for cardiovascular disease. Women need to take responsibility for themselves by modifying their risk factor profiles. This involves a healthy diet, exercise, targeted nutritional supplementation and, possibly, hormonal replacement therapy as well.

Eating a high-fiber, low-fat diet and consuming generous servings of fresh fruits and vegetables will provide the necessary flavonoids and carotenoids which combat cancer and heart disease. Research suggests that, in addition, a diet of fresh fruits and vegetables may be your best protection against lung and colo-rectal cancer. Some evidence indicates that a low-fat diet will also protect you from breast cancer. Other studies report that the saturated fat commonly found in animal foods and full fat dairy products increases a woman's risk of ovarian cancer by an average of 20 percent.

Regular daily exercise is extremely beneficial, especially in cardiovascular prevention. In addition, recent data states that women who exercise three or more hours a week in the decade following menstruation (approximately age 12) can lower their risk of breast cancer by 30 percent by the time they reach age 40. If a woman continues to exercise moderately, incorporating four hours a week into her lifestyle, she can reduce her risk of breast cancer by almost 60 percent as she approaches the middle years.

Targeted nutritional supplementation supports health and helps prevent the most dreaded maladies women face, i. e., birth defects, heart disease, cancer and bone disease. I emphasize that folic acid should be consumed by every living woman on the planet. In young women, it helps prevent birth defects. In women of all ages, it helps prevent accelerated cardiovascular aging if high homocysteine levels are found in the blood.

And again, in both younger and older women, folic acid protects against cancer of the cervix.

It is absolutely essential for every child-bearing woman to know about the feared congenital defect - spina bifida. Waiting to take prenatal vitamins until after the first prenatal visit may be too late, as these defects develop during the first few weeks of pregnancy. Unfortunately, many young women in their teenage years eat a multitude of "junk" and processed foods deficient in essential B vitamins, particularly folic acid, which is necessary for normal fetal nervous system development.

Calcium, vitamin E, magnesium, vitamin D and iron each have a special place in contributing to a woman's health at different stages of her life. In addition to vitamins, minerals and herbs, there are other particular targeted essentials that are instrumental in protecting a woman's health. Consider Co Enzyme Q_{10}, a "miracle nutrient" that I discuss many times in this book. For women, it has been tremendously successful in alleviating congestive heart failure and improving the contractile ability of the heart. In cases of cancer, it has also proved to be life-saving. Recent research confirms that breast cancer treated with high doses of Co Q_{10} (up to 390 mg) yields a regression in the cancer. Another nutrient which has also been especially helpful is L-Arginine.

L-Arginine, an amino acid, is an indispensable nutrient which has received much favorable press, not only in anti-aging strategies, but also in fighting some diseases. Several studies have documented L-Arginine's role in improving wound healing, the immune response and vasodilatory activity on blood vessels, blood clotting and cholesterol levels. Dietary L-Arginine is found mainly in plant proteins, especially cottonseed flower, pumpkin seeds and peanuts. In lower concentrations, it is found in animal proteins such as beef and halibut. Since L-Arginine has been shown to cause tumor regression in animal studies and in clinical studies of patients with breast cancer, the use of L-Arginine as a natural amino acid may have a unique role in promoting and maintaining the health of women.

Thus, there are many nutrients, herbs, vitamins, minerals and lifestyle modifications that are particularly germane in enhancing the health and longevity of women. As trite as it sounds, prevention is easier than cure. This is particularly so in promoting the health of women and children, with their specific needs and vulnerabilities. Given the array of available resources reviewed in this chapter, women and children today can place health first by implementing these simple approaches for achieving *Optimum Health*.

Twelve

MOVE!

EXERCISE - THE TONY LITTLE STORY

Tony Little succeeded against the odds.

He was a well-known bodybuilder with everything to look forward to. Then in 1985, he suffered a terrible automobile accident which nearly cost him his life, and did cost him his career. In the months that followed, Tony slipped deeper and deeper into depression and self-pity. Finally, one day Tony decided he was tired of blaming his circumstances; he realized that things would not improve until he began to act.

Tony started to work out again, to eat sensibly and, in general, to pay attention to himself. As a result, his health improved, his depression subsided, and his ability to plan was sharpened. He decided that if he could motivate himself, he could motivate others. Today, Tony has been called, "America's Number One Personal Trainer," a statement validated by the millions of exercise videotapes sold.

Like Roger Buffaloe, in the midst of a crisis, Tony Little found a new beginning. Perhaps this was his destiny, to rise above utter despair and search out some way to lead a life of dignity. In his search for finding answers about himself, Tony built a platform for a spiritual opportunity. This again is the real essence of healing. The answers are really within ourselves. We just need to listen to the messengers and events that confront us in our daily lives.

Tony's mission today is to teach millions of people about healthy forms of exercise. He has many gifts to offer. For example, on mass media, he has repeatedly told us that consistent involvement in aerobic exercise has been shown to be an important component to a healthy lifestyle, including weight management.

Exercise is crucial for weight loss. In addition to the negative energy balance resulting from exercise, many individuals feel that exercise reduces their appetite. During a strenuous work-out, the body burns carbohydrates and turns them into sugar. Therefore, a higher blood sugar in itself will assuage the appetite. However, we really don't have to exercise

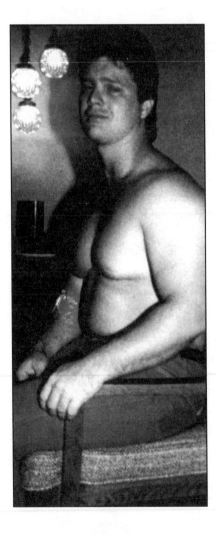
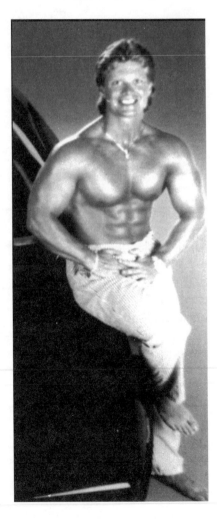

strenuously for weight loss or *Optimum Health*. This is a myth. Many cardiologists, myself included, do not recommend jogging or running.

DON'T OVERDO IT!

We have all heard of healthy people having accidents while jogging. Such occurrences may include strained muscles, tendonitis, back injuries, knee sprains and even the rare occurrence of the dissection of the aorta and sudden death. Excessive running has been reported to cause delayed menstruation and amenorrhea in women. Jogging in polluted environments, on roadways with excessive exhaust fumes, is unhealthy, as is jogging in very hot or cold weather, which may result in heat exhaustion, frostbite or even a dog-bite.

Scientific evidence has consistently linked regular physical activity to a wide range of physical and mental health benefits, as well as alleviation of occupational stress. Exercise training has been shown to benefit patients suffering from congestive heart failure as well. Regular participation in exercise has been reported to have positive psychological effects, including improved self-concept, lower levels of anxiety and depression and perhaps a halt in the deterioration that accompanies the aging process.

Demographic statistics suggest that 59 percent of the adult population engage in at least some form of exercise, with 32 percent exercising for three hours a week; 11 percent described themselves as committed runners. Long distance running has become increasingly popular as a fitness activity. However, as the age of the active runner increases, so does his or her cardiovascular risks.

We studied physiological and psychological profiles in middle-aged committed runners. Although these runners had high cardiovascular fitness, slept better and had a heightened sense of well-being, my personal observations led me to suspect a superficial "paradoxical" acceleration of the aging process. These subjects indicated they ran an average of 30 miles per week. Fifty-nine percent had participated in at least one marathon, and most of them reported having participated in an average of nine races in the previous year.

The physical demands of committed running are extreme. Evidence of a runner's "wear and tear" can be seen in the loss of hair, a receding hairline and premature wrinkling of the skin. Although averaging 40 years of age, many of the participants in our study looked much older. I was personally struck by how much pain these committed runners endured when exercising at high speed on the treadmills. There was clenching of the jaw, distortion of the face and intense wrinkling of the skin. In contrast, psychotherapists who work on softening their bodies and experiencing held-in emotions look considerably younger than their stated age.

In short, some exercise is good, but too much can be bad.

Such physically demanding aerobic exercise has also been associated with a growing number of hazards, including shin splints, tendonitis, stress fractures, neck and back injuries, sudden death and, in rare cases, rupture of the aorta. Estimates indicate that between 45 and 65 percent of the almost 20 million runners in the USA injured each year are hurt seriously enough to require them to stop running for some period of time. This raises the question - how risky is exercise? And, if regular exercise is beneficial, how great is that benefit? If regular exercise can be dangerous, how dangerous?

Although relatively few heart attacks occur during or immediately after exertion, heavy exercise does increase a person's immediate risk. However, this risk is not the same for everyone; it varies according to how much exercise is performed, and how often.

Two major studies recently answered these questions, revealing among other things that for those who engage in heavy exercise less than once a week, the risk of heart attack rose 107 times in the hour after heavy exertion. The increase in risk was 20 times greater for people who performed heavy exercise one to two times per week, and about ten times greater for those who performed exercise on a more regular basis of three or four times a week. But the risk increased only 2.4 times for the people who engaged in regular physical exertion at a level of at least six METS five times a week. A MET is a metabolic equivalent measuring work load. One MET is a minimal movement of the body, such as moving your arms. Two METS equals a very slow walk. Six METS is the equivalent of slow jogging, singles tennis, swimming or heavy gardening. So the higher the MET level, the more strenuous the activity.

The risk of heart attack after heavy exertion was similar for both men and women. The question remains, however, what is it about heavy exertion that can trigger a heart attack (myocardial infarction)?

Researchers speculate that sudden surges in blood pressure and heart rate may cause altherosclerotic plaques in coronary arteries to rupture, thus starting the cascade of clotting and eventually myocarial insufficiency. Although regular exercise has multiple health benefits, including control of blood pressure and cholesterol levels, one has to keep in mind that the heart may be more vulnerable at certain times.

Even though regular exercise has been shown to reduce the over all risk of heart attack, the minute-to-minute risk is greater during or just after physical exertion. So, perhaps the worst scenario for everyone to consider is the inactive person who occasionally engages in strenuous tasks. Obviously, most people will have moments in their lives when they must participate in heavy physical activities. But during these times, the risk of heart attack is certainly less for those who exercise regularly.

As a clinical cardiologist, I recommend exercise on at least an every other day basis. Walking, dancing and cycling, in my opinion, are still the most preferred exercise types. We also need to consider that jogging, running and other types of strenuous exercise may have negative trade-offs, particularly in the "week-end warrior" type.

Since the free radical theory has been incriminated as being related to some of the deleterious aspects of exercise, the provocative question remains: Should a healthy diet and targeted nutritional supplementation program be made an integral part of a regular exercise program? Can antioxidant manipulation reduce tissue oxidative damage?

As I previously mentioned, there are direct lines of evidence suggesting that free radicals and lipid peroxidation are normal physiological adjustments to increasing oxygen consumption with exercise. Lipid peroxidation is when harmful LDL cholesterol becomes oxidized. After oxidation, the cholesterol activates the body's white cells, causing the formation of angry foam cells called macrophages. Researchers believe that it is the foam cells that initiate the damage in the lining of blood vessels which starts the process of clogging the arteries.

We can measure elevated markers of lipid peroxidation in the blood by measuring a free radical product called serum malondialdehye (MDA). Measuring the quantity of penthane in our breath is another way of assessing free radical indices.

Clinical research has suggested that the daily ingestion of beta carotene, vitamin E and ascorbate results in a significant reduction in expired penthane and MDA levels, both at rest and after moderate and heavy activities. Since the natural endogenous enzyme antioxidant defense of the body can be overwhelmed during strenuous physical activity, secondary defense mechanisms consisting of free radical scavengers, such as vitamin E, vitamin C, beta carotene, glutathione and Co Enzyme Q_{10} may be protective against free radical damage.

Nutrition and Exercise

Glutathione, a polypeptide amino acid, has also been known to be a powerful free radical scavenger and antioxidant. As a major intracellular antioxidant, reduced glutathione prevents toxic accumulation of free radicals. Reduced glutathione (GSH) also protects cells against oxidative damage by free radicals. In a study of rats, the supplementation of glutathione protected muscular membranes and smaller blood vessels against free radicals. Thus, the supplementation of glutathione in the exercising individual may be effective in reducing the vulnerability from free radical oxidative stress.

Vitamin E is a primary lipid soluble antioxidant and can quench the singlet oxygen radical. Vitamin C is water soluble and can also quench the singlet oxygen radical. These antioxidant vitamins can react in both the aqueous phase and lipid phase, and thus protect tissues against damage by trapping free radicals.

Beta carotene is the most potent quencher of the singlet oxygen radical and is most effective at low oxygen partial pressures. Vitamin E, as a lipid soluble antioxidant, is considered to be more effective at relatively higher oxygen partial pressures. Since vitamin E levels are decreased in muscle with endurance training, it may be reasonable to consider vitamin E supplementation in the well-trained athlete. Vitamin E supplementation in situations of increased altitude, such as mountain climbing, has demonstrated decreased exhaled penthane levels.

Vitamin E may be helpful in preventing exercise-induced lipid peroxidation at high altitudes, especially in situations requiring strenuous activity. Since the oxidized form of vitamin E can be reduced by Co Enzyme Q_{10}, the interplay between vitamin E regeneration is synergistically improved.

Co Enzyme Q_{10} is an oxidant known for membrane stabilizing activities, as well as for preventing depletion of metabolites necessary for the resynthesis of ATP. Co Q_{10} has been demonstrated to scavenge free radicals, especially those produced by lipid peroxidation. In its reduced form, it is also a recycler of vitamin E. The effect of Co Enzyme Q_{10} has been studied in the animal model, demonstrating more resistance to lipid peroxidation than controlled subjects.

In another study of rats running down hill, animals which were supplemented with Co Q_{10} had decreased initial releases of muscle breakdown products. Thus, in these animal models, supplementation with Co

Q_{10} may exert a protective effect from free radical oxidative damage to membranes and tissues. Membrane lipid peroxidation is a major factor in strenuous exercise, pathological situations and even aging itself.

Since the major recycling of vitamin E appears to depend upon Co Q_{10} status, the implications for preventive use of Co Q_{10} in aging appear reasonable. This synergism of vitamin E and Co Q_{10} certainly would have special appeal to those engaged in physically demanding aerobic exercise, such as competitive runners or competitive athletes.

NUTRITION AND THE ATHLETE

As you've seen, there seems to be an accumulation of data suggesting that antioxidant supplementation may alter exercise-induced lipid peroxidation and oxidative stress. This may have special meaning to the competitive athlete. As many athletes consume low fat diets, they may be deficit in vitamin E, iron and magnesium. Since athletes are more prone to a catabolic state where tissues are constantly broken down, additional minerals and electrolytes may be required. Over utilization, coupled with a low absorption of antioxidants, can create the syndrome of "antioxidant insufficiency." This condition may occur in the athlete or in anyone who regularly performs strenuous exercise.

For example, jogging on hot, sunny polluted days to the point of exhaustion may result in tissue oxidative damage that is aggravated by poor dietary intake of antioxidants. Thus, it makes sense to optimize one's diet and to consider targeted antioxidant supplementation to minimize the cardiovascular risks and maximize the benefits of those engaged in strenuous physical exercise.

Although some studies are not yet conclusive concerning enhanced athletic performance, the supplemental use of vitamin E, magnesium, glutathione and Co Enzyme Q_{10} seem reasonable, especially to those committed to fitness as well as the competitive athlete. Co Enzyme Q_{10}, for example, has been shown to significantly increase exercise capacity.

Exercise has been shown to control several of the cardiovascular risk factors, including obesity, high blood pressure, diabetes and elevated blood lipids. In cardiovascular rehabilitation, we exercise people after heart attack and bypass surgery to improve physical endurance. Once an individual improves his physical conditioning, this may result in the heart utilizing oxygen more efficiently, thereby increasing the amount of exercise that can be done before developing chest pain. Angina is a term doctors frequently refer to as a situation of coronary insufficiency when blood flow to the heart muscle is decreased and there is insufficient oxygen supply. This condition may result in heart cramps, or in pressure or burning in the chest.

Exercise can reduce body fat and increase muscle mass. An important and beneficial metabolic result of exercise is an increase in serum HDL levels. High endurance and aerobic exercises such as cross country skiing are excellent in increasing HDL. Other biochemical considerations of exercise include a reduction in the stickiness of blood, which may prevent the blood clots that cause heart attacks. Other favorable effects on insulin and glucose metabolism occur. In women, exercise also protects against osteoporosis.

Perhaps the greatest benefit of exercise is the reduction of emotional stress. Exercise has been known to assuage the driven Type-A behavior pattern and is an alternative way to utilize the peripheral muscles instead of our precious heart muscle under situations of high stress and arousal. In this way, dynamic exercise can interrupt a chronic state of visceral-vascular readiness and assuage the overactive nervous and cardiovascular systems.

So, enough about the benefits. How much is needed and how should we go about it?

MAY I HAVE THIS DANCE?

Although there is considerable debate about how much exercise is necessary to promote optimum physical and emotional well-being, it is my feeling that *any amount of activity is better than none*. We supported this belief in a passive versus active exercise study at The New England Heart Center that was published in the *Journal of Cardiopulmonary Rehabilitation*. In approximately 94 women who were placed in various groups, i.e. control, walking, and passive exercise, any activity proved beneficial when matched against controls. Even the passive exercise toning tables appeared to be as beneficial as walking to overall health and reports of well-being. Although the walkers had better cardiovascular fitness, the women who performed on the toning tables had the same favorable metabolic and physical improvements in their health and well-being. When measured with calipers, they both lost the same amount of millimeters of fat as well.

The study was extremely provocative because it showed that even simple walking or passive exercise promotes improvement in metabolic, physiological, and psychological profiles. Therefore, it really is not necessary for *Optimum Health* to get involved in strenuous forms of exercise such as high-impact aerobics, running, or racing, for that matter. *The term "no pain, no gain" is totally untrue.* Any activity, active or passive, will have some beneficial effect.

In my opinion, walking and dancing are the best forms of exercise. Even as simple everyday activities, they can make a difference in your overall cardiovascular health. Walking is a form of aerobic exercise, strengthening the heart and improving circulation. So just by walking the dog, you can help improve your (and your dog's) health!

Isometric exercises, such as heavy weight-lifting and resistance exercises, including waterskiing, do not improve the conditioning of the heart. Rather, these types of exercise may increase strength and perhaps add extra muscle or provide additional bulk to the body. It is aerobic exercise that causes us to breath deeply, expanding the chest and thereby providing more oxygen to the heart and the rest of the body. Types of aerobic exercise include cycling, swimming, skiing and some calisthenics.

The reason why athletes have a lower heart rate than sedentary people is because the heart pumps more blood with each heartbeat. Since the average heart rate is close to 72 beats per minute, conditioning usually has occurred when the resting heart rate comes down to approximately 60 beats per minute. In some of the professional athletes I have treated, it is not uncommon to see the heart beat in the 40 to 50 range. The heart is a muscle, and like our biceps and calves, can be gradually strengthened. If the heart beats rapidly and wildly under conditions of simple aerobics, this is a sign of poor conditioning or oversympathetic arousal. In the conditioned person, the heart rate will remain steady, only gradually increasing with aerobic activity. The fit individual may even combat stress and emotional trauma better than a physically unfit person. After all, one of the greatest advantages of exercise is a release of stress and tension in the body.

If you wish to consider a more advanced exercise program than walking the dog, I recommend that you see your physician prior to beginning exercise. If you are over 40, your physician may recommend an exercise stress test to determine the possibility of any cardiovascular risk. For those who wish to exercise and raise their pulse rate to greater than 120 beats per minute, an exercise evaluation is an excellent screening tool for assessing your risk. However, if you do not wish to involve yourself in a formal exercise program, you may wish to perform daily passive exercise.

Not the Remote Control!

Passive exercise is simply accomplished by doing your normal daily activities, but instead of using machinery, you are using your own legs. Passive exercise includes such things as walking to the train station or bus station, parking the car farther away from the entrance of your place of employment, using the stairs instead of the elevators, perhaps taking a walk during lunch time and, most importantly, *throwing away the television remote control.*

For those who wish to involve themselves in a more formal program, the following are a few tips to make your fitness and exercise program more enjoyable:

1. Find a convenient time and place to exercise. (This may be before breakfast, during lunch or after work.)
2. Try to avoid the heat of the day or the nocturnal hours.
3. Set a definite goal, such as walking one mile or cycling 20 minutes three times a week.
4. If you miss an exercise session, make an agreement with yourself that you will make it up at a later time.
5. After you have lost two pounds or a half inch on your waistline, reward yourself by treating yourself to something such as a movie, a haircut, a manicure or a sports event.
6. Keep your exercise program enjoyable and varied.

Better Warm-Up First

If you feel motivated, and I hope you do, and wish to engage in more brisk aerobic forms of exercise, you will need to consider a warm-up period of stretching and breathing. The first set of exercises may include the four following maneuvers:

Exercise 1

This exercise includes abdominal breathing. Lie on the floor and bend your knees, keeping your feet on the floor. With your eyes closed and your hands over your navel, breathe out naturally and feel the abdomen push against the hands. Again, breathe nasally, with a full inspiration and expiration. This form of breathing can be practiced prior to any exercise session or even meditation.

Exercise 2

After developing a sense of abdominal breathing, lie on the floor with the pelvis extended and the knees bent. Insert a rolled up blanket in the small of the back and place the feet securely on the floor. You will feel a sensation of stretching in the abdomen that will allow fuller and deeper breathing. This is also a good stretch for the lower back. You may wish to push your buttocks into the floor to accentuate the stretch.

Exercise 3

This is a back exercise. Lie down on the floor. Bring your knees to your chest and then swing them to the right and then to the left. This frees up the lower muscles of your back. While keeping your lower back on the floor, swing your knees back to your chest. Gently rock yourself forward and backward several times so you are rocking on your lower back region. Remember not to strain yourself. Repeat this six or seven times and then gradually get up slowly.

Exercise 4

For this exercise, place your hands on your hips and bend at the waist, bringing your torso down toward your knees. Bend as far as possible without straining. While keeping your hands on your hips, you may feel a mild stretching in your lower back and then in your hamstring muscles at the backs of your calves. Now, come to the upright position. Spread your legs as wide as possible, with the toes pointed inward. Now, place your knuckles in the small of your back and lean backward as far as possible while opening up your throat by releasing a sound. This will stretch the muscles in the chest, diaphragm and neck. Remember, again, do not strain yourself. Do this five to ten times.

A PRESCRIPTION FOR EXERCISE

These warm-up exercises will take only about five minutes. They are excellent exercises to stimulate your breathing and provide stretching to the legs, abdomen, chest and lower lumbosacral spine. After you have done this warm-up, you can then choose to exercise as you like. In choosing an exercise, consider several aspects: how long, how much and how often. Now we are getting into the realm of physical fitness that includes guidelines for an exercise prescription. The following are the components:

1. Type of activity
2. Duration of activity
3. Frequency
4. Intensity
5. Progression.

Fitness experts, such as doctors in the American College of Sports Medicine, of which I am a member, have established the following recommendations for the quantity and quality of exercise in order to develop and maintain both body composition and cardiovascular fitness:

Type of Activity – *Aerobic exercise is preferable for fitness.* Aerobic activity stimulates breathing by using large muscle groups in a continuous and rhythmical form. Such exercises include jogging, running, walking, hiking, dancing, swimming, skating, rowing, cross country skiing, jumping rope and bicycling.

Duration of Activity – *Fifteen to 60 minutes of continuous or discontinuous aerobic activity* is required for health and fitness. For example, to perform 15 minutes of rope skipping continuously would be difficult. To perform this type of activity for three to five minutes, however, taking a short rest, and then continuing for a total of 20 minutes is manageable and effective. Fast walking can also be performed for a 20 minute stretch. Since walking is not as intense as rope skipping, it does not need to be discontinuous, though both are aerobic.

Frequency – *Three to five times a week* is considered by most sports experts to be an appropriate frequency for exercise.

Intensity – The intensity of activity can vary. Most fitness experts are in agreement that *between 70 to 85 percent of one's predicted maximal heart* rate is a good reliable index of intensity. For example, suppose you had an exercise stress test with your physician, and your maximal heart rate obtained during that evaluation was 150 beats per minute. If you take 70 percent of 150, this equals 105. Eighty-five percent of 150 equals 127.5. Therefore, if you exercise in an aerobic activity and wish to enhance your cardiovascular fitness, your exercise target heart rate should be between 105 and 128. Although there are other formulas that have been advocated, this is the easiest way for developing an exercise prescription. For the unfit or overweight individual, this exercise prescription is perhaps the safest, especially when constructed from an exercise treadmill evaluation. In this case, an exercise program should only be utilized with the advice of your physician.

Progression – In the unfit or overweight individual, little progression or increase is advisable. If, however, you have begun to notice improved fitness and a reduction in weight, you may *increase your total work effort by perhaps 10 percent per month*. However, recommended rates of progression varies with individuals. It is usually best to progress slowly and increase gradually in a spirit of keeping your motivation and interest intact and not torturing yourself. The old motto, "Exercise 'til exhaustion," is counterproductive.

THE EXERCISE SESSION

To safely undergo an exercise program, it is necessary to include at least three phases: Warm-up, work-out and cool-down. Each phase has a particular purpose.

The warm-up phase usually includes the stretching and breathing exercises that we already have mentioned. It may last from five to ten minutes, with the purpose of increasing the body temperature, loosening-up the joints and ligaments and relieving any undue soreness. A slight elevation in heart rate is also a benefit of the warm-up phase. Generally, *the older or the more obese the person, the longer the warm-up should be.*

The work-out phase usually lasts between 15-60 minutes, with an ideal period of approximately 20 minutes, plus five minutes to warm-up and five minutes to cool down. To improve cardiovascular fitness and body composition, as well as to lose weight, continuous aerobic activities of low to moderate intensity are recommended.

The cool-down phase, which should last from five to ten minutes, brings back the physiological system toward the resting level at a gradual pace. After a vigorous work-out, our cardiac output may be considerably elevated, perhaps two to three times the resting level for an individual. Thus, it is important to cool-down to permit a gradual re-adaptation of the body system. One of the best cooling-down exercises, again, is slow walking. After a work-out such as running, jogging or rope-skipping, a walking cool-down is all that is required. In structured rehabilitative-type exercise programs such as our hospital's Cardiovascular Rehabilitation Program, the cool-down period usually includes relaxation techniques. For example, after the clients have completed their work-out phase, many of them will walk around the room. After a brief walk, we ask them to lie down and focus on their breathing and then we lead them into a meditation to get them in touch with their bodies and their feelings about their bodies. These procedures are extremely helpful in relieving stress and tension in the cardiovascular system.

So now you know about exercise and how an exercise prescription works. But what are the forms of exercise, and what types of exercise should we do? Let me first begin this discussion with my two favorite types of exercises: Dancing and walking.

DANCING

Dancing is without a doubt the best form of exercise as it incorporates the whole body. The benefits from dancing are enormous. Have you ever seen people put their whole heart into dancing? Their bodies becomes graceful. Their movements are integrated with the music. Their hips, chest, thighs and arms are coordinated in rhythm with the music. My patients often ask me what types of dancing are best. Any form of dancing will do, whether it is square dancing, ballroom dancing, freestyle or country and western. All have a common denominator: Movement with music.

Dancing is also a great way to get over our inhibitions. One of the best features of dancing is that it gives us permission to use the pelvis, which many of us feel is taboo. The pelvic floor is a major location for the center of energy in our body. By rotating this area, we are able to move the whole body. And dancing can be done alone and at any age.

Have you ever listened to the radio and started to sway to a favorite song? Next time, get up and dance! Don't stop yourself from feeling the music and moving. We put our emotions into dancing. When you see couples close their eyes while dancing slow, do you get a feeling of tranquility and connectedness? Any exercise we put our feelings into, particularly positive feelings, enhances not only the spirit, but also the core of our beings.

By the same token, anyone who has negative energy such as anger or rage, should not, I feel, use strenuous physical exercise to work it out. Instead, I would recommend the releasing emotional exercises described earlier, such as kicking the feet on a bed or verbalizing feelings in a stationary car. Contrary to popular belief, trying to work out anger through exercise could perhaps do a disservice to the body. With rage, we have an increase in adrenaline. Coupled with strenuous exercise, it's like throwing gasoline on a fire - by overcharging the already overstimulated heart, we can overdose on our own hormones.

For example, after I resuscitated two victims of sudden death in the emergency room, they both indicated that they had been very angry and were using exercise as a way of discharging their anger. They both forced themselves to exercise these highly charged negative emotions off, thus making exercise an obligation, and not a pleasure. Exercise will not take away anger, but merely burn off some of the excess energy that is associated with it. The way to get rid of anger is to express it in a clean and straightforward manner.

WALKING

Walking is also an excellent exercise for all ages. Young and old love to walk. I encourage walking in my older population because of its safety. I rarely have heard of people hurting their legs, ligaments or knees while walking. Try to take in the surroundings when you walk. And don't worry about the pace. Most exercise enthusiasts believe that we have to walk fast or briskly in order to burn calories. This is not the case. In fact, a mile of walking burns as many calories as a mile of running. Enjoy this activity. Take time for yourself. Move your hips and get into the natural ebb and flow of a rhythmic motion. Feel your body. Feel each step. It can be very enjoyable.

I would recommend a minimum of at least 20 minutes of walking once a day. After you have progressed and feel comfortable about walking one mile, try working up to walking two miles, or better yet, walk 20 minutes twice a day. Again, this should be fun and leisurely. Remember, it costs nothing and you can do it alone. Walking with someone or perhaps in a group will offer an excellent support system.

Many of my patients have commented that walking can sometimes be boring when done day after day. On the surface, this may be true, so be creative! One can go hiking through the woods, or through the mountains, for that matter. For example, I am an avid fly fisherman and I frequently need to walk up and down river banks and through the fields to get "where the fish are." Surf fishing is another excellent exercise, moving up and down the beach while casting and reeling and recasting and reeling.

I have met numerous surf fishermen well over the age of 60, many of them with their rod in their hand. The anticipation of catching a fish is a feeling for which many fishermen develop an addiction. I know - I have it! Isn't it crazy to get up at daybreak to go fishing? Many a time, I wanted to cuddle in the sheets of my bed and not go out in that cold, early morning air, but once I started to get ready and anticipate walking and breathing in the fresh ocean spray, my priorities changed. Remember that surf fishing requires walking, and next to dancing, walking is the best form of exercise.

Other ways to incorporate walking into our lives is in the game of golf. Again, this is an activity that is good for both the young and the old. It is so heartwarming to hear of an elderly man score close to his age. I have endorsed golf as an exercise to many of my clients. Although in a cardiovascular sense the amount of exercise is minimal, golf still requires considerable walking. And if you carry your clubs or pull your golf cart, you will even burn up more calories. Although there are many exercise specialists who speak disparagingly of golf, or tennis, for that matter, I feel they are excellent activities that are good for both the mind and the body.

OTHER EXERCISES

Skiing, both cross-country and downhill, are other types of recreational activities that are excellent forms of exercise. Cross-country skiing gives all the benefits of running without any of the side effects of shin splints, ankle, knee or hip injuries. Instead of pounding on a hard surface, the cross-country skier uses rhythmic movements to gently glide across the snow. Downhill skiing is another form of exercise that again utilizes walking. Although most of us use chairlifts, many downhill skiers do lots of walking. Unfortunately, it usually occurs after losing a ski or retrieving lost equipment!

Other activities I endorse are *swimming* and *cycling.* These two non-weight bearing activities are especially good for the overweight or elderly person. Stationary cycling is preferred over outdoor cycling for the elderly or during inclement weather, especially if you live in New England as I do. I frequently tell my patients to cycle for approximately five to 15 minutes. This could even be done with a low-grade tension on the bicycle. If some of my patients get bored, I suggest they listen to the news or turn on the television; some patients even read while stationary cycling. My own recommendation is to let your mind go and just focus on the rhythmic activity of the legs.

Other indoor activities could include *climbing stairs* or using a *rowing machine.* As a former director of our Cardiac Rehabilitation Program, I suggest the rowing machine as one of our preferred forms of exercise. A good rowing machine will exercise almost all the major muscles of the body. When I row, I particularly feel a sensation in my abdomen, arms and lower back. Rowing also creates a rhythmic activity which I find enjoyable. Rowing to music is a nice way of exercising. Try rowing to classical music with your eyes closed. After a couple of minutes, you may not even realize you are exercising.

A *treadmill* is another form of exercise I recommend. We also use this piece of equipment in our Cardiac Rehab Center. Participants are asked to walk on a treadmill with a gradual increase in speed and elevation, which they use in conjunction with their exercise prescription. My suggestion here is to just use the treadmill as a walking machine, not another stress test. It is not necessary to increase the speed or raise the elevation to a high degree. For starters, it is best to start with the machine at 1.7 miles an hour, with perhaps a five percent grade. If you walk at this pace for three minutes, you are achieving approximately three METS of work, the term that cardiologists frequently use to refer to a metabolic equivalent. While simply walking at a slow pace is considered to be one to two METS, walking at a faster pace or up a slight incline is three METS. My recommendation would be to walk at a low level of activity at a low elevation for perhaps 15 to 20 minutes.

Walking on a treadmill is not as good as walking outside because the variety in terrain allows different muscles to be worked. But this can be done as an alternative, particularly when weather conditions are not permitting. Indoor exercise allows you to fit a program to your schedule as time permits, but doesn't have the benefit of support and change of scenery that outdoor exercise programs can offer.

Let me explain what I mean by *support.* I can remember how an exercise support group was extremely helpful in bringing one of my patients out of a low grade depression. He had recently lost his wife to a sudden heart attack and became very depressed. He, too, was a victim of heart disease, sustaining a massive myocardial infarction only nine months prior to his wife's sudden death. After recovering from his heart attack, he gained a new sense of self only to lose his will to live when his wife died.

Although this was a very fragile man in his 70s, with high-grade coronary artery disease, I advocated an exercise program as a way for him to strengthen his heart and develop a new vital connection. In our Phase III Cardiovascular Rehabilitative Program, he indeed made many such connections and new friendships. In short, he became an exercise enthusiast. He came to the program three times a week and walked and talked with almost everyone. Exercise not only increased the strength of his cardiovascular system, but also gave my patient a new interest in life. The establishment of new vital connections after the loss of a significant other can truly be rewarding and life-sustaining.

Another indoor exercise that I can suggest is *repetitious dynamic light weight-lifting*. This can be done alone at home or with others at a gymnasium. I am recommending it more and more to my patients, even those advancing in age. As we gradually grow older, and particularly after the age of 40, the average man loses his lean muscle mass, which is replaced by fat. Since increasing age is inevitable, it makes sense to exercise isolated muscle groups with light weights. If you prefer to exercise at home, you do not need to go out and purchase barbells, dumbbells or fancy weightlifting equipment for this exercise. I have even told my patients to try lifting magazines or heavy books after appropriate stretching. Repetitive light weight training is a good way to increase muscle tone, decrease fat and burn calories. Remember to breathe through the lift, exhaling on effort. Always avoid breath holding.

Sit-ups with the knees bent or elevated, perhaps on a bed or chair, is another good activity that can be used in conjunction with weightlifting. Sit-ups are an excellent endeavor in the strengthening of the abdominal muscles. Many of us have chronic back problems in which simple muscle toning of the abdominal wall will alleviate many of our lower back ailments. I have found *Tony Little's Ab Isolator* to be an excellent exercise aid while performing sit-ups because it helps prevent back strain.

Push-ups are also an alternative. But we need to be cautious about utilizing push-ups or sit-ups, or even low weights in individuals who are hypertensive or have heart disease. So a stress test may be in order before beginning a formal exercise program. When performing sit-ups, exhale on the effort to lift up, inhale as you slowly lie back down.

Another favorite exercise of mine is *jumping rope*. For this, you will need a good pair of padded athletic shoes and a jump rope that may be purchased in many of the sporting stores. Remember that if you jump rope, *do not jump with both feet at once*, but rather alternate one and then the other. Most of us would agree that five minutes of jumping rope can be quite fatiguing and is equivalent to perhaps ten to 15 minutes of cycling or rowing! As a wrestler, I used to jump rope for five to ten minutes as a warm-up exercise prior to our several-minute scrimmages.

There are many types of exercises we can perform. Aerobic exercise is preferred over isometric exercise. With exercise, we need to be *creative*. To avoid boredom, we may have to switch our daily routines. For example, walk one day, cycle another and perhaps roller skate or ice skate on another. If walking is the core in your routine, you can supplement it with recreational activities such as golf and tennis. The point is to try to do some light exercise every day. If you are involved in a cardiovascular fitness program, it is prudent to only exercise three to four times a week at your target heart rate.

HAVE FUN!

Exercise is a cardinal ingredient in weight reduction and *Optimum Health*. Exercise not only increases muscle tone, but also alters the metabolic rate in our bodies; a fit individual will burn more calories than a less fit one. If you are involved in high aerobic activity, I recommend that you get an exercise prescription from your doctor. Remember that exercise can be thought of as a drug or certainly as a therapy that has tremendous benefits, but also some hazards.

You may be wondering why I have not discussed taking your pulse during leisurely exercise activity such as pleasurable walking or dancing. My problem with taking your pulse rates is that it takes us out of our bodies and into our heads. It also takes the fun out of it! You can tell when you're overdoing it. You should not be gasping for breath or dizzy. Listen to your body and nurture it, don't torture it. *The important thing about exercise is to keep it safe and to have fun.*

However, if you are trying to achieve fitness in a high-level aerobic program or following a physician-oriented exercise prescription, you will need to know if the pulse rate is within your recommended guidelines.

There are many devices on the market that digitally display the user's heart rate at a glance. I feel these are oftentimes preferable to pulse-taking because they do not take the individual back "into his head" to palpate and compute heart rate. They do allow for a quick check of heart rate to ensure that exercise is within safe guidelines.

Exercise does not need to be a struggle. If you make it fun by choosing an activity you enjoy, you will more easily incorporate it into your daily living program and soon manifest the numerous physiological, psychological and biochemical benefits that exercise provides.

To summarize, regular exercise promoting flexibility and strength has been known to reduce the risk of cardiovascular disease, stroke, developing high blood pressure, osteoporosis, obesity and non-insulin dependent diabetes. In addition to increasing the strength of the heart, exercise can also increase levels of endorphins, which will produce a sense of well-being and, in most instances, will make you feel better as well. I continue to recommend various forms of exercise to my patients, since I believe the benefits far outweigh the risks.

Thirteen

NUTRITIONAL HEALING

I n 1994, the National Cancer Institute recommended five to, preferably, nine servings of fresh fruits and vegetables a day. I wholeheartedly endorse this recommendation.

A prudent diet is your best asset in weight reduction and your best defense against illness. Agreeing with the old cliche, "You are what you eat," nutritional healing utilizes a diet that makes you feel better both in body and mind. Of course, I prefer the new cliche, "You are what you absorb."

This chapter is designed to look at foods that enhance and nourish your body. We have previously discussed the advantages of complex carbohydrates and monounsaturated fats, the importance of water, along with various vitamins and minerals, and the negative aspects of both caffeine and alcohol. This chapter is about experiencing a new array of foods. In the spirit of nondeprivation, and with a slow and patient approach, we can learn to consume less of certain foods and utilize other, equally as enjoyable, new ones .

Changing your food patterns may not be easy. Since you have been building your eating habits all of your life, it may be difficult to substitute one type of food for another. But if you have an open mind, it doesn't have to be painful. To the contrary, experimenting with new recipes and foodstuffs can be fun. For example, for years I loved red meat. I then gradually switched to chicken and fish for most of my animal protein, and now I enjoy my food as much as ever. I am even eating less animal protein. The transition to a healthier diet may take some time, however. *My first exposure to seaweed was a disaster!* It tasted too fishy and I didn't like it. Gradually, it became palatable, and now I find it most enjoyable. During the transition phase I would recommend you gradually do the following:

1. Reduce the amount of red meat in the diet.
2. Reduce dairy products, particularly whole milk and high-fat cheeses and ice creams.
3. Reduce eggs.
4. Reduce saturated fats.
5. Omit refined sugars, including white table sugar.
6. Reduce refined flour and bleached flours.
7. Omit as many processed foods as possible.
8. Limit sodium intake to under three grams per day.
9. Reduce alcohol consumption and caffeine intake.
10. Increase fiber consumption.
11. Increase complex carbohydrates in terms of whole grains, pastas and beans.
12. Increase consumption of fresh fruits and vegetables.
13. Increase consumption of sea vegetables.
14. Consider miso soups and broths.

Most expert nutritionists and some physicians, particularly those interested in a macrobiotic approach, feel that an optimal diet should include approximately 40 percent whole grains. Whole grains (wheat, corn, rice, oats, millet, rye, barley and buckwheat) are those that are unrefined and are exceedingly nutritious. They contain more vitamins, minerals and fiber than their lighter, whiter and fluffier counterparts found in commercially packaged goods. In their raw form, grains contain a seed and a covering to protect the seed. With the advent of the Industrial Revolution and modern processing, it became easier to remove the germ and bran layers, making available to the general population white flour that was once reserved only for the rich.

Unfortunately, these discarded segments contain all the fiber and the vast majority of the B-complex vitamins, as well as the vitamins E and A and the minerals magnesium, potassium, zinc, iron and selenium. In refining grains, the flour is commonly bleached, giving it a lighter, seemingly more presentable image and a softer texture. Additionally, these refined grains are frequently laced with additives and preservatives. White flour used in white bread and pastries contains many empty calories. It provides carbohydrates, but little fiber. Most of the carbohydrates are not eliminated, but rather converted to glucose and stored as fats in the body.

With greater awareness, many people are now purchasing breads that favor a whole-grain concept. Wheat breads and fiber breads are now quite plentiful in supermarkets, but *the best sources of vitamins, minerals and fiber from whole-grain bread products are available in your local health food store or bakery.* Since whole grain is unrefined and contains multiple nutrients, it is the closest thing to a complete food because it contains not only carbohydrates, but also a balanced amount of protein, low-fats, multiple vitamins, minerals and sufficient fiber.

Civilizations all over the world have been utilizing grains for centuries as a diet staple. Primitive cultures are also known to have the lowest rates of cancer and heart disease. Grains, as we discussed in an earlier analysis, decrease the transitory time of waste through the bowels. In addition to having high fiber, grains also are made up of polysaccharides. These complex sugars are less quickly converted to glucose than simple sugars found in refined products and, therefore, are less available for conversion to fat. It is important to incorporate whole grains into your diet; I recommend one to two servings per day. The following is a list of good possible grains.

BROWN RICE - Brown rice may be obtained in the short, medium or long grain varieties. It is also available in a sweet version called basmati. In addition to containing many of the vitamins and minerals mentioned, brown rice contains the mineral silicon, which is a necessary element for our body. Some investigators point out that silicon helps prevent "burn-out" in high-performance individuals who drive themselves excessively in both their personal and professional lives. Brown rice is easy to cook. It can be boiled, steamed or even fried. To cook brown rice, wash the grain thoroughly and soak it in water for several minutes; rinse and drain; add one cup of grain to two cups of water and a pinch of salt in a saucepan. Bring to a boil; immediately cover the pot and turn down the heat to simmer; do not lift the lid or stir until the water has been absorbed, approximately 45-50 minutes. This is the way I prefer to cook brown rice. I frequently will cook two cups of rice at a time and then reheat it for use over the next few days. Brown rice is an excellent complex carbohydrate that goes well with almost any fish dish. When brown rice is used in combination with beans, it provides excellent sources of protein in the diet.

BARLEY - Barley is grown throughout the world and is a popular grain in America. It is chewy with a nutty taste. Barley has been used as a natural sweetener and in making beer. It is an excellent grain to use in soups, or it can be mixed with brown rice and served as a side dish. Merely add one-third cup of barley to one cup of brown rice and prepare in the same manner as brown rice.

BUCKWHEAT - Buckwheat is technically the seed of a fruit rather than a true grain. It has a rich and somewhat bitter flavor. The Eastern cultures grind buckwheat into flour to create noodles. Buckwheat flour is a good flour to use, particularly in pancakes. A pancake recipe is included in this text.

MILLET - Millet is a grain that was used traditionally for centuries by the people of Africa and China. Millet can be boiled by itself or with a variety of vegetables. It goes especially well with broccoli or cauliflower and may be substituted for brown rice or barley.

CORN - For centuries, corn has been the stable grain of the Indian cultures in North and Central America. Although not frequently considered one, corn is actually a grain. Corn can be ground into flour to make cornmeal, which may be used to make cereals, polenta and tortillas. It also makes a delicious muffin. This is an excellent substitute for people allergic to wheat. Whole corn or corn-on-the-cob contains good sources of fiber as well as vitamins and minerals, particularly beta carotene.

WHEAT - Wheat is especially rich in B vitamins and vitamin E. In its refined form, it is lacking many of the important nutrients, but in the form of whole-wheat flour or berries, it provides excellent sources of minerals and vitamins. Wheat berries, when cooked, create a tasty and nutritious dish with a hearty, chewy texture.

Other grains that can be consumed include *oats, rye* and *wild rice.* I strongly recommend any of these grains. Another highly nutritious food that I recommend to many of my clients is *soba, or the buckwheat noodles of Japan.* They are frequently used in soups but may be used as a pasta. *Pasta,* in my opinion, is one of the best foods we can consume. Not only does it taste good, but it is low in fat and contains coarse carbohydrates. It is easy to prepare and goes well with a numerous variety of sauces, vegetables, meats and fishes. I recommend my cardiovascular clients eat either pasta or rice on a daily basis.

COMMERCIAL FOR CARLA'S PASTA

In Chapter 14, I'll share several of the recipes that I use to prepare my pasta dishes. Like whole grains, pasta can be prepared in many different ways and in many styles. The herbs and spices that may accompany pasta, i.e., *basil, garlic, onions* and *parsley*, are magnificent ingredients that have a healing quality on the body, particularly the heart. Dry packaged pasta, either in its traditional form made with *semolina flour* or made from *whole-wheat flours* is an excellent high-complex carbohydrate. Fresh or frozen pasta, however, contains eggs. Fortunately, one manufacturer I asked has been able to make a fresh frozen pasta with minimal egg yolk. Usually, it takes six eggs to make one pound of fresh frozen pasta, which is greater than 1200 mg of cholesterol per pound. *Carla's Pasta* in Manchester, Connecticut, offers a fresh frozen pasta made from predominantly egg whites with only one egg yolk instead of six. It can be shipped and stored and has greater than 90 percent of the fat and cholesterol removed.

MORE RECOMMENDATIONS FOR HEALING FOODS

In this analysis, we have discussed whole grains and pastas as being healing foods in our diet. Another highly nutritious food that I would recommend on a daily basis is *beans.* Beans are high in calcium and contain twice as much protein in comparable volumes as meat and poultry or dairy food. When combined with grains, they provide all the needed essential amino acids. Beans are really the best single vegetarian source of protein. Some bean products include *black-eyed peas, chick-peas, lentils, pinto beans, split peas, adzuki and lima beans.* Any of these bean combinations are good. Lentils are a particular favorite of mine, especially in soups. They are easy to digest as well as to prepare, and they also provide an excellent source of vegetable iron.

Boiling is perhaps the best method for cooking beans. Usually, beans should be soaked overnight. When boiled, a pinch of salt and/or stalk of seaweed may be added. Cooking usually takes one and one-half to two hours. Like short-grained brown rice, beans can be cooked and reheated for later use.

Soybeans are perhaps the highest in protein and are a favorite in macrobiotic cooking. *Tofu, tempeh, tamari and miso* are all made from soybeans and are easily found in health food stores. Miso is a particular favorite of mine, and in its soup form is highly recommended to virtually all clients in our weight-reducing program as well as many of my heart patients. Miso is made from fermented soybeans, grains and sea salt and contains many of the enzymes that strengthen the body.

In a major Japanese study, *those who ate miso soup every day had a significantly lower risk of dying from cancer and heart disease compared to those who never consumed miso or did so only on occasion.* This large prospective study, in excess of over a quarter of a million people, demonstrates one of the best kept secrets of Oriental medicine. Based on my review of the medical literature, particularly with the overwhelming evidence of population studies, it appears that sea vegetables and the miso preparations do enhance health and longevity. Miso is used in the recipe for sea vegetable soup that follows in the chapter, *Recipes For Preventive Medicine.*

The next section of this chapter will include particular foods that I feel have healing properties. For example, we briefly discussed *sea vegetables,* which were reported to lower heart disease in Japan. The highest incidence of longevity is found in the village of Oki on Oki Island, whose inhabitants eat large amounts of sea vegetables. Compared with other regions of Japan, these villages also have an unusually low rate of stroke. I prefer sea vegetables not only because of the high vitamin and nutritional constituents, but also because they are protective against minor effects of nuclear radioactivity. Medical research has determined that sea vegetables contain a substance called sodium alginate that helps eliminate from the body radioactive strontium, a breakdown product of uranium. Since we constantly take in minute amounts of radiation from sources as various as the sun to x-rays and microwaves, sea vegetables are a good form of insurance.

SEA VEGETABLES

My first introduction to sea vegetables resulted from the use of miso soup. After some minor research, in which I learned that sea vegetables are highly nutritious and help eliminate unwanted fats in our bodies, I decided to use them in our weight-reducing program. After making several types of miso soups with the various combinations, I experimented with *wakame* and *kombu seaweeds*. My first exposure to these seaweeds was not good; I found them distasteful and very "fishy." Nevertheless, because of their nutritional value, I put small amounts of the seaweeds in the soups. Some of my patients, however, really savored the taste. As a matter of fact, in our group support sessions, I was amazed to see how many people really thoroughly enjoyed these miso soup preparations. Yet, I still wasn't sold on the taste.

It wasn't until my sister came to my house and made a sea vegetable soup that I learned how versatile seaweeds really are. She had recently undergone a hysterectomy and received considerable doses of radiation to the pelvis and abdomen. Due to her interest in reducing the effects of radiation, she bought Steve Schechter's book on food and radiation, *Fighting Radiation with Foods, Herbs and Vitamins - Documented Natural Remedies that Boost Your Immunity & Detoxify*. In the book she found a recipe for "Sea Vegetable Soup." To say this soup was delicious would be an understatement. It was outstanding! After consuming the sea vegetable soup on several occasions, I developed a particular affinity for it. The combination of the olive oil, miso and various herbs and garlic made it a very flavorful and satisfying concoction. I actually felt better after eating the soup. I had more energy. I felt more alive and became more clear. It wasn't just a coincidence, either. *I really believe in the "healing" properties of this broth.*

Since the time of recorded history, seaweeds have been utilized by many cultures in various areas of the world. They have been harvested from the coastal waters of Japan, Ireland, France and Canada. In our own country, for example, they have been taken from the Maine coastal waters. After doing considerable research into seaweeds, I became convinced that they have both a protective and a healing effect on the body. Sea vegetables are extremely rich in vitamins, minerals and nutrients. In fact, *they contain all 56 minerals!* As a group of foods, sea vegetables contain the highest amounts of magnesium, iron, iodine and sodium. For those individuals who have a history of congestive heart failure or high blood pressure, it is recommended that sea vegetables be consumed only once a week. It is also important to soak seaweeds for at least one-half hour before preparation. By soaking them in tap water or spring water, the sodium content will be reduced.

As seaweeds contain extremely high amounts of calcium and phosphorous, they are beneficial in situations where calcium is needed in the body, such as in osteoporosis. Seaweeds are also approximately 25 percent protein and two percent fat. They are low in calories, which makes them an extremely useful adjunct to diet therapy when one wants to limit calories from fats. Seaweeds are rich in many vitamins and trace elements, as well. For example, they are high in beta carotene, vitamin B-12, niacin, pantothenic acid (B-5) and vitamins A, C and E, as well as the mineral selenium. As I previously stated, selenium, combined with vitamins A, C, E and Q_{10}, is extremely important in the overall functioning of the heart. In the Chinese culture, selenium is found in the soil where the incidence of heart disease is markedly lower. Some investigators believe that it is the intake of selenium that offers a protective environment for the healthy functioning of the heart.

In summary, many clinical studies indicate that seaweed is one of nature's best nutritional supplements in healing. It contains virtually all of the minerals and vitamins that are useful in preventing "free radical formation." Sea vegetables have been utilized in treating cancer, lowering blood cholesterol, thinning the blood and even preventing ulcers. Sea vegetables are also known for their effect on dissolving fat deposits and eliminating heavy metal contaminants from the body, including radiation, cadmium and other environmental toxins. Oriental folklore and fact shows that consumption of sea vegetables offers a nutritional package that is simple, inexpensive and easy to prepare. It is a dietary supplement that should be used by everyone. Seaweed is one of nature's wonders!

VEGETABLES

Although some of my macrobiotic colleagues may disagree, I believe that most vegetables are healthful to our bodies. My only restrictions at this point are *avocados* and *olives*. *Avocados and olives contain abundant sources of fat*, and olives contain considerable quantities of sodium as well. Most vegetables, however, have an abundant source of vitamins, including beta carotene. *Vegetables should make up approximately 25-40 percent of the calories in our diet, including leafy green, round and root vegetables.* For example, *daikon*, a root vegetable resembling a long white radish, has a high calcium content and is extremely useful in healing. Roots are also rich in complex carbohydrates as well as vitamins and minerals. *Carrots* and *parsnips* are excellent root vegetables to consume. In general, most of the "nonstarchy" vegetables, from asparagus to zucchini, contain approximately two grams of protein and five grams of carbohydrate per one-half cup serving. The more starchy vegetables such as corn-on-the-cob, lima beans or potatoes, have approximately 15 grams of carbohydrate and two grams of protein per one-half cup serving. Vegetables make excellent choices in our diet.

Green vegetables, including cabbage, kale, leeks, broccoli, watercress, Brussels sprouts, parsley, turnip greens and bok choy, offer tremendous sources of vitamins A and C. Kale is abundant in calcium, yielding approximately 300 mg per cup, which is similar to four ounces of daikon or a cup of milk. Remember that vegetables contain no cholesterol and are virtually free of fat. They are also rich in fiber and easy to digest.

The round vegetables include turnips, cabbage, pumpkins, potatoes, beets, garlic and onions, to mention a few.

Cabbage is a most exciting gift from the divine. Like broccoli, it is a cruciferous vegetable that contains major amounts of compounds called isothiocyanates. These compounds have a particular affinity in preventing cancer. Cabbage also contains indole-3-carbinol, another anti-carcinogen. As a class, the cruciferous vegetables are perhaps the best weapon in combating cancers.

Vegetables can be cooked in many ways, such as boiling, steaming, stir frying, baking or pressure cooking, as well as simmering them in stews and soups. Raw vegetables are preferred when possible, especially with the skins intact.

Almost every vegetable is good for you. Some have particular advantages. Turnips are exceedingly high in vitamin A. Artichokes are abundant in iron; asparagus is high in chlorophyll. Chlorophyll, found in the tops of vegetables, alfalfa sprouts and green leaves, contains an abundance of iron and is a red cell builder. Chlorophyll compounds such as chlorella, wheat grass, green barley or magna, not only provide multiple vital nutrients and support one's energy, but also are quite helpful in the natural healing approach to arthritis. I also believe that these compounds, in general, possess anti-aging properties.

If you prefer lettuce, try leaf lettuce over iceberg head lettuce. Leaf lettuce has almost as much as a hundred times of iron as head lettuce. You really can't go wrong by consuming as many vegetables as possible. The list is endless and far beyond the scope of this text. Try as many vegetables as you can.

I do have a preference for organically grown vegetables. Remember that organic vegetables are not cultivated with pesticides, herbicides or fertilizers.

FRUITS

Most fruits contain potassium and vitamin C. As a clinical cardiologist, I prefer my clients to ingest one to two servings of fruit a day, especially if on diuretics, which deplete potassium. Even though fruits are high in natural sugars that eventually turn into glucose, they also contain abundant sources of fiber, as well as beta carotene and pectin. *Grapefruit* is the highest in pectin, and from a previous analysis, we know that pectin yields a favorable blood cholesterol profile. In an article in *Cardiology World News*, September 1991, animal research indicates that pectin may not only reduce cholesterol, but also may lower the incidence of cancer. It was demonstrated that grapefruit pectin, even in the face of a high-fat diet, restricted the development of atherosclerosis. It is important to remember to eat fruits in their fresh state. Fruits grown locally and in season are the best. Dried fruits also need to be considered. I frequently recommend my clients *eat dates, currants, raisins and figs one to two times a week*. Again, though they are high in natural sugar, they are a source of calcium as well as vitamins and fiber.

Fruits and vegetables are an excellent source of bioflavonoids, carotenoids and flavonoids. Because of the risks of heart disease, cancer and other health conditions, individuals are encouraged to consume more fruits and vegetables. Scientific evidence shows us that one's diet may play a broader role in heart disease than simply affecting cholesterol levels.

Consider that countries with a low fruit and vegetable intake, like Scotland, have a higher rate of cardiovascular disease than do countries with a high intake of fresh fruits and vegetables, like Greece. Southern Europeans consume significantly greater amounts of fresh fruits and vegetables (foods containing high amounts of carotenoids) than do Northern Europeans, and this high intake correlates with lower coronary artery disease.

In addition to antioxidants, fresh fruits and vegetables may contain vital nutrients such as flavonoids, polyphenols and quercetin (which we already discussed). Carotenoids represent the yellow and green pigments found in fresh fruits and vegetables and have been extensively studied in both heart disease and cancer. About 200 papers in the medical literature show the reduced incidence of cancer in people eating fresh fruits and vegetables containing flavonoids and carotenoids.

Carotenoids are found predominantly in fresh fruits and vegetables, with carrots being the primary source of beta carotene and tomatoes being the best source of lycopene. Lycopene has twice the antioxidant activity of beta carotene. Lycopene has been touted to be particularly effective in cancer of the pancreas and cervix. However, beta carotene has been the primary focus in studies, probably because of its potential vitamin A activity. Several studies of dietary intake of beta carotene have been shown to be inversely related to cardiovascular disease. For example, one study showed that increased beta carotene content of subcutaneous fat was directly related to lower risk of heart attack.

Other carotenoids that are present in substantial concentrations in human plasma include alpha carotene, lutein, lycopene and beta cryptoxanthin. There are approximately 600 carotenoids. Some have greater antioxidant activity than others. In a recent study of 3,806 men with increased fat and cholesterol in the blood, participants with higher carotenoid levels in the blood had a decreased risk of coronary heart disease. This finding was stronger among men who never smoked.

At the present time, there are many controlled interventional trials with antioxidants that are being carried out worldwide. During the next several years, results from observational studies and randomized trials may permit specific public health recommendations that go beyond eating a healthy diet of fresh fruits and vegetables. For now, it is a simple and established fact that the prevention of heart disease can be modified by a healthy lifestyle, utilizing a healthy intake of fresh fruits and vegetables. So eat your spinach and kiwi!

SEEDS AND NUTS

Although a small amount of seeds and nuts may provide a crunchy and tasty part of the diet, most contain high quantities of saturated fat. Most of the calories in peanut butter are derived from fat. It is my recommendation that *peanut butter be strictly avoided in all diets but those of growing children.*

THE PEANUT BUTTER STORY

Peanut butter can be a mortal sin. One of my patients, unbeknownst to me, was a peanut butter addict. George consumed approximately two jars of peanut butter a week and a jar or two of peanuts, also. He believed that peanut butter was a healthy food. After his first four-vessel bypass ten years ago, I struggled with him to reduce his serum cholesterol.

He continuously told me that his diet was healthy, consuming more fruits and vegetables, and eating less meat and dairy products. After his second four-vessel bypass, when he was 58, I gave him my book, *Lose to Win*, as a present, if he agreed to read it. He did.

He returned, shocked and chagrined, indicating that he did not know that peanut butter and peanuts were taboos. He did not realize that peanut butter and peanuts not only contain saturated fat, but other fats as well. If the peanut butter is hydrogenated, which it usually is, it contains cis-trans isomers. After George stopped the peanut butter, we were both amazed at how his cholesterol fell. He accepted his destiny and omitted these mortal sins from his diet and life. Fortunately, my patient is doing well and the story has a happy ending.

Walnuts also contain approximately 80 percent fat. Almonds, on the other hand, are more favorable, and in some clinical studies have been shown to improve cholesterol levels. *Chestnuts* are the lowest in fat and are good eaten raw or roasted. *Sesame seeds*, although containing some fat, are exceedingly high in vitamins C and E, as well as calcium and protein. Toasted sesame may be ground as an exceptional condiment called tahini, which can be used in salad dressings and soups. Tahini can be purchased at health food stores or in some supermarkets. Remember, the unhulled seeds have a longer shelf life than hulled seeds, which are more prone to spoilage after losing their protective coating.

SOUPS AND SHITAKE

Soups can be made with a wide variety of vegetables, beans, grains and, particularly, sea vegetables. Keep in mind that sea vegetables, especially *kelp*, are exceedingly abundant in magnesium and have 150 times more iodine than any of the commonly used land vegetables. Soups are also another way to incorporate *Shitake* (Shi-tah-kee) *mushrooms* in our diet. These Japanese mushrooms have been used for centuries as an ancient Oriental medicine said to promote vitality and youth. As studies have shown, they build resistance against viruses and have been used in the treatment of some cancers. They have also been used to treat fatigue. When preparing the dry Shitake mushrooms, it is best to cut them up into small pieces and place them in soups. They have a distinct flavor and can be easily assimilated into the diet. I try to consume Shitake mushrooms at least one time per week. If I don't go to my favorite Japanese restaurant (*Shogun*) around the corner, I make my quick and easy recipe of shitake, garlic and artichoke hearts. All you have to do is sauté freshly chopped garlic with a little olive oil in a pan, add shitake mushrooms and artichoke hearts from a jar. Sauté over a low heat. Add freshly chopped parsley, and you think you died and went to heaven.

SWEETENERS

As we have seen in the previous analysis, *the use of table sugar should be strictly avoided* in the diet. Other natural sweeteners are preferred. For example, *barley malt, rice syrup and apple juice* make excellent sweeteners. Although I may be going out on a limb, I will recommend *honey*. Some of my colleagues may have difficulty with this recommendation, but after much research and scrutiny into honey, I do believe this is an acceptable food that we need to consider in our diet. Since honey contains several amino acids and large amounts of B-complex vitamins, as well as C, D, E and minerals, honey is not considered an empty-calorie food like sugar. And because it is twice as sweet as most other sugars, smaller amounts can be used.

Honey comes from the nectar of flowers, which is collected in the bee's honey sac. One tiny worker bee is known to produce approximately one-half teaspoon of honey during its lifetime. Honey occurs naturally and is not produced artificially. It is made up of water, dextrose, levulose and other substances, including resins, gums and pollen. The therapeutic uses of honey as a healing agent have been passed on by multiple civilizations over the ages. Honey is an outstanding energy food. I remember our coaches telling us to swallow honey prior to our athletic bouts. It is a far better sweetener than monosaccharides such as glucose, and it doesn't require additional metabolic energy to digest.

Honey has also been used as a remedy in hayfever, allergies, sleep disorders and sore throats and colds. I am particularly impressed with Dr. Jarvis' Vermont's *Folk Medicine,* in which he discusses the therapeutic and healing effects of honey. I have tried some of his recommendations on myself, such as his cold remedy of one tablespoon of honey and one tablespoon of apple cider vinegar, with four ounces of warm water. I found it quite nurturing and healing. Since honey quickly enters the blood, however, it needs to be utilized with caution by diabetics. Because honey is a raw food, it also should not be given to infants since their immune systems are not fully developed.

Another food related to honey is *bee pollen* which, like honey, contains an abundance of vitamins and nutrients. The human consumption of bee pollen dates back to antiquity and was frequently used in the Olympic games in Greece. Today, bee pollen is gaining increasing popularity as being effective protection against many of the common pollutants in the environment, including carbon monoxide, lead, mercury and nitrites. Bee pollen is used in the treatment of allergies, similar to an allergy shot, as it desensitizes the individual. There have also been studies showing that bee pollen strengthens the resistance of immune systems in both cancer and radiation studies. This is one particular product that may become more popular because of its nutritional and high protein values.

GARLIC AND ONIONS

Garlic and onions are considered by cardiologists to be some of the most healing foods. I have discussed with you the healing properties of quercetin found in onions. In addition, many clinical studies show that garlic and onions contain an active anticoagulant that acts very similar to aspirin. Garlic has been known to lower blood pressure and inhibit platelet aggregation, thus reducing the possibility of blood clotting.

As knowledge about the benefits of garlic continues to spread from antiquity and folklore to mainstream medicine, recent research conducted around the world has substantiated that garlic may be a significant aid in lowering blood cholesterol levels, thereby lowering the risk of coronary disease. The best evidence available suggests that swallowing one half to one clove of garlic per day reduces one's cholesterol levels by nine percent. Thus, the rhyme variation of *"one garlic clove a day will keep heart disease away"* is definitely worth remembering.

Research indicates that, in addition to lowering the blood cholesterol levels, garlic provides even more protection against heart disease by preventing the formation of blood clots that can block arteries and lead to heart attack and stroke. The reported health benefits of garlic date back thousands of years. Garlic was used in Greece, Egypt, Rome, China and Japan for many centuries. In Africa, garlic was even used to treat typhus and cholera. Today, more than 600 studies are online, supporting the medicinal values of garlic.

One clove of garlic contains a meager four calories and a variety of vitamins, minerals and nutrients. For example, garlic contains selenium, a powerful antioxidant. Garlic also contains allicin, a powerful natural antibiotic that helps combat many bacteria, fungi and viruses. Allicin is capable of killing 23 kinds of bacteria - including salmonella - and at least 60 types of fungi and yeasts - including candida. Thus, garlic has been touted as a potent immune stimulant as well. This is why fresh garlic is the best way to take garlic, as much of the allicin is destroyed in cooking.

An allicin breakdown product, ajolene, is a major factor in blood clotting. This chemical plays a role in preventing red blood cells from clumping together. Researchers also believe that ajolene may have an effect on cholesterol synthesis. Clinical studies have demonstrated that garlic not only lowers cholesterol, triglycerides and LDL, but also increases the beneficial cholesterol, HDL, ratio. Several studies worldwide demonstrate similar results. These results occur in patients with coronary heart disease and in patients with high cholesterol levels.

But how does garlic fight cholesterol? According to researchers in France, the ajolene which affects blood clotting mechanisms may also prevent the digestive system from turning fat into cholesterol. It does this by inhibiting the production of human gastric lipase, an enzyme involved in the metabolism of dietary fats. If the production of cholesterol is reduced, we can surmise that the incidence of coronary disease will be reduced as well. This hypothesis has been supported in experimental animal studies showing a regression of atherosclerosis in garlic-fed animals.

By now you probably see the need for garlic in your daily diet, especially if you have a history of coronary artery disease. But how do you deal with the infamous smell of "garlic breath?" (I have patients who consume considerable quantities of garlic. They often come into my office with such a strong odor that it permeates the whole office space.)

Let's face it, having garlic breath isn't exactly the best way to make friends. The sulphur smell not only can be distributed by the breath, but also can come out of the skin. And where does the odor come from? Let me explain. To receive the benefits of garlic, our bodies activate the internal enzyme allicinase to act on a sulphur-containing amino acid to produce the reactive sulphur compound allicin. It is this sulphur component that causes the herb smell to be so repungently strong.

To counteract garlic breath, try chewing on fresh parsley or rosemary. A piece of grapefruit or orange peel may also be helpful, or you can rinse your entire mouth with a mixture of fresh squeezed lemon and water. Some people have found that chewing on fennel and raw carrots can also eliminate the symptoms. If everything fails, try taking a hot bath with oils to help get the sulphur smell out of your skin.

Raw garlic or commercially produced garlic with aged garlic extract contains significant "allicin potential" and can be a tremendous asset to lowering one's cholesterol. Besides the odor, the only problems that may occur with overuse of garlic is an upset stomach or an occasional allergic reaction.

Garlic and onions constitute a major portion of my diet as I frequently use them in many of my sauces and salad dressings. Garlic is great to use with fish, particularly when marinating. It works well with swordfish, bluefish and flounder. I will frequently marinate a fish with a dressing of chopped garlic, small amounts of white wine, freshly squeezed lemon and freshly ground basil, with one to two tablespoons of olive oil. Pour this over fish and sprinkle with fresh parsley. Marinate in the refrigerator for several hours or perhaps overnight. This type of marinade works well to take the "fishy taste" out of bluefish. When cooking, garlic can be chopped into fine pieces or can be used as whole cloves. Like onions, garlic makes a fine choice for nutritional healing.

PARSLEY

You are probably wondering why I recommend garnishing with parsley in most of my recipes. Parsley contains a high concentration of chlorophyll, which is similar to the red blood cell structure called hemoglobin. Parsley is an excellent vegetable protein and, in addition to chlorophyll, contains high quantities of iron as well as vitamins A and C. It is also interesting to note that chlorophyll combats the effects of radiation in experimental animal studies. This may be why it is considered an anti-cancer agent. Fresh parsley not only tastes great, but also yields a beautiful green color to freshly prepared foods, and green is the color associated with good health. Like several other food supplements, parsley does enhance healing. I also recommend chlorophyll derivatives in my natural healing approach toward arthritis, as well as my nutritional remedies to support patients undergoing chemotherapy or radiation therapy.

A NATURAL APPROACH TOWARD HEALING ARTHRITIS

Begin this program with the 24-hour juice and veggie fast (See enclosed recipes).

After the initial 24-hour fast, follow the schedule:

1. Consume an alkalizing diet consisting of one glass of carrot juice, apple juice or frozen wheat grass juice daily. Consume only fresh fruits and vegetables, avoiding "nightshades" such as peppers, eggplant, tomatoes and potatoes. Do not drink sodas, caffeine or chocolate. Increase yams in the diet and consume a cup of miso soup daily. Increase selection of high-fiber, low-fat foods. Decrease use of citrus, dairy and animal proteins (meat and fish).

2. Use one small Certo package or one tablespoon of Certo in apple juice daily.

3. Drink one cup of ginger tea daily.

4. Drink one chlorella, green barley or wheat grass daily.

5. The following supplements should be taken daily:
   Flax oil 1000 mg capsule after each meal
   One Optimum Health Multivitamin after each meal
   One Immuboost with bioflavonoid complex after each meal
   One cayenne 40,000 heat units after one meal

Note: Cayenne pepper is an excellent herb for coronary heart disease and cholesterol-lowering, but it may irritate your stomach. If you cannot tolerate hot chili, you will not be able to take cayenne. For a "hot stomach," the antidote is bread, a few crackers or even ginger.

NUTRITIONAL HEALING FOR INDIVIDUALS ON CHEMOTHERAPY OR RADIATION THERAPY

Begin this program with a 24-hour juice and veggie fast. (See recipe section)

After the initial 24-hour fast, follow the schedule:

1. Consume a vegan diet which consists of no dairy or animal proteins.
2. Drink ginseng tea daily.
3. Consume one cup of miso soup garnished with parsley and shitake mushrooms daily.
4. Take one frozen wheat grass, one green barley or magna extract daily.
5. The following supplements should be taken daily:
   Glutathione 100 mg daily
   One Optimum Health Multivitamin after each meal
   One Immuboost with bioflavonoid complex after each meal
   Co Enzyme Q10, 30 mg after each meal

Fourteen

RECIPES FOR
PREVENTIVE MEDICINE

The following recipes that you are about to consider are recipes that I use in my daily life. Over the years my diet has mainly been of a Mediterranean nature. I eat rice and pasta often - I really could eat pasta every day - and I use whole grains, breads, soups and vegetable stews as a staple in my diet. The pasta recipes are, for the most part, my own creation. When I don't have pasta, I usually have brown rice. I seldom eat red meat and infrequently have chicken or turkey. For the most part, I try to have fish at least one to two times a week.

I usually accompany my meals with a simple salad of *lettuce* and *tomatoes* or *vegetables* marinated in *olive oil*. I am, however, not perfect. I do "indulge" now and then and eat less healthy foods when they are prepared for me by someone else (a friend, restaurant, party, etc.). I enjoy them, too. My point here is that I have discovered ways to eat healthy foods more often and unhealthy foods less often without feeling deprived.

In the following recipes, note the frequent use of olive oil. Although it is best to use as little oil as possible, I wholeheartedly endorse the use of olive oil for salads and cooking. Since many of the recipes require two tablespoons of olive oil and most of the recipes are for a family of four or five, the grams of fat per person is still quite reasonable. For example, two tablespoons of olive oil, having 28 grams of fat divided by four people, would be seven grams of fat, the equivalent of a large tablespoon of ice cream. Even though there are seven grams of fat in the portion of olive oil, the grams of fat in the other constituents are quite low, yielding recipes that are low-fat and, in most instances, high-fiber.

Whenever possible, use fresh ingredients when preparing food, particularly *lemons, basil, parsley, watercress* and lots of *garlic* and *onions,* all of which are heart-healing. Try to *steam* as many items as you can. When cooking with oil, use *low heat* and *short cooking times* to prevent "over cooking and oxidation" of oil. Always try to minimize the use of salt and pepper.

DR. SINATRA'S LIQUID FASTING DIET
(Follow with Physician Supervision Only.)

This program has been designed to aid with weight loss in a safe, high-fiber, nonfat, nutritionally sound program. This liquid diet contains approximately 15 grams of fiber, 56 grams of protein, 139 grams of carbohydrate and about 800 calories, as well as the essential vitamins, minerals, nutritionals and herbs needed for weight loss and energy.

Through my many years of supervising weight loss programs, I have concluded that the secret to weight reduction and dissipating hunger is to avoid eating solid food. If an individual maintains a liquid program and does not put solid food in his mouth, hunger will cease, allowing for quick, healthy weight loss.

Begin this program with the 24-hour Juice and Veggie Fast, then follow the program for up to 21 days, depending upon the amount of weight you need to lose. (**This program should be followed only under the supervision of your physician.**)

Upon Awakening:	Begin each day with one-half fresh lemon squeezed into a glass of bottled water. Add one teaspoon of maple syrup for flavor.
Breakfast:	Two scoops of Great Earth Fat-Away or Ultra Energie with one glass skim milk.

Lunch:	One glass carrot juice and either frozen wheat grass, green barley or chlorella with water and one glass very veggie juice (Knudsen's Brand).
Dinner:	Two scoops Great Earth Fat-Away or Ultra Energie with one glass skim milk. One bowl of miso broth and one glass of papaya juice.
Bedtime:	One cup of either chamomile, ginger or uva ursi tea.

In addition to the above, drink four glasses of water per day, take three of the Optimum Health Multivitamin/Mineral Formula per day, one after each meal, and take the Perfect 7 psyllium herbal combination once every other day. Please note that your fiber totals will be a few grams lower on the days you are not using Perfect 7. Most of the above products can be found in your local health food stores.

24 HOUR FRUIT AND VEGGIE FAST

Begin the fast by squeezing one-half fresh lemon in a glass of bottled water and adding one teaspoon of maple syrup.

Breakfast:	Drink one glass of cranberry juice.
Lunch:	Drink one glass of apple or carrot juice with either frozen wheat grass, green barley or chlorella added. Drink one cup of ginger tea.
Dinner:	Drink one glass of papaya juice and two bowls of Hot Miso Broth.
Bedtime:	One cup of either chamomile, ginger or echinacea tea.

In addition to the above, drink eight glasses of water per day. You will find the majority of the products listed above at your local health food store.

VEGETABLE MISO HOT BROTH RECIPE

Ingredients

　2 quarts water
　4–5 carrots
　2 potatoes with skins
　1 onion
　4 Shitake mushrooms
　3 celery stalks
　1 garlic clove
　½ bunch parsley
　½ cabbage or ½ cup of Brussels sprouts
　½ bunch of broccoli
　½ inch of ginger root

Directions

Simmer all ingredients for 30 minutes, then discard all solids. Add two tablespoons of miso. Stir and simmer at a low heat.

MISO-VEGETABLE SOUP

Ingredients

1 tablespoon toasted sesame seed oil
3 quarts of water
2 onions, chopped
3 carrots, sliced
1 clove garlic, crushed
10-15 mushrooms, cut in quarters
4 teaspoons of miso
½ cup of cooked, short-grain brown rice, barley or uncooked
lentils, peas, millet, wheatberries or adzuki beans (optional)
Sea salt and freshly ground pepper
Fresh parsley, or optional watercress or scallions, chopped

Directions

Bring water to boil and add chopped onions, one clove garlic and carrots; cover and simmer until vegetables are tender. Add mushrooms which have been sautéed gently in sesame seed oil. Add the miso and simmer for approximately five to ten minutes. Do not boil. You may wish to add minimal freshly ground pepper and sea salt to taste, one bay leaf and a dash of sesame or olive oil. *You may be creative!* For example, you may add kale, string beans, spinach or other vegetables. Add one-half cup of cooked rice or other grains or beans. Garnish with freshly chopped parsley, scallions or watercress.

SEA VEGETABLE SOUP - NATURE'S WONDER

Ingredients

1 cup various sea vegetables (dulse, kelp, wakame, kombu, etc.)
3 quarts spring water
3 tablespoons toasted sesame seed oil
1 large onion, chopped
1 carrot, chopped
1½ cups broccoli, chopped
2 cloves garlic, minced
1 teaspoon thyme
1 teaspoon marjoram
Dash of cayenne pepper, freshly ground pepper, or ginger
2 tablespoons miso
Fresh parsley, chopped
Optional ingredients: mushrooms, potatoes, brown rice

Directions

Soak sea vegetables for 30 minutes and discard water (this takes out the excess sodium). Now place in spring water and simmer. Sauté onion, carrot, broccoli and garlic for five minutes, or until onions are partially translucent. Add vegetables to spring water with remaining ingredients except miso. Simmer for 30 minutes. Turn off heat. Remove one-half cup of liquid and dissolve miso in it. Return to soup and heat for three minutes, do not boil. Adjust seasonings to taste. Garnish with parsley.

This recipe, with slight modification, was taken from *Fighting Radiation with Foods, Herbs and Vitamins - Documented Natural Remedies that Boost Your Immunity & Detoxify* (Vitality, Ink., 1990) by Steven R. Schechter, N.D.

ANTIGUAN BLACK BEAN SOUP

Ingredients

2 tablespoons olive oil
½ green pepper, chopped
1 onion, chopped
½ clove garlic, minced
½ pound dried black beans cooked according to
package directions or substitute 2 one pound
cans of black beans
2 quarts water
Fresh ground pepper
2 tablespoons red wine vinegar
1 dried bay leaf
1 cup short-grain brown rice (see brown rice recipe)
Fresh parsley, chopped

Directions

In large saucepan, combine olive oil, green pepper, onion and garlic. Sauté until tender.

Add precooked or canned black beans to two quarts of water. Add remaining ingredients and simmer for 30 to 40 minutes with bay leaf. Remove bay leaf before serving and top with chopped onion, short-grain brown rice or both. Garnish with chopped parsley.

BEET SALAD WITH LEMON AND HONEY

Ingredients

    3 medium beets
    1 tablespoon olive oil
    1 tablespoon red wine vinegar
    ½ cup fresh squeezed lemon
    1 tablespoon honey
    1 teaspoon tamari
    Fresh chopped parsley

Directions

Peel and chop the fresh medium-sized beets into fine pieces, or use a food processor if desired. Make the dressing by first combining the olive oil and red wine vinegar. Add the lemon, honey and tamari to this and stir briskly. Pour over beets and toss. Sprinkle with freshly chopped parsley.

BOSTON LETTUCE AND WATERCRESS SALAD

Ingredients

1 head Boston lettuce
1 bunch watercress
1 teaspoon whole grain mustard
Sea salt and fresh ground pepper
2 teaspoons finely chopped garlic
1 tablespoon red wine vinegar
½ tablespoon balsamic vinegar
2 tablespoons extra virgin olive oil
Fresh parsley

Directions

Remove the core of the lettuce, pull the leaves apart. Cut off the tough ends of the watercress, rinse greens well and pat dry.

Put the mustard in a salad bowl with sea salt and pepper. Add the garlic and vinegar and beat with a wire whisk. Gradually add the oil, beating briskly with the wire whisk until well blended. Add the lettuce and watercress. Toss well and serve. Garnish with parsley if desired.

DAD'S ITALIAN STYLE TOMATOES

Ingredients

1 tablespoon olive oil
4 medium to large tomatoes
1 clove garlic, finely chopped
1 tablespoon balsamic vinegar
Sea salt and freshly ground pepper
Fresh basil OR crushed oregano to taste

Directions

Wash and dry tomatoes and place in the refrigerator to chill. Slice tomatoes into one-quarter inch pieces and place on a plate. Sprinkle drops of olive oil, pieces of garlic, balsamic vinegar, sea salt and pepper over the tomatoes. Sprinkle with freshly chopped basil or crushed oregano, but do not use both oregano and basil together.

EASY ITALIAN STYLE TOMATO SAUCE

Ingredients

2 tablespoons olive oil
3 cloves garlic, chopped fine
2 medium onions
2 cans Italian style plum tomatoes, or
2 pounds fresh plum or cherry tomatoes
1 ounce red or white wine
1 tablespoon freshly chopped basil
1 teaspoon freshly crushed oregano
Sea salt and freshly ground pepper
Fresh parsley, chopped

Directions

Place the olive oil in a pan and sauté with garlic and onion; cook for approximately 30 seconds to one minute. If you are using canned tomatoes, crush, chop or use a blender. For fresh tomatoes, chop them up in small cubes. Add red or white wine and sauté for three to four minutes. Add basil, oregano, sea salt and pepper to taste. Serve over spaghetti or linguini and sprinkle with freshly chopped parsley.

LINGUINI WITH GARLIC, MUSHROOMS AND PARSLEY

Ingredients

2 tablespoons olive oil
6 garlic cloves
1 12 ounce carton mushrooms
1 large bunch of parsley
1 ounce white wine
Freshly ground pepper
Freshly grated parmesan cheese

Directions

Into a pan place the olive oil and finely chopped garlic. Gently sauté for a couple of minutes. Add finely chopped mushrooms and chopped parsley. You may wish to use a food processor if available. Simmer. Add white wine. Serve over a bed of white linguini or fettucine. Sprinkle with fresh parsley and add grated parmesan cheese. Use freshly ground pepper to taste.

PASTA A LA SINATRA

Ingredients

2 tablespoons olive oil
4 chopped garlic cloves
3 small onions
1 eight-ounce jar sun-dried tomatoes
2 medium summer squash, finely chopped
Basil and fresh ground pepper to taste
Fettucine (¼ pound per person)
Grated parmesan cheese
Chopped parsley

Directions

Place two tablespoons of olive oil in a saucepan. Add chopped cloves of garlic and onions, chopped up in fine pieces. Sauté the garlic and olive oil in the pan for a few minutes.

Add a jar of sun-dried tomatoes mixed with olive oil in the blender or food processor and process to desired consistency. Place this in the saucepan over the onions and garlic. Take two to three mid-sized summer squash and chop them in fine pieces. Place into pan and sauté over a low heat. Add fresh basil and pepper. Place this sauce over a bed of fettucine. Add grated cheese and garnish with chopped parsley.

SPINACH FETTUCINE WITH A FRESH, MILD TOMATO

Ingredients

2 tablespoons olive oil
1 clove garlic, chopped
2 medium onions
6 medium tomatoes (skinned)
Fresh basil, one small bunch, cut
Freshly grated parmesan cheese
Freshly ground pepper
¼ pound pasta per person

Directions

Place olive oil, finely chopped garlic and onions in a pan and gently sauté. To remove the skin from tomatoes, place the tomatoes in a pot, cover with water and bring to gentle boil. After the water has boiled, take tomatoes out and peel skins, which should remove easily. Don't over boil. Slice tomatoes into fine pieces and add to the mixture of garlic, onion and olive oil. Sauté in pan for a few minutes. Add freshly cut strips of basil. Cook the pasta in a pot for two to three minutes and drain. Place fresh basil-tomato sauce on top. Sprinkle with grated cheese and freshly ground pepper to taste. This is a dry pasta dish, yielding little extra sauce.

PASTA SHELLS WITH ORGANIC SPINACH

Ingredients

2 tablespoons olive oil
3 cloves garlic, diced
1 dozen mushrooms, finely sliced
2 bunches organically grown spinach
1 pound pasta shells
2 tablespoons parmesan cheese
Fresh ground pepper

Directions

Into large pan put two tablespoons olive oil. Add diced garlic (or substitute one tablespoon dried flaked garlic) and sliced mushrooms. Sauté over medium heat for a couple of minutes. Add spinach. Cover pan and steam spinach for two minutes. Toss before serving. Spoon over pasta, one-quarter pound servings per person. Garnish with grated parmesan cheese and add freshly ground pepper to taste.

PASTA WITH FENNEL AND TUNA

Ingredients

1 pound fresh fennel
2 tablespoons olive oil
1 large onion
½ cup tomato sauce
½ tablespoon pine nuts
3 tablespoons dried black currants
Sea salt and fresh ground pepper
1 pound fresh tuna cut in one inch pieces
6 threads saffron
Fresh parsley, chopped

Directions

Boil the fennel until tender; drain and chop. Sauté the tuna and onion in olive oil and brown. Add tomato sauce and simmer. Add fennel, pine nuts, currants, sea salt and pepper to taste. Cook over a low heat. Continue to simmer for approximately 20 minutes.

Prepare pasta to taste and dissolve saffron into two tablespoons of warm water. Add saffron to dried cooked pasta and mix thoroughly. Spoon tuna sauce over pasta and serve with freshly chopped parsley as desired.

RICE WITH STEAMED AND STIR FRIED VEGETABLES

Ingredients

2-3 ounces of water
2-3 medium sliced carrots
2 medium zucchini, chopped
1 small bunch of broccoli, chopped
2 medium summer squash, chopped
1 dozen mushrooms, chopped
¼ head of cauliflower, chopped
1 tablespoon dried garlic or 3 cloves fresh garlic (minced)
2 teaspoons dried basil
2 tablespoons olive oil
2 tablespoons parmesan cheese
1½ cups short-grain brown rice (see brown rice recipe)
Fresh chopped parsley

Directions

Place into a wok or fry pan with two to three ounces of water. Use a steaming rack if available. Place the chopped vegetables into the wok or fry pan and cover. Sprinkle garlic and crushed dried basil on top. Stir frequently if not using a rack. Heat and steam for several minutes until the vegetables are tender. When tender, sprinkle two tablespoons olive oil over the mixture and add fresh ground pepper to taste. Sprinkle freshly grated parmesan cheese and freshly chopped parsley over the steamed vegetables and serve with short-grain brown rice.

FRIED RICE

Ingredients

1 tablespoon dark sesame oil
1 medium onion, sliced
1 dozen mushrooms, sliced
½ package frozen peas
1 tablespoon shredded daikon
4 cups cooked short-grain brown rice
½ tablespoon tamari soy sauce
Chopped scallions or fresh chopped parsley

Directions

Brush skillet with sesame oil. Heat for a minute or less but do not let oil start to smoke. Add onion, mushrooms, peas and daikon; place rice on top. If rice is dry, moisten with a few drops of water. Cover skillet and cook on low heat for 10 to 15 minutes. Add tamari soy sauce and cook for another five minutes. Stir to mix before serving.

Garnish with scallions or chopped parsley.

BUCKWHEAT PANCAKES WITH BLUEBERRIES

Ingredients

   1 cup buckwheat flour
   1 cup other whole grain flour
   1 teaspoon baking powder
   2 cups soymilk or water
   2 egg whites
   1 tablespoon canola oil
   1 tablespoon honey
   ½ cup fresh unsweetened blueberries

Directions

Stir dry ingredients together. Add soymilk, egg whites, oil and honey and mix briefly. Add blueberries and stir gently. Cook on hot, lightly-oiled griddle.

This is my version of a recipe taken from *Fighting Radiation with Foods, Herbs, and Vitamins* - Documented Natural Remedies that Boost Your Immunity and Detoxify (Vitality, Ink., 1990) by Steven R. Schechter, N.D.

Blueberry/Apple Cinnamon Bran Muffins

Ingredients

2 cups bran cereal
1 cup skim milk
1½ cup whole-wheat flour or
wheat germ white flour
2 tablespoons baking powder
2 tablespoons canola oil
2 egg whites
⅓ cup molasses
1 tablespoon honey
½ tablespoon sea salt
1 cup blueberries OR
1 grated apple and 1 teaspoon cinnamon

Directions

Mix bran and milk and let stand five minutes.
Add oil, egg whites, honey and molasses.
Add flour, baking powder mixture and sea salt.
Add blueberries or apple cinnamon mixture.
Stir until just mixed.
Bake at 400 degrees for 15 minutes.
Makes one dozen muffins.

CHICKEN WITH PEAPODS AND ZUCCHINI

Ingredients

8 oz. boneless breast of chicken
2 tablespoons peanut or olive oil
12 sliced mushrooms
1 teaspoon dried basil, crushed
2 cloves garlic, crushed, or one tablespoon dried garlic
1 tablespoon dried onion
1 medium zucchini, chopped
1 cup peapods
1 ounce white wine
Grated parmesan cheese
Brown rice (see brown rice recipe)
Fresh parsley, chopped

Directions

Slice boneless breast of chicken into two inch by one-half inch strips. Heat two tablespoons of peanut or olive oil in wok or fry pan. Add chicken, mushrooms, dried basil, garlic, onion, zucchini and peapods. Spoon-sauté until chicken is done. Add one ounce of white wine (optional). Simmer gently until zucchini and peapods are tender. Serve over pasta with grated cheese, or serve with brown rice. Garnish with parsley.

CHICKEN WITH ARTICHOKES

Ingredients

8 oz. boneless breast of chicken
2 tablespoons olive oil
1 teaspoon crushed dried basil
2 cloves garlic or one tablespoon dried garlic
12 thinly sliced mushrooms
1 ounce white wine
1 large or two small jar(s) marinated artichoke hearts (drained)
½ lemon
Fresh parsley, chopped

Directions

Slice boneless breast of chicken in two inch by one-half inch strips. Heat two tablespoons peanut or olive oil in wok or fry pan. Add chicken, one teaspoon crushed dried basil and two cloves garlic or dried garlic. Spoon-sauté. Add one dozen thinly sliced mushrooms, one ounce white wine (optional) and one large or two small jar(s) artichokes. Squeeze one-half lemon on top and mix. Garnish with fresh parsley and serve.

Variation

Additional ingredients
    Bread crumbs
    Fresh ground pepper

Directions

Slice chicken into larger pieces, four inch by two inch strips. Sprinkle with olive oil, chopped parsley, chopped garlic, bread crumbs and pepper. Grill one and one-half minutes on charcoal grill or until bread crumbs are brown. Place in bowl and squeeze lemon juice over it; add artichokes and serve.

SANTIAGO'S CHICKEN

Ingredients

4 boneless breasts of chicken
4 cloves of garlic, chopped
½ cup dry sherry or white wine
1 fresh lime
1 teaspoon paprika
½ teaspoon coriander
½ teaspoon cumin
½ teaspoon ginger
Sea salt and freshly ground pepper to taste
Fresh parsley, chopped

Directions

Place the boneless breasts of chicken in a dish and add remaining ingredients, excluding parsley, to form a marinade. Place in refrigerator for at least one to two hours. Turn the chicken every so often to coat evenly with marinade.

Cook over a charcoal or mesquite fire; grill chicken until it is tender continuing to baste with marinade while cooking. Garnish with freshly chopped parsley.

BREADED SOLE, FLOUNDER OR FLUKE

Ingredients

2 tablespoons olive oil
1 ounce white wine
Fish fillets
Italian style bread crumbs
1 lemon
½ teaspoon basil
Sea salt and freshly ground pepper
Watercress
Fresh parsley, chopped

Directions

Prepare marinade using the olive oil, wine, the juice of one lemon, basil and parsley; sea salt and pepper to taste. Dip fish in this marinade and then gently role it in bread crumbs. Grill the fish over a hot charcoal fire for only a minute or two on each side. Serve with lemon slices and garnish with chopped parsley and/or watercress.

GRILLED TUNA OR SWORDFISH WITH SPINACH

Ingredients

1 tablespoon olive oil
1 bunch of spinach
1 fresh lemon
1 pound fresh tuna or swordfish
1 teaspoon basil
Sea salt and fresh ground pepper
Fresh parsley, chopped

Directions

Into a saucepan add one tablespoon of olive oil. Rinse the spinach, discarding the stems, and place it wet into the pan and cover. Simmer for a few minutes but do not over cook. Squeeze lemon over fish and sprinkle with sea salt, pepper and crushed basil. On a hot charcoal grill, place the tuna and cook only two to three minutes per side. Tuna should be slightly red in the middle. Remember that tuna does not need to be uniform throughout in its color. Rare tuna, like rare meat, tastes very good. If you grill a swordfish, you will need to grill longer, at least until there is uniform color throughout the meat. After the fish is cooked, take the spinach out of the pan and place on a platter. Place the fish on top of the spinach, squeeze some fresh lemon over it. Sprinkle with fresh parsley and serve.

MARINATED BLUEFISH

Ingredients

2 medium sized bluefish steaks
½ lemon
2 tablespoons olive oil
1 ounce white wine
½ teaspoon crushed dried basil
3 cloves garlic, finely chopped
Sea salt and fresh ground pepper
Fresh parsley, chopped

Directions

Place bluefish steaks on a platter and squeeze fresh lemon on top. Mix olive oil, white wine, basil, garlic, sea salt and pepper. Pour over fish. Marinate for several hours or overnight if desired. Sauté fish in a lightly oiled pan or grill on an open fire. Add marinade to the sauté. Sprinkle with fresh parsley and serve. This dish is served nicely over rice accompanied by a watercress salad.

EYE OF ROUND ROAST WITH ROSEMARY AND POTATOES

Ingredients

2 pound eye of the round roast
Rosemary, crushed in a small bowl
Sea salt
Freshly ground pepper
8 small red potatoes cut in half
2 onions, sliced
2 tomatoes, sliced
Fresh parsley, chopped

Directions

Trim off excess fat from the roast and sprinkle with crushed rosemary, sea salt, and freshly ground pepper to taste. Place the roast on a rack in roasting pan and add one ounce of water. Place potatoes around roast and sprinkle with rosemary. Preheat oven to 350 degrees and then roast till tender, approximately one and a half hours. Slice thin and serve with raw sliced onions and tomatoes sprinkled with fresh parsley.

LOW-FAT EXCEPTIONAL HAMBURGERS

Ingredients

> 2 pounds top round steak or London broil, ground
> Few drops extra virgin olive oil
> Sea salt and freshly ground pepper
> Fresh parsley, chopped

Directions

Ask the butcher to weigh the meat and then trim off all the fat. Grind the round steak or roast. Knead the meat into quarter-pound hamburgers.

Into a cast iron or steel fry pan, add a few drops of extra virgin olive oil and place the hamburgers over a high heat. Sprinkle with sea salt and fresh ground pepper to taste. When cooked, serve with freshly chopped parsley.

This is the most nutritious way to have meat. Each quarter pound of the steak includes only four to five grams of fat per serving. This is an excellent recipe for those who desire red meat.

SALAD DRESSINGS

SOUR CREAM AND CHIVE DRESSING

½ cup	Light sour cream
1 clove	Garlic, crushed
1 tablespoon	Apple cider vinegar
1 teaspoon	Dijon mustard
2 teaspoons	Dried or fresh chopped chives or finely chopped fresh parsley

4 servings

LEMON-HONEY DRESSING

Juice of one large lemon

2 tablespoons	Honey
2 tablespoons	Olive Oil
½ teaspoon	Dried, crushed basil

Shake or beat in a glass jar.

4 servings

OLIVE OIL – BALSAMIC DRESSING

| 2 tablespoons | Olive Oil |
| 1 tablespoon | Balsamic vinegar |

Pinch of garlic powder and black pepper; finely chopped fresh parsley

BASICS

FLUIDS:

8 glasses of water a day
OR
6 glasses of water minimum and 2 glasses other -
    unsweetened apple juice
    mineral water
    vegetable juice (check sodium content)
    seltzer water (no sodium)
1 caffeinated coffee, tea or
2 decaffeinated coffees, teas

VEGETABLE RECIPES:

Asparagus: Boil asparagus until almost tender. Place in pan; add one teaspoon olive oil. Squeeze lemon and sprinkle garlic powder to taste. *Steamed Spinach:* Use wok or covered pan. Sauté one to two cloves garlic and one teaspoon olive oil; add spinach with two ounces water and cook until tender. Squeeze lemon and sprinkle garlic powder to taste.

Brown Rice: Wash one cup brown rice, drain water and add two cups water with a pinch of sea salt. Boil five minutes; stir. Place lid on pot and simmer for 40–45 minutes. Do not pick up lid (rice will become mushy).

Baked Potato: May use one tablespoon light sour cream, chives, scallions and parsley. May use all the raw onion, garlic and scallions you want!

Foods to Avoid

Lard, margarines, coconut oil, palm oil, salt pork, suet, bacon, meat drippings, gravies, cream sauces, catsup, mayonnaise and butter. Whole milk, cream, sour cream, non-dairy coffee creamer, whipped toppings and, particularly, cheese.

Red meat, fatty meats, spareribs, pork, ham, corned beef, regular ground meat, cold cuts, hot dogs, sausages, bacon, meats canned or frozen in sauces or gravies, frozen packaged dinners, fried fish, fried meats, egg yolk, duck, poultry skin, shrimp, sardines, fish roe and, most importantly, organ meats and peanut butter.

White flour and its commercial products, including biscuits, muffins, sweet rolls, doughnuts, waffles and french toast. Also to be avoided are french fries, potato chips, junk foods, popcorn with salt or butter.

Olives, creamed or fried vegetables and avocado.

Cream soups, dehydrated soups and commercial bouillon.

All beverages with added sweeteners, alcohol and caffeine. (coffee one cup/day)

Pies, cakes, cookies, chocolate, coconut, cashew and macadamia nuts, candies, jams, jellies, granulated sugar, molasses and especially ice cream.

Avoid the five mortal sins:

1. Margarine
2. Ice cream
3. Butter
4. White table sugar
5. Peanut butter

Foods to Substitute

Cold-pressed extra virgin olive oil, canola oil, flax linseed oil, safflower oil, corn oil, unsaturated margarines in small amounts and meat juices.

One-percent milk, low-fat cottage cheese, skim milk cheese, ricotta cheese.

Fresh fish one to two times per week, lean beef one to two times per week only, egg whites, one whole egg (250 mg cholesterol) per week, lean veal and lamb, lobster, scallops, crab in small amounts, chicken, turkey, wild goose, tuna fish (water packed), dried beans, lentils, pasta, rice, potatoes, barley, buckwheat, millet, peas, seaweed and tofu.

Graham crackers, whole-wheat and rye bread, pita bread, baked goods containing no whole milk, egg yolk or sugar, unsweetened cereals, unsalted and unbuttered popcorn.

Celery, cauliflower, zucchini, daikon (white radish), green beans, broccoli, squash, kale, onions, garlic, cabbage, parsley, mushrooms, watercress, spinach.

Chicken soup (no fat), clear broth, fat-free vegetable soup and, most importantly, miso soup.

Fresh squeezed juice, or unsweetened frozen or canned juice, mineral water, herbal teas.

Angelfood cake, puddings made with skim milk, frozen yogurt, cooked apples, all fresh fruit, unsweetened frozen or canned fruit (drained), rice pudding, chestnuts and almonds.

Fifteen

THE AGONY AND ECSTASY OF CHANGE

This chapter will deal with the many repercussions, both positive and negative, of weight loss. The text will support you in handling the multitude of new challenges you will now face, including keeping the weight off.

Since any change often brings up deep emotions and feelings, losing a great deal of weight may create some unforeseen problems. As these feelings and situations arise, it will be tempting for you to go back to your previous maladaptive, yet familiar, ways of handling them. Remember, we often use food as a substitute when we are really hungry for something else. We eat when we are alone, sad, depressed, frustrated or even happy, for that matter, as we often turn to food unconsciously. The toxic effects of repressed anger can also drive us to eat voraciously, yet without awareness.

As I mentioned before, the unconscious drives are what really motivate us and, at times, control us. This is the reason why outside feedback and support is so helpful in learning about ourselves. There are similar threads of experience that overweight people face and share. In emotional support groups, we can experience the sharing and caring of others who have the same pain and conscious struggles over obesity. While we may not be aware of our own unconscious issues, group support can sometimes bring them out. As we relate and react to others' issues, we may then realize are ours as well. Through others we can see ourselves. Mood swings, for example, are common after losing a considerable amount of weight. You may feel elated, proud of yourself, excited about your future - or *sexy*, as well as sad, scared, defensive and lost. These feelings will modify in time, but meanwhile, it helps to have someone who understands what you are going through to encourage and support you.

Not only will *You* have a reaction to your new self, but people you have known for years who are accustomed to you as a fat person are going to have various reactions to "The New You." This will range from total support and an expression of being happy, to becoming jealous of you, judging you, possibly rejecting you or, perhaps, even coming on sexually to you. *Get ready*! If you are oversensitive to others' opinions of you, their forces can be counterproductive to all your hard work. No one is able to be consistent all the time. We all have our ups and downs. You might have a friend who validates you often. If you begin to rely on her for a sense of yourself, what happens when she is having a terrible day, or week, or even year? What happens when she is feeling particularly insecure or angry? She can inadvertently pull that validation away, and if you are dependent on her for validation, you may start feeling negated and worthless.

When you stop basing your value on having or not having a particular attribute, you will feel 100 percent better about everything. *You must begin to realize that your self-worth is not about anything you do.* You are worthy simply because you exist. It is wonderful to grow and heal and change for the better, but it is not as if you will be more worthy when you do it. This kind of *conditional acceptance* sets up relentless expectations of what you *have* to change in order to be loved, lovable, happy or worthy. Unfortunately, our society programs us to believe in this destructive setup. Thus, the man who is incredibly sensitive, creative, loving, hardworking and earning a moderate yet respectable living can be seen as less valuable than the millionaire CEO of a major corporation who may have little integrity and be ruthless and uncaring, destroying the morale of his personnel, or the environment for that matter. This is a trap. *Only you can change yourself* - your beliefs and perceptions. It will take longer for society to change its faulty belief systems.

Having a stronger sense of self, of who you are and what's great about you, without validation from the outside, is important to all people - fat and thin. While support groups can help you establish these beliefs about yourself, you have to take over the helm at some point. It is particularly crucial for you to be self-directed if you are going to keep the weight off, because old foes and friends alike may tempt you to go back to the way you were, to the person they "knew or loved," that is, someone with whom they felt comfortable and unthreatened. *You can't stay stuck for anyone.* You may indeed become threatening, but this may be a gift to others. You might elicit feelings that cause them to look at themselves and their behavior just as you have. You may have a close friend who is still overweight express happiness for you, and yet, you feel the opposite energy coming toward you from "underneath," which usually is that person's unconscious or subconscious feelings. He or she may not mean to be rejecting or cruel, but when a person gets frightened or jealous, triggering the emotions on a deep level, that person can act out on you and/or attack you in one way or another.

Any strong negative reaction is an indication that *they* very much want to change for the better, too, but feel stuck, or believe they can't, or are terrified to do so. Don't fall into the trap of then feeling guilty for your own good fortune. You've worked hard for this new body. You deserve it. You are not a bad person if they experience pain due to your healthier self. Stop feeling that it is your job to protect people from their pain. There is potential for change, growth and healing through this pain. Let others grow.

WEIGHT LOSS IS GREAT - CHANGE IS HARD

There are going to be many other changes and shifts that accompany your weight loss. You might be asking yourself the following questions:

Should I go out and buy a different wardrobe?
Do I have enough money to buy the clothes I need?
What if I gain the weight back after I buy all these clothes?
Should I change my image?
With my new image, should I change my hairstyle?
With my dress size diminishing, do I look too sexy?

Many of these questions will come up and many decisions will need to be made. My advice here is to *take your time.* When you are clear, the changes will come automatically. The new you is becoming more integrated and developing a deeper sense of self, meaning that you can trust your instincts to know what you want. With new awareness, you will start to get a new sense of what to do. Although you may change your look two or three times before you find the one that feels right, take the struggle out and enjoy this process.

You may begin to feel more sexual energy. With the loss of weight, your body may look more appealing. This may cause you to feel more alive and happy, or perhaps even guilty and frightened. But sexuality is a healthy part of life, and once viewed as such can bring much pleasure and satisfaction. If you feel a new sexual energy being directed at you, use it as a tool. If it frightens you, you may want to explore it with a professional counselor. If, on the other hand, it excites you, move with it. Flirt, play, have fun. Do not try to suppress these feelings for fear that something uncontrollable will happen to you. Your body is awakening and moving toward its natural urges. Accept it and allow it to happen.

Realize, though, that a husband or wife may go into fear of losing you because you are looking so terrific. Do your best to express your love and commitment to them. Accentuate the positive effects your transformation has on them as well as you. Go out dancing. Create more romance. This could be an opportunity to ignite a delightful fire in your marriage. If, on the other hand, you are in an unfulfilling relationship, this may be the time to explore it. While I don't recommend taking on too many emotional issues at one time, neither do I suggest remaining stuck in a bad relationship. It is often difficult to let go of relationships, even destructive ones. It takes a certain conviction to heal your life, in wanting to surround yourself with people who are there for you most of the time, not trying to manipulate or control you, or use you to satisfy their needs at your expense. People hold on to destructive relationships for various reasons, sometimes out of fear of being alone. If you have connections that no longer work for you, that hurt you, then you owe it to yourself to see if you want to let them go or to work on them by restructuring the dynamics of the connection.

Be aware that in any recovery aspect, you need to take more responsibility for your actions and look at the negative patterns that you would like to change in your relationships as well as yourself. If you have a tendency to manipulate loved ones with your weight, the old pattern can show up if tensions are high at home. For example, if your spouse wanted you to lose weight and is now thrilled that you did, be careful not to reach for food if he or she upsets you. Remind yourself that you are the one who ultimately is punished by this action. Continue to find and utilize healthier ways to handle your strong emotions. If you are feeling angry and your old pattern was to eat, take note of the anger. Once you are in charge of it, instead of it being in charge of you, you can channel it in a different direction. You can go out and *take a walk, go into the woods and scream, turn on some music and dance, walk the dog, go to a movie, or call a friend and share your feelings. Remember, patterns change with repetition of new behavior.* The more you take different action, the more you acknowledge your commitment to yourself. When you care enough to change, the new behavior will strengthen, becoming easier to follow.

Let's say you go home to visit your family. At dinner, your mother tries to serve you many items that your awareness knows is harmful. If, when you say, "No, thank you," you hear "But, I made this especially for you," you will know that you need to change your usual way of interacting with her. You may feel enraged. You may feel guilty and compelled to eat what you don't want to eat. But it is better to perhaps disappoint your mother than to betray yourself. If your mother expresses love through pushing food, and saying, "No," indicates in her mind that you don't love her, you might try expressing that you appreciate the time she took to cook for you and that you love her, but that you have worked so very hard to change your eating habits that you must honor your commitments.

Be a Friend to You!

This brings to mind the case of Sally, a school teacher who was in the weight-loss program I supervised. Sally weighed about 225 pounds when she started. At five feet three inches, she was round, to say the least. Over the course of the program, she lost 70 pounds and really felt great about herself. In the two years since the program ended, Sally has kept off at least 50 pounds of the original weight, fluctuating within a 10-15 pound range. I spoke with her recently, and she is still determined to lose more. Her twin sister, on the other hand, was also in the program and, while losing weight then, has put all of it back on. Now the relationship between the sisters is strained. Sally sometimes feels responsible for the tension, for having succeeded where her sister didn't, yet she knows she must honor herself and not go back to the old way of punishing herself. After she lost the weight, Sally wrote me the following letter. You might be able to relate to it.

> "Smile 'tho your heart is aching," a corny song I suppose, and the rest of it just gets worse. What happens if you actually lived that line all your life?
>
> There have been a multitude of lines ingrained into my being over the past 38 years, lines such as, "keep busy, don't make waves; a quitter never wins; SMILE, it will be okay; what you give you gather; do for

others even if it means sacrifice; do your best; make believe you are happy and you will be; show everyone you can cope as well as deal with everything for everyone else; never never say no or I'm too busy right now; always ask how you can help." Do things you really don't want to do, Sally, just to please others so they will give you praise, a pat on the shoulder, a hug and/or compliment. But hugs, compliments, smiles and words of encouragement aren't quite enough right now. I've got to do more.

Smile. Smile. Smile. Try to help others. Feel sorry for them instead. Be a candle, burn yourself out lighting the way for everyone else, and then sit home in the dark and smile and EAT, EAT, EAT. That was my cure. Who needs help? Keep busy, it will cover the loneliness, emptiness, lack of self-worth, self-doubt, insecurity, the side of me I won't accept as part of me right now. Stop wondering who will help me when I need it. Forget it. Tuck the thought away. I'll never need help. What a joke! I do need help.

I was taught how to love everyone, it helps build self-confidence and self-esteem in others, but wait, what about me? These characteristics are now growing within me with the weight-loss. I now have more energy to do more for others - WRONG! That's the energy I need to turn inward toward myself. That's part of becoming the WHOLE me, not just the me who's becoming thinner. I have to do this for me, the person who needs to learn to relax and do things just for me. *If I take the time to love and nurture myself,* people will love me and I will love me, even though I have faults. People won't love me because I'm the person who can do it all.

I need to take little steps instead of diving into this concept. I am starting to chip away at my smiling facade and peeking inside, discovering that there really is a beautiful person underneath who is slowly learning to become satisfied.

What am I doing for 10 weeks this summer? No more two aspirin or Band-Aid cures! I wouldn't think of doing that to others or, God forbid, to the children I teach. I want to dig into who I really am and find those roots to help ground me. What's wrong with not smiling for awhile? Not a thing because I AM growing with patience, love, caring, intelligence, dedication, time, sharing, God's help, and all the energy that I take pleasure in giving to others every day of my life. I'm not only going to have strong roots and growth, I'm going to BLOOM!

God didn't and won't sponsor any junk."

Love, as we can see, has incredible healing powers. Filling yourself up with food or even someone else's love will not fill the emptiness. But loving yourself will. And if you become upset with yourself or suffer a setback and go through some turmoil that results in overeating, be careful not to turn your self-love into self-hate. If this does occur, catch it as soon as possible and *apologize for turning against yourself.* This may sound silly, but it works. Self-hate, or anger turned within, will only cause you to feel even more turmoil and possibly prolong or create another binge. If you slip up, remember to forgive yourself. Understand that it takes time to change these old patterns completely, and don't become greedy. If you have lost 25 pounds or have toned your stomach, but your legs still need work, look in the mirror with approval. Don't knock those legs. They need you now to love them as they are. In all the therapy I've done with women, their biggest issue was the size and shape of their legs. Perhaps this is because women feel that men place too much emphasis on legs. However, in the Men's Self-Awareness Group that I run, I've learned this is not the case.

FRIENDS OR FOOD POLICE?

Weight reduction is recovery and self-healing. Perfection is not the key to happiness. Be patient, but keep the momentum going. Take a few moments here and there to praise yourself and express gratitude. Look in the mirror and thank yourself out loud. This may sound silly, but your mind needs this type of reinforcement, and speaking to yourself while looking into your own eyes is a powerful exercise. While others may support you or even unconsciously try to undermine you, you are the one who is ultimately responsible for your own feelings, your growth, your behavior, your happiness and your body.

Friends may think they are being encouraging by being "food police," suggesting what you eat or don't eat. You can choose to respond to each situation accordingly. If they do indeed care, you can thank them for their suggestion, knowing in your heart that you are "recovering." On the other hand, a friend may think that something you are eating is bad for you while you know that in your program of awareness, you can balance the food with other less caloric items. You are responsible for your own choices. Only you know what truly is best for you. And if you are doing something that is not in your best interest, you will know it, and a gentle reminder may be all that you need to put you back on track. You are writing your own program and can create it according to your own taste and preferences. Support from friends is fine. Intrusion is not. While you may want an occasional reality check, be aware that others' reality may not be your own. And you must stay firmly within your own boundaries.

Checking your real feelings is a good way of staying in touch with yourself. When someone makes a comment that you know is true about yourself, you feel it in your gut. When they try to force their reality on you, however, you will feel an assault to your being and can tell them so. This is self-actualization and it requires a vigilance that many people would rather not face. These are exactly the confrontations that some people back away from by padding themselves with fat or acquiescing to everyone else's wants and needs. While this may or may not have been your old behavior, it certainly isn't part of a new self-worth investment in *Optimum Health.*

Other friends may be consciously or unconsciously jealous of you, trying to undermine you. Friends, co-workers and family members close to you, who do not respond well at first to your transformation, are resisting change. They were comfortable with you the way you were, so they may be reacting to losing the familiar. In due time, they will come back around and accept you.

As a matter of fact, you may be feeling a loss yourself. If you have been overweight for many, many years, or you have lost 60-100 pounds, it may feel as though you have lost a friend. Or if you have been using your weight to hide, you may feel a sense of fear in terms of how you will survive. This is when it is especially beneficial to look yourself in the eyes in the mirror and find comfort where you once may have seen rejection. In time, you will adjust and develop healthy ways to feel safe.

Again, taking quiet time to acknowledge that you love yourself is one such way to do this. Rejoicing in your weight loss is another. You may reward yourself by buying clothes in the regular-size department instead of the "big-is-beautiful" department. If you have been leading a reclusive life and begin to feel more alive and want to go out more often, do so. Or, like Roger Buffaloe, if you had trouble fitting into cars before, you may now physically and metaphorically love the pleasure of riding comfortably. As you participate in more activities that satisfy you and occupy your thoughts, you will be relieved of your preoccupation with your body. Allow yourself to enjoy your meals; put love into your food, especially when you prepare it for yourself and others. Food made with love tastes better. I know. My father taught me this, and his meals were always outstanding. I've never had a weight problem. I appreciate food and the love that goes into it, but I know it is only a symbol for the love of the people behind it.

As you adopt a new lifestyle that supports you in making changes, losing weight and keeping it off, you will have helped everyone around you. You will have more energy available to give to others because you first gave to yourself; and you will give authentically only when and what you are able. You may be an inspiration to those who are close to you, exuding a positive energy that says "I've changed for the better. You can too." Our society desperately needs role models who offer hope. We can look back on that old person in the mirror and see our growth reflected in the symbol of our new image - an image of integration and self-love. As trite as it may sound, I genuinely feel, *we all need hope, faith and love.*

Sixteen

THE SEARCH FOR THE FOUNTAIN OF YOUTH

Greek mythology discussed the "myth of aging" in one of the most famous and ancient riddles of the Sphinx. The question was, *What is it that has one voice and yet becomes four-footed, two-footed and three-footed?*

Oedipus provided the "obvious" answer: the human being. The human being crawls on all fours in infancy, walks on two legs as an adult and then leans on a cane as he approaches old age. The assumption in the riddle of the Sphinx indicates that as we grow older, we become stiff and debilitated.

As we age, a gradual degenerative process occurs. Aging becomes synonymous with degeneration. Scientific medicine has shown that many of our hormone systems decline with age.

But, do we really have to age? Can we interrupt the gradual deterioration of the body? Many people in every generation age, yet continue to function without developing degenerative diseases. Geriatric analysis shows that humans age in very different ways. Perhaps some age successfully while others don't. The question we need to ask ourselves is, *What is it that makes one person age quicker than another?*

AGING GRACEFULLY

Certainly, people are different. I have often asked myself why some of my very old patients look younger than their age and some of my younger patients look older than their age. Recently, a Russian gerontologist tried to answer this question. He examined 15,000 individuals, ages 80 and above, in the Soviet Union.

He found four common denominators for longevity:

1. These people worked outside with lots of physical activity.
2. They ate a diet of grains, fresh fruits and vegetables. Many sometimes lacked for food, which obviously caused calorie restrictions.
3. They enjoyed good relationships with love, intimacy and support in their lives.
4. Many of these individuals continued to have an active sex life, even in their 80s and 90s.

Thus, the common denominators for longevity appear to include a low-fat, high-fiber diet, exercise and supportive, loving relationships. In addition, these people had an optimistic outlook on life. There is nothing like intimacy, support and an emotional connection to keep life worthwhile.

On the other hand, a pessimistic outlook on life with negative emotions of hostility, anger and resentment, depresses not only one's personality, but also one's immune response. Therefore, when considering longevity, you have to include mind/body interactions.

Before we discuss aging, we need to be clear about the symptoms of aging. The most obvious symptom of aging is disease. Diseases related to aging include coronary artery disease, arthritis, osteoporosis, low back pain, Alzheimer's and cancer. We need to ask ourselves the question, *Is modern medicine really useful in curing these illnesses?*

As a physician, I have to say that the answer is *No*.

Other symptoms of aging can be very subtle, like diminished sexual activity, poor sleep habits, constipation, joint stiffness or poor skin tone. More obvious symptoms include memory loss, diminished immunity and susceptibility to infections, allergies and/or diseases.

Many of my patients really don't understand that the older we get, the more weight we gain because our metabolic rate falls. Ask any man in his 40s and he will tell you that his waist size is increasing. I know it is happening to me! Many of us also get little exercise after the age of 40.

And then there is the most obvious symptom of aging that I see: the patient who comes into my office taking multiple drugs for various symptoms and illnesses.

Although many of my patients don't specifically ask me to prescribe anti-aging therapies, many would like an increase in sexual libido, would prefer a better memory and would like to sleep better.

WE CAN BE FRIENDS WITH AGE

Age does not have to be an enemy. The only enemies that I see are illnesses like cancer, severe depression, resignation and despair. So, what can we do to delay or prevent aging? Is there anything that we can do to give us a better quality of life, full of vitality, energy and enthusiasm for living? The answer is *Yes!*

There are many ways to attack the aging process. There are nutritional and food therapies, vitamins, minerals and enzyme therapies; herbal therapies, exercise therapies and other recommendations, including good personal hygiene and minimum exposure to sunlight, microwaves and x-rays. Maintaining a normal or even less than normal body weight will also help prevent aging.

More advanced aging therapies include the use of hormones, amino acids and powerful antioxidants. Later in this chapter, I will give you my prescription for health, healing and longevity which combines all of these therapies.

Previously in this book, we discussed important health maintainers. We talked about cholesterol levels, preferably low LDL and high HDL as good markers. We talked about iron overload and about the harmful effects of homocysteine. But there are also two other exciting markers of health. They include the protein serum albumin in your body and the hormone called DHEA (Dehydroepiandosterone).

Think of the ice man that was found in the European Alps. Although he had some arthritis and possibly even some vascular disease, he was a very healthy individual. They found a grain pouch on him. He probably ate seeds, grains, plants and roots. Biochemically, the ice man was in good shape. He had high levels of DHEA and low levels of insulin. This is modern man in reverse. We have low DHEA and high insulin levels, making us prone to the degenerative diseases I just mentioned.

What causes degenerative disease and aging? The answer is free radical oxidative stress, causing cellular oxidative stress and deterioration. What can we do to protect ourselves from unnecessary free radical damage and optimize our health? Read on.

Although I've mentioned DHEA, I really didn't tell you what it was. Dehydroepiandrosterone is the mother steroid precursor to some 18 hormones in the body. As we age, our DHEA levels fall. Remember when you were 18? Do you remember how much energy you had? We find the highest hormonal levels of DHEA during this time.

If our DHEA levels decline too rapidly with age, we get sick more often. For example, there was a recent article in *Circulation - A Journal for Cardiologists*, indicating that lower levels of DHEA were found in patients with premature coronary heart disease. Declining levels have also been noted in cancer and the HIV positive syndrome. And, when DHEA levels fall to very low levels, HIV turns into the actual AIDS syndrome.

In animal studies, animals supplemented with DHEA showed an increased life span, reduced degenerative diseases and reduced body fat. DHEA is also known to be a factor in weight reduction. Other uses of DHEA include enhancing immunity by increasing the antibody effect. It also reduces undesirable blood clotting. DHEA increases sex hormones in men and women, which may help to activate sexual libido.

WILD YAM EXTRACT

Wild yam extract is a natural form of DHEA. As mentioned previously, Wild yam is dioscorea villosa. Wild yam extract actually contains very low doses of DHEA. However, remember that before taking any of these agents, whether DHEA, wild yam extract or pregneolone (a precursor of DHEA), you should consult your physician, as these therapies may cause some side effects. With DHEA, men should be evaluated periodically for prostate size and gland activity. In women, excessive DHEA may increase facial hair. Discussing these concerns with your physician should eliminate any problems when contemplating these treatments.

STRESS AND HEALTH

It's also interesting to note that DHEA levels have an inverse relationship with our emotional stress. That is, the more stress we are under, the more serum cortisol (the body's natural hormone response to stress coming from the adrenal glands) increases. As cortisol increases, DHEA levels decrease. It isn't any wonder, when we're under stress, our immunity decreases.

Frequently, one may get a cold, an infection or even a heart attack under situations of acute emotional stress. Sometimes when we're under stress, our memory fails. Research seems to indicate that higher serum cortisol levels can be associated with structural changes in brain cells, causing cell death. As a result, our memory fails. Since the effects of stress can be cumulative over time, our memory, as well as our brain, is affected. It is true that severe, unrelenting stress may be a risk factor for Alzheimer's disease and premature death. There is a lot of credibility in the expression, "Don't worry, be happy."

Recently, I heard an exciting lecture at the second annual conference on Anti-aging Medicine and Biomedical Technology for the Year 2010. The lecture was about how simple meditation can be used in reducing stress and vigilance. Vigilance is being fearful that something could happen. It is waiting for the other shoe to drop or waiting for some disaster to occur. The presenter, Darma Singh Khalsa, a meditator for years, shared vital information on meditation, as a way to lower serum cortisol levels, thereby improving memory. Meditation not only enhances mental and physical health; it also supports memory. In Alzheimer's disease, as memory decreases, DHEA levels fall and albumin (the body's master protein) levels deteriorate.

YOU AND YOUR ALBUMIM

Multiple studies have indicated that lower levels of albumim are also a predictor of health and disease. In Alzheimer's disease, for example, the lower the serum albumim, the more severe the dementia. Albumim is the most abundant serum protein found in the cerebral spinal fluid as well as other tissues. Albumim is our most versatile antioxidant. It stabilizes and strengthens our immunity and transports vitamins A, D and C, along with minerals zinc, copper and magnesium throughout the body. It is important to keep your albumim as high as possible. If the body contains at least 48 grams per liter, this demonstrates excellent health.

Although increasing nutritional defenses by eating a healthy diet and taking vitamins, minerals and herbs will help maintain our albumim, increasing our personal hygiene is one of the best ways of keeping our albumim level elevated. Antibodies claim a large percentage of the body's plasma proteins. In response to immune system challenges such as bacteria and allergies, the percentage of antibodies rises while the albumim drops. It works something like this. Plasma proteins are maintained at approximately 75 grams per liter in the body. Albumim makes up 60 percent of the protein, antibodies 20 percent and carrier proteins another 20 percent. If we are under stress, have an acute infection or an allergy, our antibodies rise to the offending invaders. As antibodies get higher, albumim must get lower.

If albumim gets lower, this creates an overall weakened condition. So why is it vital during situations of infection and high allergy states to increase our personal hygiene? By cleaning our fingernails, eyes, nose, skin and nasal cavities, it helps to eliminate sources of bacterial contamination. This reduced stress on the immune system allows the albumim levels to be maintained.

Albumim and DHEA are certainly terrific partners in maintaining health and delaying aging. But we still have not defined the biochemistry of aging. In other words, we haven't gone into detail as to why aging occurs in the first place.

HOW AGING OCCURS

I believe that aging is really a disease. Although there are many theories, including hormonal, neuroendocrine and immunologic, perhaps the best and most reasonable theory is the free radical theory. Aging, in simple terms, is related to the accumulated damage to membranes and cells as a consequence of oxidative stress.

Remember that oxidative stress occurs in a cellular environment, characterized by an elevation and steady state concentration of free radicals and other reactive oxygen species. Oxidative stress occurs if the delicate balance between cellular endogenous antioxidant defenses and the offending agents triggering these oxidative conditions is overwhelmed. Thus, if the biochemical war is in favor of oxidative stress, we tend to interrupt and impair cellular membranes.

The destruction of cellular membranes is, therefore, the sinequanon of the aging process. If cellular membranes are kept intact, cellular functions remain intact. However, if cellular membranes receive permanent damage due to free radical attacks, our health deteriorates to degenerative diseases and aging. In a previous analysis, I gave you a simple explanation of the free radical theory. For a more comprehensive evaluation of aging, however, I should discuss the free radical theory in deeper detail.

Although oxygen is necessary for aerobic life, the metabolism of oxygen has an ominous consequence - the formation of free radicals. A free radical is a molecule with an odd number of electrons (negatively charged particles). Stable compounds such as oxygen contain paired electrons. In contrast, highly unstable and reactive compounds (free radicals) contain unpaired electrons. The normal metabolism of oxygen by cells in the body proceeds via a pathway known as reduction.

During this process, oxygen is "reduced" to water by the addition of four electrons by a sequential transfer. The oxygen molecule acquires electrons one at a time, thereby forming at each stage molecular fragments (free radicals) with unpaired electrons having very high chemical reactivity. As unpaired electrons are transferred to a nonradical, another free radical is created, setting up a chain of reactions of electron transfer. Such chain reactions may occur thousands of times before the reaction is terminated.

Under normal conditions, 95 to 98 percent of molecular oxygen consumed by cells is reduced to water. The remaining two to five percent, however, give rise to reactive free radicals, even under the best conditions. Free radical generation reaches much higher levels during situations of extraordinary radical flux such as infection, inflammation, radiation exposure and high oxygen tension states that occur during vigorous exercise. It also occurs in situations in which one has a heart attack and the occluded vessel doing the damage is opened by a "clot buster." By using an agent that dissolves the blood clot, the heart attack is usually much smaller and the patient survives.

However, even though a patient receives a "clot buster," a small residual heart attack remains. The reason is the result of massive free radicals causing the heart damage. Although research shows that free radicals may play a fundamental role in supporting some basic life processes, such as hormone synthesis, these unstable and deleterious highly charged particles have been incriminated to cause extensive damage to cell membranes, cell contents (called organelles) and even DNA itself. This paradox of free radical chemistry has generated considerable interest among health care professionals, especially those interested in preventive medicine.

I have already told you that free radicals, over time, cause biological changes which may lead to the acceleration of aging and the development of a variety of chronic diseases such as heart disease, cancer and cataracts. Fortunately, the body has its own complex antioxidant defense systems against free radicals. If it were not for these antioxidant defense systems, thousands of chain reactions of free radicals generated within seconds could quickly cripple and destroy cellular functions. Most of these natural body antioxidant enzymes deactivate free radicals by using them to generate safer chemical reactions. However, these antioxidant systems can be overwhelmed during extraordinary oxidative stress such as an acute heart attack, or after the ingestion of a heavy fat-laden meal. Another key factor in free radical damage is one's intrinsic metabolic rate.

A definite correlation exists between cancer, aging and aging-related disorders because of oxidative damage related to the breakdown of food and the energy one consumes due to the breathing process. This is the so-called metabolic rate in mammals. The higher the metabolic rate, the greater the number of free radicals released by oxygen reduction. The metabolic rate and free radical damage which follows can be slowed by caloric or protein restriction. This has been demonstrated in the animal model by rodents on a restricted diet. A similar finding was noted among survivors of World War II. Individuals who were starved or were survivors of concentration camp conditions had a significantly lower incidence of coronary artery disease later in life. This was a by-product of sharply restricted caloric intake.

The basal metabolic rate is variable for different species, including man. Professor Ames and other investigators estimate that 100,000 oxidative hits to DNA occur per day in a rat. Since oxidative lesions in DNA accumulate with age, by the time the rat is two years old, it has had approximately two million DNA lesions. Since mutations associated with DNA damage also accumulate with age, a two-year-old rat is more susceptible to degenerative diseases like cancer than a younger rat. Although the basic metabolic rate of the rat is seven times higher than that of a human, similar reasoning may be applied. Thus, the older we get, the more susceptible we are to cancer and other degenerative diseases because of this free radical induced DNA damage.

The most potent free radical invader in these oxidative processes is the hydroxyl radical (OH). The hydroxyl radical is a key factor in the chain reaction formation of polyunsaturated fatty acids (PUFA). PUFA peroxides are extremely toxic and damaging to the cardiovascular system. They also play a role in the aging of the eye, causing lens opacity and cataract formation. They are also related to nerve degeneration.

PUFAs, like free radicals, present a paradox. Although they are essential building blocks for providing cellular elasticity and pliability, they are easily broken down by free radicals. I have previously recommended that you avoid polyunsaturated fatty acids. Since PUFA peroxides play a major role in the development of atherosclerosis and cancer, I would avoid the polyunsaturated fats found in the diet, such as margarines and unsaturated oils. Again, the safest oil that you can consume from the cardiac point of view to prevent heart disease is olive oil, a monounsaturated fat.

OTHER ANTI-AGING STRATEGIES

L-Arginine

I previously discussed anti-aging strategies, using calorie restriction, vitamin and mineral supplementation, DHEA and wild yam. A newer agent on the horizon is L-Arginine. Briefly introduced in my chapter on cholesterol and women, L-Arginine has received favorable press in preventing both heart disease and cancer.

To refresh your memory, animal studies have shown that the amino acid L-Arginine reduces cholesterol blockages in the thoracic aorta. It works like nitrous oxide, which is a substance that keeps blood vessels open. Physicians call this vasodilatation.

Although L-Arginine may be used for people with refractory elevations of cholesterol, a recent article in surgical literature also advocates high dosages of L-Arginine for stimulating immune function. In one review, L-Arginine was said to increase immune function in patients with breast cancer. The authors recommended 30 grams of L-Arginine per day as adjuvant therapy in breast cancer, in combination with the traditional approaches. Melatonin, another anti-aging prospect, has also shown promise in treating similar tissue cancers.

Melatonin

Melatonin is another powerful antioxidant. This naturally occurring substance comes from the pineal gland situated in the brain and from areas of the retina and gastrointestinal tract. Melatonin is secreted in response to light. If people do not get enough light, they may suffer from a seasonal affective disorder (SAD). When you do not get out in the light or if your eyes are not exposed to daylight, melatonin is not properly secreted by the pineal gland or the retina. Such low levels of melatonin have been discovered in people with seasonal affective disorders; resulting in an increase in depression and fatigue.

Melatonin is a powerful free radical scavenger. It helps to eliminate the hydroxyl radical, one of the most devastating free radicals in the body. Like DHEA and Albumin, the natural production of melatonin decreases with age, particularly for those over the age of 40. Fasting and dieting increase the natural body stores of melatonin. This is in itself a bonus when we lose weight.

Raising melatonin levels may be one method to slow aging. In animal studies, melatonin definitely produced an increase in longevity in populations of rats and mice. In addition to stimulating immunity, increasing antibodies and promoting lymphocyte function, melatonin has also been shown to enhance sleeping.

Many physicians and researchers take melatonin at night because it has no side effects. I can personally attest to the benefits of taking melatonin for the relief of jet lag. Since I began using melatonin while flying across the country to give lectures, jet lag has become virtually non-existent.

DMAE

Another interesting compound to consider is DMAE, called Dimethyaminoethanol. This substance is found in anchovies and sardines - the famous "brain foods." A precursor of choline, DMAE increases production and alters levels of acetylcholine in the brain. Acetylcholine is needed for learning and memory. DMAE preserves memory by stabilizing and building cellular membranes. When these membranes are destroyed, accelerated aging occurs. DMAE can be taken as a supplement of as little as 100 mg daily and has been found to increase mood, memory, learning, sleep and energy.

L-Deprenyl

Lately, I have been writing more and more prescriptions for the agent L-Deprenyl, marketed as Eldepryl in this country. This drug was originally discovered in Europe, perhaps as recently as twenty years ago. Deprenyl has tremendous merits.

As we age we produce a substance called monoamine oxidase (MAO). In patients with Alzheimer's disease, monoamine oxidase levels are extremely high. To lower the body's amount of monoamine oxidase, we must inhibit its development. This is where L-Deprenyl comes in.

Deprenyl is actually a monoamine oxidase inhibitor, lowering the levels of MAO while increasing the body's levels of dopamine. In fact, as a monoamine oxidase B-inhibitor, Deprenyl works to increase not only dopamine in the brain, but also levels of norepinephrine and phenylethylamine, the so-called "love hormone."

Dopamine is one of the most important hormonal transmitters of our brains. Without dopamine, people become stiff, immobile, severely aged and unable to function on a musculoskeletal level. In Parkinson's disease, dopamine levels often become nonexistent as the disease progresses. This lack of dopamine is why patients with Parkinson's have a "stare," resting tremors, rigidity of limbs and often a shuffling walk which they cannot stop.

In addition to its therapeutic effects in Parkinson's disease, some investigators believe that Deprenyl may be useful in treating Alzheimer's disease as well. By stimulating the body's natural level of dopamine, Deprenyl has been said to enhance mental alertness and memory. It has also been touted to increase libido by raising the amounts of central nervous transmitters in the brain. Thus, Deprenyl may not only heighten one's overall energy and mental alertness, but also may effect one's sexual libido as well.

The production of dopamine in our brain decreases with advancing age, usually after the age of 45. The word on this drug is not out yet. Unfortunately, L-Deprenyl is not popular in the United States. Nevertheless, Europeans, who have much more experience with L-Deprenyl, prescribe it frequently. I have met a few researchers and physicians, for example, who not only prescribe Deprenyl for their patients for an array of depressive and mental disorders, but also use this anti-aging remedy on themselves. Many physicians also take pycnogenols - a class of powerful antioxidants.

Proanthocyanidins

I am very comfortable with taking Proanthocyanidins.

Proanthocyanidins are remarkable plant-derived substances originating from standardized extracts of rapeseed and pine bark. Arguably, they are the most powerful natural antioxidants available. The Proanthocyanidins go by popular names such as pycnogenol and OPC (Oligomeric Proanthocyanidin). These registered trademarks are patented and distributed in Canada, Western Europe and North America.

Pycnogenol

The French researcher Professor Jacques Masquelier is credited with the discovery of the compound he named pycnogenol. In 1987, he patented pycnogenol as a free radical scavenger, licensing his patent to Horphag Research Ltd. in the United Kingdom.

The history of pycnogenol, however, dates back to the North American Indian medicine man. He used pycnogenol as a way of curing the devastating disease called scurvy. In 1535, the French explorer Jacques Cardia and his crew of 110 men were almost wiped out by scurvy. The crew had been existing on sea biscuits and meats instead of fresh fruits and vegetables. As members of his expedition continued to die, Cardia met a Quebec Indian who gave him a remedy for scurvy. The Indian brewed a tea from the Anneda Tree, described by Cardia and his comrades as a large tree with evergreen leaves and easily removable bark. Cardia fed his crew and himself the bark, pine needles and leaves. Fortunately, many of them survived, including Cardia.

Years later, Jacques Masquelier discovered this information, returned to France and found similar potent bioflavonoids from the Pinus Maritima Tree of Southern France. Consequently, the proanthocyanidins, a life saving cure for scurvy, exploded in the later part of the 20th Century as the most potent antioxidant available.

Proanthocyanidins contain many bioflavonoids like catechins and epicatechins, as well as organic acids. We have already discussed the polyphenolic compounds quercetin and other flavonoids that are extremely important in preventing both coronary heart disease and cancer.

In addition to proanthocyanidins, pycnogenol contains catechin, epicatechin and small organic acids like caffeic acid. These components include a strong family of flavonoids which are capable of enhancing health and healing. They are also very powerful antioxidants, which enhance memory, stimulate immunity and improve circulation (particularly capillary permeability). They also may be used in diabetic retinopathy.

Pycnogenol also improves skin smoothness and elasticity, reduces phlebitis and assuages the inflammation from allergic disorders. Furthermore, pycnogenol serves an important function for the brain. Since it is one of the few dietary antioxidants that can readily cross the blood-brain barrier, pycnogenol is able to protect brain cells, resulting in stimulated memory and retarded aging. Because of this ability, I believe pycnogenol has considerable potential in anti-aging strategies.

When implementing pycnogenol, be aware that your body may respond negatively at first. Although there have been no reports of toxicity with pycnogenol's compounds, the body may react with a detoxification response. This occurs when the body quickly interacts with the nutrient, and, in an effort to cleanse out any junk or toxins, may become "allergic" for a short period of time. The detoxification effect is for the body's protection; the short allergic situation soon dissipates. Actually, this process can be a very positive sign that this talented nutrient is working.

There are literally dozens of public studies on pycnogenol's safety and benefits. It has been used for three decades, with no signs of toxicity. I, too, like pycnogenol and have used it personally. I even included it in one of my Immuboost formulas for stimulating immunity and for anti-aging (brain membrane stabilizing) strategies.

In conclusion, I feel that pycnogenol, L-Deprenyl, melatonin, wild yam extract (DHEA), L-Arginine, proanthocyanidins, Co Enzyme Q_{10} and many other vitamin and mineral supplements enhance health and healing, and may even work as anti-aging agents. Before considering DHEA, melatonin, DMAE or L-Arginine you must get approval from a physician.

AGENTS NOT RECOMMENDED

There are, however, several agents I do not recommend at this time. Human growth hormone, although promising, needs more research. Another popular agent is GH3, or gerovital, discovered by Romanian scientists. This anti-aging formula's chemical derivatives are procaine and PABA. Although gerovital demonstrates a mild anti-inflammatory and mild anti-depressant effect in the elderly, I would not use this hormone until further research confirms its safety and effectiveness.

A STRATEGY OF PREVENTION

The search for the fountain of youth has been going on for centuries. Today, people are especially concerned with delaying the process of aging. In my mind, the best method for halting disease and delaying aging is prevention. A good prescription for disease prevention and anti-aging tactics includes a healthy diet, targeted nutritional supplementation with vitamins, minerals and herbs, green chorophyll-type foods and mild to moderate exercise regimens. Those seeking a more aggressive approach may consider the leading hormonal and protein therapies.

When fighting age and disease, we must not forget the environment. I am genuinely concerned about the deterioration of the water supply in this country. In my office and home, we use bottled water and central water filters to filter out chlorine, heavy metals and harmful bacteria. I also advocate air filters, which extract carbon monoxide, pollens and other impurities from the air.

Futuristic lighting is another area of interest for me. Remember that full spectrum lighting is much more natural and safe. It also helps to nurture the body, particularly the eye and pineal gland, which stimulates natural body sources of melatonin. Recently, I placed full spectrum lighting in my home and office. Healthy air, water and light are essential components of any anti-aging program.

In summary, I believe that futuristic medicine will be one that engages the anti-aging process, because if you can delay aging, you can delay disease. For instance, take the problem of cataracts. If cataracts could be delayed a mere ten years, the country could perhaps save billions of dollars in reduced health care costs.

Searching for the fountain of youth can be very exciting, when done in a way that supports one's continuing vitality and promotes living a satisfied and enthusiastic life. Getting old is not bad - it's inevitable. Premature aging with its accompanying degenerative diseases is an unnecessary hardship. This pathological aging process certainly can be a tragedy. But we have the opportunity to delay and even prevent it! Think about it!

My Recommendations for Health, Healing and Longevity

1. Nutritional and Food Therapy

1. Consume a high-fiber (greater than 30 grams), low-fat diet (less than 30 grams) per day.
2. Increase consumption of fresh fruits and vegetables, organic preferred (5 to 9 servings per day).

3. Consume more grains, complex carbohydrates, pastas, beans, rice, etc.
4. Consume less animal protein and dairy products.
5. *Omit* granulated white table sugar, margarine, butter, ice cream and peanut butter.
6. Use more monounsaturated fats such as olive oil, canola oil or almond oil.
7. Avoid polyunsaturated fatty acids such as corn oil, safflower oil, etc.
8. Use more Omega #3 oil such as organic flax oil containing Linolenic Acid, an essential fatty acid.
9. Use miso preparations one to two times per week.
10. Increase garlic and onion in the diet; consider sea vegetables.
11. Substitute tea in place of coffee.
12. Maintain an adequate calcium intake of greater than 1000 mg per day.
13. Use less alcohol and caffeine. Drink six to eight glasses of bottled water daily.
14. Limit sodium intake to less than 3 grams per day.
15. Take targeted nutritional supplements daily.

2. **Vitamin, Mineral, Enzyme & Nutritional Supplementation**

Multi-vitamin/multi-mineral combinations should be ingested on a daily basis with the following essential 15 ingredients:

Beta Carotene	12.5 - 25,000 units
Vitamin C	300 - 600 units
Vitamin E	200 - 400 IU
Selenium	100 - 200 mcg
Folic Acid	400 - 800 mcg
Vitamin B-6	20 - 40 mg
Pantothenic Acid	25 - 50 mg
Vitamin B-12	20 - 40 mcg
Magnesium	140 - 280 mg
Chromium Picolinate	50 - 100 mcg
Co Enzyme Q_{10}	20 - 60 mg
Quercetin	10 - 40 mg
Vanadium	200 - 400 mcg
Bromelain	50 - 100 mg
L-Glutathione	15 - 25 mg

3. **Herbal Therapy (optional)**

Ginger - Enhances immunity, anti-nausea
Garlic - cholesterol lowering, anti-inflammatory,anti-thrombolytic
Ginseng - Enhances immunity & energy
Gotu kola - Enhances memory
Ginkgo biloba - Enhances memory, improves dizziness, CNS
Cayenne pepper - Energy, heat, cholesterol, arthritis
Echinacea extract - Enhances immunity, T-Lymphocytes
Goldenseal - Enhances immunity, T-Lymphocytes
Hawthorne berry - Heart
Wild yam extract - DHEA

4. **Green Chlorophyll Therapy (optional)**

Chlorella, Wheat grass, Green barley, or Magna extract; one dose per day.

5. **Other Recommendations**

1. Maintain normal or less than normal body weight.
2. Consider a juice-cleansing fast once a month. (See enclosed instructions)
3. Avoid heavy metals, pollutants, toxins and smoking.
4. Exercise regularly.
5. Avoid prolonged exposure to sunlight, microwaves, televisions and computers (electromagnetic contamination). Avoid unnecessary x-rays.
6. Use good personal hygiene for eyes, nose, fingers and fingernails, especially during infection or allergy season, i.e., hayfever.
7. Consider installing water filters, air filters and full spectrum lighting.

General Markers of Health

1. DHEA levels greater than 800 ng/dl.
2. Serum albumin levels greater than 48 gm/liter　　(4.8g/dL)
3. Cholesterol levels less than 180.
    HDL greater than 45.
    LDL less than 130.
4. Serum ferritin, iron, TIBC within normal range
5. Serum homocysteine levels lower than 14umol.

Seventeen

OPTIMUM HEALTH

This book has been a collection of chapters that can enable you to actively participate in your health and nutrition as well as your awareness in life. Although attitudes and belief systems are influential in establishing ideals, understand that every one of us can be open to change. Being able to change our prejudices, our negative habits and our lifelong self-defeating patterns opens us up to growth. It is truly growth that makes life rewarding and worth living.

The goal of this book is to help you integrate your body, mind and spirit as you seek true aliveness and satisfaction in life. We are each responsible for our own health and happiness. While "Life" may strike us unexpected blows, we can do as much as possible to turn around bad situations and, also, try to prevent them. Healthy eating, exercise and emotional release can be considered preventive medicine. These are habits that will be with us for the rest of our lives once we begin the pattern. They do not require much self-sacrifice, merely awareness.

A low-fat, high-fiber diet is but the first step. Throughout the book I have stressed that we cannot deprive ourselves of good tasting meals and foods that we like. I included several of my personal recipes that were created with a healthy heart and trim, fit body in mind. I recommended eliminating very few products completely from the diet, but rather simply using less of them and substituting low-fat versions of old comfort-foods for those ones that no longer fit a healthy lifestyle.

Enough said. You now know my favorite foods and my personal and professional recommendations for a healthy diet. Much, if not everything I have written in this book, I have incorporated into my own life. For me, life has been a continuous journey.

THE BEST OFFENSE IS A GOOD DEFENSE

Our lives are governed and influenced by thoughts, beliefs and lifestyle patterns that can be equally damaging to the mind and body. My waiting room is full of clients who have both chronic and acute illnesses. With their lifestyles of "All-American" diets, maladaptive habits and overweight tendencies, some have waited too long. They come into my office wanting to be cured, yet they rarely take responsibility for their own condition or attempt to change it. My clients want me to give them relief. But I am not a magician, nor do I have any powers that can induce healing. I can't make a new body with pharmacological agents. I can't replace a heart that is ravaged with disease with a new healthy one. It all has to come through lifestyle patterns - the way you live in the world now. Granted, many people who now have heart disease were not taught how to take care of themselves. It's hard to believe, but *preventive medicine in this country is not a major component of medical training, instruction or energy.* Much of my generation, for example, grew up on junk foods. As a medical student, I was never taught about junk foods. Fortunately, this is changing somewhat.

I was delighted to see in the *Archives of Internal Medicine,* June 1991, an article recommending a national effort to educate the public on the benefits of nutritional healing. The panel of physicians urged the medical community, as well as the government, media, educational systems and food industry to collaborate in this effort.

The doctors who have made the recommendations for the National Education Cholesterol Program believe that not only health professionals should be concerned with making efforts to improve the state of public health, but also *other* professionals. They are calling upon government to coordinate nutrition statements and policies emphasizing low-fat and healthy eating; they are asking the media to report these findings and to explain nutritional terms and information; they are asking food manufacturers to research and develop tasty, low-fat and high-fiber food products.

TABLE 22

RECOMMENDATIONS OF THE NATIONAL EDUCATION CHOLESTEROL PROGRAM

RECOMMENDATION B.1 — The panel recommends that healthy Americans, both adults and children, select, prepare, and consume foods that contain lower amounts of SFAs, total fat, and cholesterol.

RECOMMENDATION E.1 — The panel recommends that health professionals advise patients and the public to adopt the recommended eating patterns.

RECOMMENDATION F.1 — The panel recommends that food producers, manufacturers, and distributors increase the availability of good-tasting foods that are lower in SFAs, total fat, and cholesterol.

RECOMMENDATION F.2 — The panel recommends that the food industry participate actively in helping the public attain desirable eating patterns through labeling and advertising activities.

RECOMMENDATION F.3 — The panel recommends that food vendors and other food distribution sites participate actively in the national effort.

RECOMMENDATION F.4 — The panel recommends that the food industry, including food and animal scientists, food technologists, and nutritionists, continue to develop and modify foods to help the public meet the recommended eating patterns.

RECOMMENDATION G.1 — The panel recommends that the mass media provide information on a lower SFA, lower total fat, and lower cholesterol eating pattern.

RECOMMENDATION H.1 — The panel recommends that government facilitate attainment of healthful eating patterns by modifying policies and approaches.

RECOMMENDATION I.1 — The panel recommends that all public and private educational systems become active partners by disseminating information about the role of eating patterns in CHD prevention.

From My Heart to Yours

This text has been a collection of facts, thoughts, scientific papers and folklore, explaining in simple terms how to follow a lifestyle-awareness program utilizing nutritional and dietary approaches, with an emphasis on nutritional, emotional and spiritual healing.

The physicians of the future will be consistently involved in environmental matters concerning multiple-chemical sensitivities, air pollution and water pollution. *Radiation is something I am genuinely concerned about.* Manufactured toxins that ravage the earth are slowly and insidiously infiltrating our bodies and our planet. Our mother earth and our seas are being continuously contaminated by oil spills, radiation leakage and man-made toxic wastes.

The evils of nature are prevailing, and we are not winning the war against disease. The environmental toxicities, the receding ozone layer of the atmosphere, the polluted water, the viral epidemic of AIDS and other malignant, life-threatening viruses that abound are subjects that every human being needs to be concerned about. It is true that our planet is on the verge of a biological Armageddon. Although I ponder these things, I have greater dread about what my children's children will face.

However, I do have some hope for the future.

There is a new generation of people and a new generation of doctors who have taken responsibility for ourselves, the environment and the planet. As a physician and a healer, I have worked in a microcosm, offering my knowledge and experience to individuals and groups. My path now has taken me to a different level: into the mass media - publishing books and newsletters, as well as lecturing throughout the country. My experience as a cardiologist has given me the opportunity to observe people digging deeper into their emotional and spiritual selves. I've seen people afflicted with heart disease transform and adopt new ways of living.

The Core of Our Being

As a clinical cardiologist, I know the heart is the place where everything comes together. After all, the heart is the core of our being. *Unfortunately, the hearts of many of us have been broken.* We all have experienced heartbreak on some level or another. Many of us are lonesome and need to be fed on many different levels. Some of us need to be touched. Some need to give. Others need to receive. We are all searching for solutions, happiness and joy. We all want cures.

But the best remedy, in my opinion, comes from within. It comes from deep within our core. It comes with intuition, awareness, insight and a genuine feeling of knowing.

Are you hungry? Are you hungry for a healthier, happier and more productive life? The possibilities for self-healing are endless. Like you, I have fantasies. My search continues, and my path has taken me to a higher emotional and spiritual level. It is my hope that this text will stimulate your inner self to utilize your highest power to obtain satisfaction and growth in your life.

My patients have taught me that life is so precious and ever so short. I have learned so much from them. Health is not just a condition of the physical matter but also a condition of the mind, divine spirit, love and truth. This is the basis and essence of *Optimum Health*.

TABLE 23
THE AMERICAN HEART ASSOCIATION

Dietary Guidelines

1. Dietary fat intake should be less than 30 percent of total calories (I prefer 20 percent).
2. Saturated fat (SFA) intake should be less than 10 percent of total calories.
3. Polyunsaturated fat (PUFA) should not exceed 10 percent of total daily calories.
4. Cholesterol intake should not exceed 300 mg per day.
5. Carbohydrate intake should represent 50 percent or more total calories with emphasis on complex carbohydrates (I prefer 65-70 percent complex carbohydrates).
6. Protein intake should constitute the remainder of the calories.
7. Sodium intake should be limited to less than three grams per day.
8. Alcohol consumption is not recommended, but if consumed, should not exceed one ounce a day of ethanol or eight ounces of wine or 24 ounces of regular beer.
9. Total calories should be consumed with the goal of achieving and maintaining a person's recommended body weight.
10. Consumption of a wide variety of foods is encouraged.

Are you ready to choose *Optimum Health* for your life? Are you emotionally and spiritually connected? Is this the body in which you really wish to live? We need to continually ask ourselves these questions, because

IF YOU WEAR OUT THIS BODY, WHERE ARE YOU GOING TO LIVE NEXT?

APPENDIX

Following, is an eating regimen that I have prepared for increased health and subsequent weight loss. Since it is not a "diet," it may be repeated over and over or mixed with other foods recommended in this book. The asterisks mark those recipes that I include in the *Recipes for Preventive Medicine* Chapter, so called because these are foods I have eaten for years without significant weight-gain nor continual loss. This is a balanced program of merely eating with awareness.

BREAKFASTS

1 glass fruit juice
1 frozen waffle
Spreadable fruit
½ grapefruit
1 bran muffin
2 whole-grain pancakes*
Pure maple syrup, blueberries

1 bowl oatmeal
1 cup low-fat yogurt
1 piece whole wheat toast
1 bowl whole grain cereal
1 cup 1% milk
Rice cake with honey
Banana

LUNCHES

Leaf lettuce, tomato salad
Low-fat goat or cottage cheese
 (lemon and olive oil dressing)
Salad of greens, turkey,
Feta cheese, raw carrots
Bowl of pasta and vegetables
Served hot or cold
Salad of greens and cold veggies
Cold new potatoes and/or beans
Tuna packed in water

1 cup soup
½ sandwich
(tuna, hummus, turkey)
Miso Soup*
2 8-oz. glasses water
1 cup yogurt, fresh fruit
Whole-grain toasted bagel
Spinach, raw or sauteed
Tomatoes, mushrooms
(olive oil and lemon)

DINNERS

Fish

Steamed broccoli

Baked potato

Santiago's Chicken*

Basmati rice

Green salad

Stir-fried vegetables

Brown Rice

Soup

Salad and bread

Pasta

Salad of greens

Dad's Tomatoes*

Fish

Sauteed spinach

Yellow and green zucchini

Pasta

Salad

Chicken

Salad

FINDING YOUR IDEAL WEIGHT

The next two pages may be used to determine your ideal weight. First, find your height in the left-hand column. Then move across the page to the body frame that best describes you. For the purpose of this table, your body frame is "small" if you can wrap your left thumb and middle finger around your right wrist and have these two digits overlap. If the thumb and finger barely touch, then you have a "medium" body frame. If they don't touch at all, you have a "large" build.

Courtesy of Metropolitan Life Insurance Company

HEIGHT/WEIGHT TABLE

MEN

Height Inches	Small Frame	Medium Frame	Large Frame
62	128-134	131-141	138-150
63	130-136	133-143	140-153
64	132-138	135-145	142-156
65	134-140	137-148	144-160
66	136-142	139-151	146-164
67	138-145	142-154	149-168
68	140-148	145-157	152-172
69	142-151	148-160	155-176
70	144-154	151-163	158-180
71	146-157	154-166	161-184
72	149-160	157-170	164-188
73	152-164	160-174	168-192
74	155-168	164-178	172-197
75	158-172	167-182	176-202
76	162-176	171-187	181-207

HEIGHT/WEIGHT TABLE

WOMEN

Height Inches	Small Frame	Medium Frame	Large Frame
58	102-111	109-121	118-131
59	103-113	111-123	120-134
60	104-115	113-126	122-137
61	106-118	115-129	125-140
62	108-121	118-132	128-143
63	111-124	121-135	131-147
64	114-127	124-138	134-151
65	117-130	127-141	137-155
66	120-133	130-144	140-159
67	123-136	133-147	143-163
68	126-139	136-150	146-167
69	129-142	139-153	149-170
70	132-145	142-156	152-173
71	135-148	145-159	155-176
72	138-151	148-162	158-179

BEVERAGES

	Serving Size	Calories	Sodium
Club Soda	12 ounces	0	75 (mg)
Cola, regular	12 ounces	150	14
Gatorade	12 ounces	39	123
Ginger Ale	12 ounces	125	25
Root Beer	12 ounces	150	49
Beer, regular	12 ounces	145	19
Beer, light	12 ounces	100	10
Wine, dessert	3.5 ounces	70	10
Wine, red	3.5 ounces	75	6
Wine, white	3.5 ounces	70	5
Apple juice	4.0 ounces	58	3.5
Apricot nectar	4.0 ounces	70.5	4.5
Carrot juice	4.0 ounces	55	36
Cranberry	4.0 ounces	75	5
Pineapple juice	4.0 ounces	70	1
Prune juice	4.0 ounces	90	5.5
Tomato juice	4.0 ounces	21	438
V-8	4.0 ounces	25	378
Grapefruit juice	4.0 ounces	50	1
Grape juice	4.0 ounces	80	3.5
Orange juice	4.0 ounces	55	1

BEANS/NUTS/SEEDS

Food	Serving Size	Cal.	Fat (g)	%cal/fat	Chol.	Fiber
Soybeans (Tofu) (cooked)	1 cup	234	10	38%	0	
Soybean curd	1 piece	86	5	52%	0	
Peanuts, roasted	¼ cup	210	18	77%	0	
Peanut Butter	2 Tbsp	188	16	76%	0	
Almonds, roasted	¼ cup	246	23	84%	0	
Walnuts, black (shelled and chopped)	¼ cup	196	18	82%	0	
Chick-peas	½ cup	135	2	45%	0	6.2
Kidney Beans	½ cup	110	TR		0	5.8
Lentils	½ cup	115	TR		0	2.0
Pinto Beans	½ cup	115	TR		0	5.3
Split Peas	½ cup	115	TR		0	5.1
Pork and Beans in tomato sauce	1 cup	311	6.6	19%	6	
Lima Beans (frozen cooked)	1 cup	168	0.2	1%	0	
Lima Beans (canned)	1 cup	163	0.5	2%	0	
Green Beans (fresh, frozen)	1 cup	34	0.1	2%	0	
Green Beans (canned)	1 cup	32	0.3	8%	0	
White Beans, navy (cooked)	1 cup	212	1.1	4%	0	
Yellow Beans, wax (frozen)	1 cup	28	0.3	9%	0	
Yellow Beans (canned)	1 cup	32	0.4	11%	0	
Sunflower Seeds (hulled)	1 Tbsp	51	4.3	75%	0	
Water Chestnuts	4 nuts	20	0.1	4%	0	
Macadamia Nuts	1 ounce	196	20.3	93%	0	
Pecans (chopped or pieces)	1 Tbsp	51	5.2	91%	0	

CEREAL

Food	Serving Size	Cal.	Fat (g)	%cal/fat	Chol.	Fiber
All Bran	⅓ cup	70	1	13%	0	8.6
Bran (unprocessed)	1 ounce	91	.4		0	NA
Bran Buds	1 cup	144	1.8	11%	0	NA
Cheerios	1¼ cup	110	2	16%	0	1.6
Corn Flakes	1¼ cup	110	Trace		0	.4
Corn Grits	1 cup	125	.2		0	NA
Cream of Wheat	¾ cup	105	Trace		0	.6
40% Bran Flakes	¾ cup	95	1	.9%	0	6.0
Fruit Loops	1 cup	110	1	.9%	0	.3
Granola	⅓ cup	125	5	36%	0	NA
Grape Nuts	¼ cup	100	Trace		0	2.2
Oatmeal	¾ cup	108	2	17%	0	2.8
Product 19	¾ cup	110	Trace		0	1.2
Puffed Rice	1 cup	55	Trace		0	.2
Raisin Bran	¾ cup	90	1	1%	0	3.6
Rice Krispies	1 cup	110	Trace		0	Trace
Shredded Wheat	⅔ cup	100	Trace		0	3.3
Special K	⅓ cup	110	Trace		0	.4
Sugar Frosted Flakes	¾ cup	110	Trace		0	.2
Total	1 cup	100	1	.9%	0	2.5
Wheat Chex	⅓ cup	110	1	.8%	0	NA
Wheat Germ	1 Tbsp	23	.7	27%	0	NA
Wheaties	1 cup	100	1	.9%	0	2.6

CURED MEATS

Food	Serving Size	Cal.	Fat (g)	%cal/fat	Chol.
Bacon	3 slices	110	9	73%	16
Bologna	1 ounce	90	8	80%	16
Corned Beef Brisket	3 ounces	215	16	66%	83
Frankfurter	1	145	13	80%	23
Ham	3 ounces	205	14	61%	52
Ham/lean only	3 ounces	135	5	33%	47
Liverwurst	1 slice	60	5	75%	45
Pork Sausage	1 link	50	4	72%	11
Salami/cooked	1 ounce	70	6	77%	18
Salami/hard	1 slice	42	3	64%	8

DAIRY

Food	Serving Size	Calories	Grams Fat	% cal/ fat	Chol-mg
CHEESES					
Parmesan, grated	1 Tbsp	25	2	72%	3 (mg)
Ricotta (part skim milk)	½ cup	170	10	53%	38
Ricotta (whole milk)	½ cup	215	16	67%	62
Swiss	1 ounce	105	8	68%	26
American	1 ounce	105	9	77%	27
American (spread)	1 Tbsp	47	3	57%	9
Brie	1 ounce	95	8	76%	28
Cheddar	1 ounce	115	9	70%	30
Cottage cheese (creamed)	½ cup	110	5	41%	16
Cream cheese	1 ounce	100	10	90%	31
Mozzarella (part skim milk)	1 ounce	80	5	56%	15
Mozzarella (whole milk)	1 ounce	80	6	68%	22

Food	Serving Size	Calories	Grams Fat	% cal/ fat	Chol-mg
CHEESES (*CONTINUED*)					
Blue cheese	1 ounce	100	8.2	74%	21(mg)
Feta	1 ounce	75	6.0	72%	25
Romano	1 ounce	110	7.6	62%	29
Velveeta	1 ounce	82	3.8	42%	16
MILK, CREAMS, AND MILK PRODUCTS					
Milk, nonfat (dry)	¾ cup	81	.2		0
Milk, skim	1 cup	85	Trace		4
Milk, 1%	1 cup	102	2.6	23%	10
Milk, 2% fat	1 cup	120	5	37%	18
Milk, Whole	1 cup	150	8	48%	33
Milk, evaporated (canned, whole)	1 cup	338	19.1	51%	74
Milk, evaporated (canned, skim)	1 cup	200	.6	2.7%	10
Buttermilk	1 cup	100	2	18%	9
Chocolate milk	1 cup	210	8	34%	30
Cocoa mix w/water	1 cup	100	1	.9%	1
Condensed Milk (sweetened)	1 cup	980	27	25%	104
Cream, light	1 Tbsp	29	2.9	90%	10
Cream, whipping (light)	1 cup	699	73.9	95%	265
Cream, whipping (heavy)	1 cup	821	88.1	96%	326
Cream, half & half	1 Tbsp	20	2	90%	6
Cream, heavy	1 Tbsp	50	6	90%	21
Creamer (non-dairy)	1 Tbsp	33	2.1	57%	0
Sour cream	1 Tbsp	25	3	95%	5
Dessert Topping	1 Tbls	33	2.1	69%	0
Yogurt, Low-fat (plain)	8 ounces	145	4	25%	14
Yogurt, Low-fat (with fruit)	8 ounces	230	2	7.8%	10

MILK, CREAMS, AND MILK PRODUCTS *(CONTINUED)*

Food	Serving Size	Calories	Grams Fat	% cal/ fat	Chol-mg
Yogurt (whole milk)	8 ounces	139	7.4	48%	29 (mg)
Yogurt, Frozen	8 ounces	244	3.0	11%	10
Milk Shake (Vanilla)	10 ounces	315	9	26%	33
Ice Cream (rich)	1 cup	349	23.7	61%	88
Ice Cream (reg)	1 cup	269	14.3	48%	59
Ice Cream (Eskimo Pie)	1	270	19.1	64%	35
Ice Cream (Sandwich 3 oz)	1	238	8.5	32%	34
Ice Milk (soft-serve)	1 cup	223	4.6	19%	13
Ice Milk (Hard)	1 cup	131	5.6	38%	18
Pudding mix (whole milk)	1 cup	322	7.8	22%	36
Pudding (instant) (whole milk)	1 cup	325	6.5	18%	36
Pudding mix (dry, low-cal)	4 ounces	100	–	–	–
EGGS					
Egg, boiled	1 large	80	6	68%	274
Egg, fried	1 large	95	7	66%	278
Egg, scrambled	1 large	110	8	65%	282
Egg white	1 large	15	Trace	–	0
Egg yolk	1 large	65	6	83%	272

DESSERTS

Food	Serving Size	Cal.	Fat (g)	%cal/fat	Chol.
COOKIES					
Brownie with Nuts and Frosting	1 small	100	4	36%	14
Butter Cookie	1 small	25	1	36%	NA
Chocolate Chip Cookie	1 medium	45	2	40%	1
Fig Bars	1 bar	55	1	16%	7
Gingersnap	3 small	50	1	16%	NA
Marshmallow with chocolate coating	1 cookie	55	2	38%	NA
Oatmeal Raisin	1 medium	60	2	30%	Trace
Sandwich Cookie	1 medium	50	2	36%	0
Sugar Cookie	1 medium	60	3	45%	7
ICE CREAMS (SEE DAIRY)					

PIES (9" PIE)

Food	Serving Size	Cal.	Fat (g)	%cal/fat	Chol.
Apple Pie	⅙ pie	405	18	40%	0
Banana Custard Pie	⅙ pie	335	14	38%	NA
Blueberry Pie	⅙ pie	380	17	40%	0
Cherry Pie	⅙ pie	410	18	39%	0
Lemon Meringue Pie	⅙ pie	355	14	35%	143
Mincemeat Pie	⅙ pie	430	18	38%	0
Pecan Pie	⅙ pie	575	32	50%	95
Pumpkin Pie	⅙ pie	320	17	48%	109
PUDDINGS					
Butterscotch	½ cup	170	4	21%	17
Chocolate	½ cup	150	4	24%	15
Custard	½ cup	150	8	48%	139
Rice Pudding	½ cup	155	4	23%	15
Tapioca Pudding	½ cup	145	4	25%	15

CAKES

Food	Serving Size	Cal.	Fat (g)	%cal/fat	Chol.
Angel Food	1/12	125	Trace		0
Carrot with cream cheese icing	1/16	385	21	49%	74
Cheesecake, plain	1/12	280	18	58%	170
Chocolate w/icing	1/16	235	8	31%	37
Danish, plain	1 medium	220	12	49%	49
Doughnut, yeast	1 medium	235	13	50%	21
Poundcake	1/8 loaf	246	10	39%	33
Spice w/icing	1/16	270	8	26%	NA

FATS/VEGETABLE OILS

Food	Serving Size	Calories	Grams Fat	% cal/ fat	Chol-mg
Butter	1 Tbsp	100	13	100%	31
Lard (animal shortening)	1 Tbsp	115	13	100%	12
Chicken Fat	1 Tbsp	126	14	100%	9
Margarine (imitation/diet)	1 Tbsp	50	5	90%	0
Margarine (regular/soft)	1 Tbsp	100	11	100%	0
Coconut Oil	1 Tbsp	120	14	100%	0
Corn Oil	1 Tbsp	125	14	100%	0
Cottonseed Oil	1 Tbsp	120	14	100%	0
Olive Oil	1 Tbsp	125	14	100%	0
Palm Kernel Oil	1 Tbsp	120	13.6	100%	0
Peanut Oil	1 Tbsp	125	14	100%	0
Soybean Oil	1 Tbsp	120	14	100%	0
Sunflower Oil	1 Tbsp	125	14	100%	0
Vegetable Shortening	1 Tbsp	115	13	100%	0

FISH/SHELLFISH

Food	Serving Size	Cal.	Fat (g)	%cal/fat	Chol.
Bluefish	3 ounces	135	4	26%	59
Clams, raw	2 clams	25	1	36%	59
Cod	3 ounces	100	3	27%	50
Crab, softshell (fried)	1 medium	215	13	54%	87
Crab, steamed	3 ounces	80	2	22%	79
Crabmeat, canned	3 ounces	85	2	21%	84
Flounder	3 ounces	100	6	54%	50
Herring, pickled	3 ounces	190	13	61%	85
Lobster Tail, (steamed)	1 medium	100	1	9%	88
Mackerel	3 ounces	215	15	62%	94
Mussels, steamed	3 ounces	80	2	22%	42
Oysters, raw	3 ounces	55	1	16%	42
Salmon, canned	3 ounces	120	5	37%	34
Salmon	3 ounces	150	7	42%	36
Sardines, canned (in oil)	3 ounces	175	9	46%	85
Scallops, steamed	3 ounces	95	1	9%	45
Shrimp	7 medium	200	10	45%	168
Swordfish	3 ounces	150	7	42%	56
Trout	3 ounces	215	14	58%	55
Tuna, chunk in oil (drained)	3 ounces	169	7	37%	NA
Anchovies	5 fillets	135	2	13%	NA
Herring, Pacific	3 ounces	153	8	47%	NA
Catfish	1 ounce	29	1	31%	0
Halibut, broiled	1 ounce	28	.3	9%	14
Sole	1 ounce	26	.3	10%	0

FRUITS

Food	Serving Size	Cal.	Fat(g)	%cal/fat	Chol.	Fiber
Apple	1 medium	90	Trace	–	0	2.8
Applesauce	½ cup	95	Trace	–	0	2
Apricots	3 apricots	50	Trace	–	0	2.2
Avocado	1 medium	325	31	86%	0	4.5
Banana	1 medium	105	1	–	0	2.1
Blueberries	½ cup	40	Trace	–	0	2.5
Cantaloupe	½ medium	95	1	–	0	2.7
Cherries, Canned	½ cup	105	Trace	–	0	1.7
Coconut	1 cup	277	282	91%	0	NA
Cranberry Sauce (canned)	¼ cup	105	Trace	–	0	NA
Dates	10 dates	219	.4	–	0	NA
Figs, dried	1 fig	50	Trace	–	0	3.7
Fruit cocktail (canned, water)	1 cup	91	.2	–	0	NA
Grapefruit	½ medium	40	Trace	–	0	1.7
Grapes, seedless	10 grapes	35	Trace	–	0	.4
Honeydew cubes	1 cup	60	Trace	–	0	1.2
Lemon	1 medium	15	Trace		0	NA
Mango	1 medium	135	Trace	–	0	2.9
Nectarine	1 medium	65	1	–	0	1.9
Orange	1 medium	60	Trace	–	0	1.6
Peach	1 medium	35	Trace	–	0	1.4
Pear	1 medium	100	1	–	0	5
Pineapple	½ cup	40	Trace	–	0	1.2
Plum	1 medium	35	Trace	–	0	1.4
Prunes, dried	5 large	115	Trace	–	0	7.9
Raisins	½ cup	220	Trace	–	0	4.9
Raspberries, raw	1 cup	70	.6	–	0	NA
Rhubarb, frozen (sweetened)	1 cup	381	.3	–	0	NA
Strawberries	1 cup	55	.7	–	0	NA
Tangerine	1 large	46	.2	–	0	NA
Watermelon (diced pieces)	1 cup	42	.3	–	0	NA

GRAIN PRODUCTS - BREADS, PASTA, RICE

Food	Serving Size	Cal.	Fat(g)	%cal/fat	Chol.	Fiber
Bagel	1 bagel	200	2	9%	0	NA
Corn Bread	1 piece	200	7	31%	0	1.7
Frank/Burger Bun	1	115	2	15%	Trace	NA
French Bread	1 slice	100	1	9%	0	1.3
French Toast	1 slice	155	7	40%	112	NA
Hard Roll	1	155	2	11%	Trace	NA
Pancake, plain	1	60	2	30%	16	NA
Rye Bread	1 slice	65	1	13%	0	.9
Taco Shell	1	50	2	36%	NA	NA
Tortilla, corn	1 cake	65	1	13%	NA	NA
White Bread	1 slice	65	1	13%	0	.5
Whole Wheat Bread	1 slice	70	1	12%	0	1.4
Graham Crackers	2	60	1	15%	0	2.1
Melba Toast	1	20	Trace		0	NA
Saltine Crackers	4	50	1	18%	5	.5
Blueberry Muffin	1	135	5	33%	19	NA
Bran Muffin	1	125	6	43%	24	NA
Corn Muffin	1	145	5	31%	23	NA
English Muffin	1	140	1	6%	0	NA
Egg Noodles	1 cup	200	2	9%	50	1.7
Macaroni	1 cup	190	1	4%	0	1.2
Spaghetti	1 cup	190	1	4%	0	1.6
Rice, brown	½ cup	115	1	7%	0	2.4
Rice, white	½ cup	110	Trace		0	.1

MISCELLANEOUS

Food	Serving Size	Cal.	Fat (g)	%cal/fat	Chol.
Beef - vegetable stew	1 cup	220	11	45%	71
Chili with beans	1 cup	340	16	42%	28
Corned Beef Hash	1 cup	290	10	31%	NA
Macaroni and Cheese	1 cup	340	22	46%	44
Spaghetti, canned	1 cup	260	9	31%	8
Biscuit with sausage and egg	1	555	37	60%	259
Cheeseburger Patty	4 ounces	525	31	53%	104
Chicken Nuggets	6	265	16	54%	60
Chicken Sandwich	1	615	34	49%	68
Enchilada	1	235	16	61%	19
Fish Sandwich with cheese	1	420	23	49%	56
Frankfurter	1	280	16	51%	45
French Fries	1 serving	230	12	46%	NA
Ham and Cheese Sandwich	1	400	22	49%	60
Hamburger Patty	4 ounces	445	21	42%	71
Onion Rings	1 serving	260	15	51%	NA
Pizza with cheese	1 slice	290	9	27%	55
Roast Beef Sandwich	1	345	13	33%	55
Taco	1	195	11	50%	21
Bacon Bits	1 tsp	14	0.6	38%	0
M & M Candy	¼ cup	230	9.7	37%	3
Potato Chips	10 chips	114	7	63%	
Olives, green	10	33	4	99%	
Beef Tongue	1 slice	49	3.3	60%	18
Beef Liver	1 ounce	40	1.1	24%	86
Beef Tallow, suet	1 Tbsp	120	13.2	99%	11
Pork-Deviled Ham	¼ cup	198	18.2	82%	5
Sausage, Vienna (canned)	1 whole	56	5.2	3%	10

POULTRY

Food	Serving Size	Cal.	Fat (g)	%cal/fat	Chol.
Chicken, dark meat (with skin)	4 ounces	286	17	54%	103
Chicken, dark meat (no skin)	4 ounces	233	11	41%	105
Chicken, lt meat (with skin)	4 ounces	253	12	42%	96
Chicken, lt meat (no skin)	4 ounces	193	5	24%	96
Chicken breast (no skin)	½ breast	140	3	19%	73
Chicken breast (no skin, fried)	½ breast	160	4	22%	78
Chicken drumstick (with skin)	one	110	6	49%	48
Chicken drumstick (no skin)	one	75	2	24%	41
Duck with skin	4 ounces	380	32	75%	101
Duck no skin	4 ounces	227	13	52%	95
Turkey, dark meat (with skin)	4 ounces	253	13	47%	101
Turkey, dark meat (no skin)	4 ounces	213	8	33%	96
Turkey, lt meat (with skin)	4 ounces	220	9	38%	86
Turkey, lt meat (no skin)	4 ounces	180	4	20%	79
Chicken gizzard	4 ounces	108	2.4	20%	142

RED MEAT

Food	Serving Size	Calories	Grams Fat	% cal/fat	Chol-mg
Beef chuck roast	4 oz.	413	32	69%	117
Beef flank steak	4 oz.	306	17	57%	80
Beef rib roast	4 oz.	433	36	74%	96
Beef top round*	4 oz.	210	5	21%	70
Beef shortribs	4 oz.	533	48	81%	107
Beef sirloin*	4 oz.	233	9	36%	101
Beef T-bone*	4 oz.	240	12	45%	91
Beef tenderloin	4 oz.	233	10	41%	96
Hamburger (lean)	4 oz.	326	21	58%	112
Porterhouse steak*	4 oz.	246	12	43%	90
Lamb leg	4 oz.	213	8	33%	80
Lamb loin chop*	1 large	250	14	50%	60
Lamb rib chop*	1 large	290	22.5	70%	75
Pork loin chop*	1 med.	275	19	62%	84
Pork tenderloin	4 oz.	186	5	25%	87
Spareribs	4 oz.	453	37	68%	137
Veal cutlet	4 oz.	207	5.3	23%	112
Veal loin chop	4 oz.	246	13	34%	116
Veal rib roast	4 oz.	344	24	63%	119

Most preferred

Top round
Pork tenderloin
Veal cutlet
*All visible fat removed before cooking

Soup Canned, Condensed

Food	Serving Size	Cal.	Fat (g)	%cal/fat	Chol.
Bean w/bacon	1 cup	170	6	31%	3
Beef Consomme	1 cup	15	1	60%	Trace
Chicken Broth	1 cup	40	1	22%	1
Chicken Noodle	1 cup	75	2	24%	7
Chicken Rice	1 cup	60	2	30%	7
Clam Chowder (red)	1 cup	80	2	22%	2
Clam Chowder (white)	1 cup	165	7	38%	22
Minestrone	1 cup	85	3	31%	2
Mushrooms w/milk	1 cup	205	14	61%	20
Split Pea w/ham	1 cup	190	4	18%	8
Tomato	1 cup	85	2	21%	0
Vegetable/vegetarian	1 cup	70	2	25%	0
Vegetable w/beef	1 cup	80	2	22%	5
Cream of Celery with water	1 cup	86	5.5	57%	7
Cream of Chicken with water	1 cup	94	5.8	55%	8
Canned Onion w/water	1 cup	65	2.4	33%	6
Dehydrated Onion	1 pack	150	4.6	27%	0

VEGETABLES

Food	Serving Size	Cal.	Fat(g)	%cal/fat	Chol.	Fiber
Artichoke, bud or globe (frozen)	1 whole	52	0.2	3%	0	
Asparagus	6 spears	20	Trace	–	0	2.2
Beets	½ cup	25	Trace	–	0	2.2
Broccoli	1 spear	55	Trace	–	0	4.5
Brussels Sprouts	1 cup	51	0.3	5%	0	
Cabbage, cooked	½ cup	15	Trace	–	0	2
Cabbage, raw (shredded)	½ cup	10	Trace	–	0	0.7
Carrot, raw	1 medium	30	Trace	–	0	2.4
Carrot, sliced (cooked)	½ cup	35	Trace	–	0	2.3
Cauliflower	½ cup	15	Trace	–	0	1.6
Celery, raw	1 stalk	5	Trace	–	0	0.7
Corn	½ cup	90	1	1%	0	3.9
Corn, creamed	½ cup	210	2.8	12%	0	
Cucumber, raw	½ cup	5	Trace	–	0	0.5
Eggplant, cubes	1 cup	25	Trace	–	0	4
Greens, Collard	1 cup	51	0.7	12%	0	
Lettuce, Iceberg	1 cup	5	Trace	–	0	0.5
Lettuce, Leaf	1 cup	10	Trace	–	0	1.2
Mushrooms, raw (sliced)	½ cup	10	Trace	–	0	0.9
Okra, frozen (cooked)	1 cup	70	0.2	2%	0	
Onion, raw (chopped)	½ cup	25	Trace	–	0	2.6
Peas, Chinese	½ cup	35	Trace	–	0	1.3
Peas, Green	½ cup	65	Trace	–	0	4.1
Pepper, Green (raw)	1 medium	20	Trace	–	0	0.8
Pepper, Jalapeno (raw)	1	7	0	–	0	
Pepper, Jalapeno (canned)	1	5	0	–	0	

Food	Serving Size	Cal.	Fat(g)	%cal/fat	Chol.	Fiber
Pickles, Dill	1 large	15	0.3	18%	0	
Pickles, Sweet	2 slices	11	0	–	0	
Potato, baked (no skin)	1 medium	145	Trace	–	0	3.7
Potato, boiled	1 medium	115	Trace	–	0	2.7
Radishes	4 medium	5	Trace	–	0	0.5
Sauerkraut (canned)	½ cup	20	Trace	–	0	2.4
Spinach, frozen	½ cup	30	Trace	–	0	2.1
Squash, Summer	1 cup	25	0.2	7%	0	
Squash, Winter	½ cup	40	1 gram	22%	0	3.6
Sweet Potato (mashed)	½ cup	170	Trace	–	0	3.8
Tomato, raw	1 medium	25	Trace	–	0	1
Tomato Juice	½ cup	20	Trace	–	0	NA
Tomato Puree	½ cup	50	Trace	–	0	NA
Turnip, green	1 cup	38	0.5	11%	0	
Yam, cubes	½ cup	80	Trace	–	0	2.6
Vegetable Juice Cocktail	½ cup	20	Trace	–	0	NA
Zucchini, sliced (cooked)	½ cup	15	Trace	–	0	2.7

GLOSSARY

VITAMINS

VITAMIN A (Beta Carotene) - Beta carotene is a powerful antioxidant involved with enhancing the immunity of the body. It is particularly important in the growth and maintenance of healthy skin, hair and eyes. Multiple clinical studies have shown the positive impact on heart disease, stroke and cancer.

VITAMIN D - Vitamin D is crucial in building strong bones and teeth. It is extremely important in calcium metabolism. Children and pregnant or nursing women will need additional vitamin D.

VITAMIN E - Like vitamin A, vitamin E is a potent antioxidant. It is particularly important in the prevention of atherosclerosis. Vitamin E aids in the healing of wounds and protects the respiratory system from pollution. When combined with selenium, it is known to be a potent immune stimulant.

VITAMIN C - Vitamin C must be taken in the diet as we cannot synthesize it in our bodies. It is extremely effective in enhancing immunity and building resistance to infections and fatigue. It helps protect blood vessels and improves healing after surgery. It favorably affects cholesterol in the blood and is extremely important in delaying cataract formation. Multiple clinical studies also show its unique effectiveness in combating heart disease and cancer.

VITAMIN B-1 - Vitamin B-1 helps strengthen the nervous system and is necessary in the treatment of beriberi and alcoholism. It is extremely important in the burning of sugar. It also can be effective in improving one's memory.

VITAMIN B-2 (**Riboflavin**) - Riboflavin is important in healing and in digesting fats, proteins and carbohydrates. It aids in growth and reproduction.

VITAMIN B3 (**Niacin**) - Niacin is important in the healthy functioning of the nervous system. It is essential in the production of male and female sex hormones. It improves circulation and lowers cholesterol.

VITAMIN B-6 - Vitamin B-6 is crucial in the proper chemical balance of the body. It helps convert fats and proteins into energy. Combined with vitamin B-1, it may be helpful in seasickness. It is particularly important in relieving premenstrual swelling. It has been touted in enhancing the immune system and alleviating depression.

VITAMIN B-12 - Vitamin B-12 is extremely important as a supplement for strict vegetarians. It helps to prevent anemia, and to improve digestion and memory. It supports the immune system and the nervous system.

BIOTIN - Biotin is necessary in the synthesis of protein, fats and carbohydrates. It helps prevent skin disorders, especially eczema, and builds resistance in allergic situations.

PANTHOTHENIC ACID - Panthothenic acid is frequently referred to as a "stress" vitamin. This is necessary in the proper functioning of the adrenal glands. It also helps stimulate the immune system.

FOLIC ACID - Folic acid is crucial in supporting the immune system. It has particular utility in the nervous system and has been used in the treatment of "senility." Folic acid helps prevent anemia and has recently been reported in medical literature to help in the prevention of cervical cancer as well as coronary heart disease. It prevents malformation of the nervous system in newborns.

MINERALS

CALCIUM AND PHOSPHORUS - Calcium and phosphorus are extremely important in the proper functioning and healthy maintenance of bones and teeth. Calcium is also particularly useful in the regulation of the irritability of nerves and muscles. Calcium supplements are useful in helping prevent osteoporosis.

MAGNESIUM - Magnesium is involved in over 300 enzymatic reactions in the body. It has particular utility in the prevention of cardiovascular disorders. It is useful in the PMS syndrome, especially when combined with Vitamins B-6 and E. It is also useful in the chronic fatigue syndrome because it enhances energy.

MANGANESE - Manganese is a powerful antioxidant which helps in the prevention of atherosclerosis. It helps improve fatigue and memory. It also helps in regulating blood sugar.

IODINE - Iodine is crucial in the proper synthesis of thyroxine in the thyroid gland. It aids in maintaining mental alertness and irritability. It is important in the overall functioning of the immune system.

SELENIUM - Selenium is a powerful antioxidant which has been touted in the prevention of heart disease and cancer. It is particularly important as an immune system stimulant. It is helpful in combating harmful metals in the environment.

ZINC - Zinc is crucial in wound healing as well as immunity of various infections. It has utility in healthy sexual functioning of the male as it supports the prostate gland.

CHROMIUM PICOLINATE - Chromium plays a vital role in the body's utilization of sugar. It has been reported in cholesterol-lowering. Clinical studies have also demonstrated the utility of chromium as a "fat buster," especially when used in combination with L-Carnitine. Some researchers indicate that chromium is useful in increasing longevity and up to 90 percent of us may be deficient in chromium. It is the most easily absorbable form of chromium. Chromium may also reduce triglycerides.

POTASSIUM - Potassium is particularly crucial in the overall functioning of nerves, muscles and especially the heart. It helps counteract the blood pressure-raising effects of sodium. It is useful in allergies and in maintaining proper heart rhythms.

BORON - Boron has particular usefulness in the musculoskeletal functioning of the body. Some investigators indicate that it is especially helpful in combination with calcium in preventing osteoporosis.

VANADIUM - Vanadium has been touted as an anti-aging mineral. A deficiency in vanadium has been associated with heart disease. It has been shown to have a cholesterol-lowering ability.

LIPOTROPIC FACTORS

CHOLINE - Choline is particularly important in cholesterol metabolism and in protecting the liver against toxic chemicals. Choline supplements have also been suggested to improve memory.

INOSITOL - Like choline, inositol helps protect the liver and nervous system. It regulates cholesterol levels and aids in the treatment of atherosclerosis. It has been known to counteract the negative effects of caffeine.

TAURINE - Taurine is an amino acid which has been known to alleviate insomnia, anxiety and hyperactivity. Recent work also indicates that Taurine serves as an antioxidant and membrane stabilizer.

METHIONINE - Methionine, like choline, inositol and betaine, is a lipotropic factor which helps prevent excessive fat in the liver. It also helps prevent cholesterol buildup. It is an antioxidant and free radical scavenger. It is an important amino acid, particularly for those who consume high levels of alcohol and sugar.

BETAINE HCL - Betaine HCL is important in stimulating hydrochloric acid in the gut. This is useful in the digestion of proteins.

L-CARNITINE - L-Carnitine is particularly helpful in fat metabolism. Although L-Carnitine can be manufactured by the body, adequate quantities of the amino acids lysine and methionine are required for L-Carnitine synthesis. A deficiency of L-Carnitine may result in fatty liver, weakened immune system, muscle wasting and perhaps even heart failure.

ENZYMES

PAPAIN AND BROMELAIN - Papaya and pineapple extracts not only aid in digestion, but these enzymes have also been reported to reduce the soreness and increase healing of bruises and swelling after minor trauma.

ALOE VERA - Aloe vera is a healing remedy that has been used in the healing of mucous membrane and skin. It is especially helpful in healing ulcers and has been effective in helping burns to heal.

ACIDOPHILUS - Acidophilus is a friendly bacteria in our bowel. It protects the colon from cancer and aids digestion of food. Acidophilus can be destroyed by caffeine, antibiotics and birth control pills. It also reduces putrefication in the bowel.

NUTRITIONALS

CO ENZYME Q_{10} - Co Enzyme Q_{10} is helpful in enhancing the energy of the organism. It does this by stimulating energy production in the so-called mitochondria, or power houses, of cells. It has particular utility in heart efficiency and exercise tolerance. It is used as a treatment for heart failure and angina and is believed to enhance immunity and to prevent cancer. Co Q_{10} is now being utilized in the AIDS syndrome. It has been referred to by some researchers as the "Miracle Nutrient."

L-GLUTATHIONE - L-Glutathione is a powerful antioxidant. As a free radical scavenger, it has been known to bolster immunity. It is now receiving considerable scrutiny as an effective agent in reducing HIV (AIDS) activity. It also has been reported to be useful in converting oxidized vitamin C back to a form which can serve again as an antioxidant. Glutathione also combines with selenium to form glutathione peroxidase, a potent radical scavenger.

SELECTED REFERENCES

BOOKS

Achterberg J, Dossey, B, et al. *Rituals of Healing: Using Imagery for Health and Wellness.* New York: Bantam Books, 1994.

Achterberg J, Lawlis GF. *Imagery and Disease.* Champaign, IL: The Institute for Personality and Ability Testing, 1978.

American College of Sports Medicine. *Guidelines for Exercise Testing and Prescription.* Philadelphia: Lea & Febiger, 1986.

Bailey C. *Fit or Fat?* Boston: Houghton Mifflin Co, 1978.

Balch JF and Balch PA. *Prescription for Nutritional Healing.* Garden City Park, NY: Avery Publishing Group Inc, 1990.

Bass E, Davis C. *The Courage to Heal.* New York: Harper & Row, 1988.

Bland J. *Medical Applications of Clinical Nutrition.* New Canaan, CT: Keats Publishing, 1983.

Bliznakof EG, Hunt GL. *The Miracle Nutrient Co Enzyme Q10.* New York: Bantam Books, 1986.

Bruch H. *Eating Disorders.* New York: Basic Books, 1973.

Carper J. *The Food Pharmacy. Dramatic New Evidence That Food Is Your Best Medicine.* New York: Bantam Books, 1988.

Cortis B. *Heart & Soul.* New York: Villard Books, 1995.

Cowmeadow O. *An Introduction to Macrobiotics - The Natural Way to Health and Happiness.* Wellingborough, Northamptonstine, Eng: Thorsons Publishers Limited, 1987.

Eastwood MA, Brydon WG, Tadesse K. "Effects of fiber on colon continence." *Medical Aspects of Dietary Fiber.* Spiller GA, McP Kay R, eds. New York and London: Plenum Medical Books, 1980.

Eddy MB. *Science and Health with Key to the Scriptures.* Boston, MA: Publishers Agent, 1934.

Eliot RS, Breo DL. *Is It Worth Dying For?* New York: Bantam Books, 1986.

Fletcher AM. "How to Put More Fish and Omega-3 Fish Oils into Your Diet for a Longer, Healthier Life." *Eat Fish, Live Better.* New York: Harper and Row, 1989.

Folkers K, Ed. *Biomedical and Clinical Aspects of Co Enzyme Q10* Vol 3. Elsevier, Amsterdam, 1981.

Gillespie C. Hormones, *Hot Flashes and Mood Swings, The Menopausal Survival Guide.* New York: Harper Perennial, 1994.

Goodwin J, et al. *Sexual Abuse.* Chicago: Year Book Medical Publishers, 1989.

Hirschmann JR, Munter CH. *Overcoming Overeating.* New York: Fawcett Columbine, 1988.

Hirschmann JR, Zaphiropoulos L. *Are You Hungry.* New York: Random House, 1985.

Hubert E, Soben A. "Properties and fatty acid composition of fats and oils." *Handbook of Biochemistry.* pp E-20-21. Cleveland: CRC Press, 1970.

Jarvis DC. *Folk Medicine.* New York: Fawcett Crest, 1958.

Jensen B. *Food Healing for Man.* Escondido, CA: Bernard Jensen Publisher, 1983.

Johnston IM and Johnston JR. Passwater RS, ed. and Mindell E. *Flaxseed (Linseed) Oil and the Power of Omega-3. How to Make Nature's Cholesterol Fighters Work for You.* New Canaan, CT: Keats Publishing Inc, 1990.

Keul J, Doll E. & Koppler D. *Energy Metabolism of Human Muscle.* Basel, Switzerland: S. Karger, 1972.

Kushi M with Jack A. *Diet for a Strong Heart.* New York: St. Martin's Press, 1985.

Lark SM. *PMS, Premenstrual Syndrome Self-Help Book.* Berkeley, CA: Celestial Arts, 1984.

Lesser M. *Nutrition and Vitamin Therapy.* New York: Grove Press Inc, 1980.

Lowen A. *Bioenergetics.* New York: Pelican Publishing Company, 1976.

Lowen A. *Fear of Life.* New York: MacMillan Publishing Company, 1980.

Lowen A. *Love, Sex and Your Heart.* New York: MacMillan Publishing Company, 1988, Penguin/Arkana Publishing Company, 1994.

Lowen A. *Stress and Illness - A Bioenergetic View.* New York. 1980: 1-29.

Lowen A. *The Way to Vibrant Health.* New York: Harper & Row, 1977.

Masquelier J. "The bactericidal action of certain phenolics of grapes and wine." *The Pharmacology of Plant Phenolics.* New York: Academic Press;1959.

Meiselman K. *Incest.* San Francisco: Jossey-Bass, 1986.

Miller A. *For Your Own Good.* New York: Farrar, Straus, Giroux, 1983.

Miller A. *Prisoners of Childhood.* New York: Basic Books, 1981.

Miquel J. Theoretical and experimental support for an "oxygen radical-mitochondrial injury" hypothesis of cell aging, in *Free Radicals, Aging, and Degenerative Diseases.* Johnson J.E., Walford R., Harmon D. and Miquel J., Eds. New York: Aland R. Liss, 1986, 51.

National Academy of Sciences. *Diet and Health: Implications for Reducing Chronic Disease Risk.* Washington: National Academy Press, 1989.

Niazi SK. *The Omega Connection. The Facts About Fish Oils and Human Health.* Chicago: Esquire Books Inc, 1987.

Ornish D. *Dr. Dean Ornish's Program for Reversing Heart Disease. The Only System Scientifically Proven to Reverse Heart Disease Without Drugs or Surgery.* New York: Random House, 1990.

Ornstein R., Swencionis C. *The Healing Brain: A Scientific Reader.* New York: Guilford Press, 1990.

Passwater RA, Kanddaswami C. Pycnogenol, *The Super "Protector" Nutrient.* New Canaan, CT: Keats Publishing, Inc., 1994.

Pearson D, Shaw S. *Life Extension, a Practical Scientific Approach.* New York: Warner Books, 1982.

Pennington JAT. *Food Values of Portions Commonly Used.* New York: Harper & Row, 1989.

Pfeiffer CC, et al. *Mental and Elemental Nutrients - A Physician's Guide to Nutrition and Health Care*. New Canaan, CT: Keats Publishing Inc, 1975.

Porter NA. Prostaglandin endoperoxides, *Free Radicals in Biology*. Vol. 4. Academic Press, 1980.

Poston C, Lison K. *Reclaiming Our Lives*. New York: Little Brown & Co, 1989.

Pritikin N with McGrady PM Jr. *The Pritikin Program for Diet and Exercise*. New York: Bantam Books, 1979.

Rector LG. *Healthy Healing: An Alternative Healing Reference*. Healthy Healing Publishing, 1992.

Reich W. *Character Analysis*. New York: Farrar, Straus, Giroux, 1945.

Reich W. *The Function of the Orgasm*. New York: Simon & Schuster, 1973.

Remington D, Fisher G, Parent E. *How to Lower Your Fat Thermostat. The No-Diet Reprogramming Plan for Lifelong Weight Control*. Provo, Utah: Vitality House International Inc, 1983.

Ross R. The pathogenesis of atherosclerosis. In: Braunwald E., ed. *Heart Disease: A Textbook of Cardiovascular Medicine*. 4th ed. Philadelphia, PA: WB Saunders Company. 1106-1124, 1992.

Rush R. *The Best Kept Secret*. New York: McGraw-Hill Book Co, 1980.

Sattilaro AJ with Monte T. *Living Well Naturally*. Boston: Houghton Mifflin Co, 1984.

Schechter SR with Monte T. *Fighting Radiation With Foods, Herbs, and Vitamins*. Brookline, MA: East West Health Books, 1988.

Seibin and Teruko Arasaki. "Dietary and medical applications." *Vegetables from the Sea*. Tokyo: Japan Publications,1983:32-60.

Siegel BS. *Peace, Love, and Healing*. New York: Harper and Row, 1989.

Sinatra ST. "Stress management and cardiovascular rehabilitation." *The Exercising Adult*. Cantu R, ed. New York: MacMillan, 1987.

Somer E. *Nutrition for Women, The Complete Guide*. New York: Henry Holt and Co., Inc., 1993.

Story JA. "Dietary fiber and lipid metabolism: an update." *Medical Aspects of Dietary Fiber*. Spiller GA and McP Kay R, eds. p.137. New York and London: Plenum Medical Books, 1980.

Tarnower H, Baker SS. *The Complete Scarsdale Medical Diet plus Dr. Tarnower's Lifetime Keep-Slim Program.* New York: Bantam Books, 1978.

PERIODICALS

Alession HM and Goldfarb AH. "Lipid peroxidation and scavenger enzymes during exercise: adaptive response to training." *J Appl Physiol.* 1988;64:1333-1336.

Alession HM, Goldfarb AH, Cutler RC. "MDA content increases in fast and slow-twitch skeletal muscle with intensity of exercise in a rat." *Am J Physiol.* 1988;C874-C877.

"The alpha-tocopherol, beta carotene cancer prevention study group; The effect of vitamin E and beta carotene on the incidence of lung cancer and other cancers in male smokers." *NEJM.* 1994;330:1029-1035.

Ames B, Shigenaga M., Hagent T. "Oxidants, antioxidants, and the degenerative diseases of aging." *Proc. Natl. Acad. Sci, USA.* 1993;90:7915-7922.

Anderson JW, Gustafson NJ, Bryant CA, Tietyen-Clark J. "Dietary fiber and diabetes: a comprehensive review and practical application." *J Am Diet Assoc.* 1987;87:1189-97.

Anderson JW, et al. "Dietary fiber: hyperlipidemia, hypertension, and coronary heart disease." *Am J Gastroenterology.* 1986;81(10):907-19.

Anderson JW, Gustafson NJ. "High-carbohydrate, high-fiber diet. Is it practical and effective in treating hyperlipidemia?" *Postgraduate Medicine.* 1987;82(4):40.

Anderson KM, et al. "An updated coronary risk profile: a statement for health professionals." *Circulation.* 1991;83:356-352.

Aro A, et al. "Adipose tissue isomeric trans fatty acids and risk of myocardial infarction in nine countries: the EURAMIC study." *The Lancet.* 1995;345:273-278.

Augusti KT, et al. "Partial identification of the fibrinolytic activators in onion." *Atherosclerosis.* 1975;21:409-16.

Babior MB, "Oxygen-dependent microbial killing of phagocytes." NEJM. 1978; 298, 659.

Becker AB, et al. "The bronchodilator effects and pharmacokinetics of caffeine in asthma." *NEJM.* March 22, 1984;310(12):743-46.

Bell LP, Hectome K, Reynolds H, et al. "Cholesterol-lowering effects of psyllium hydrophilic mucilloid: adjunct therapy to a prudent diet for patients with mild to moderate hypercholesterolemia." *JAMA*. 1989;261:3419-23.

Benfante R, Reed D. "Is elevated serum cholesterol a risk factor for coronary heart disease in the elderly?" *JAMA*. 1990;263:393-96.

Benson JA Jr, et al. "Simple chronic constipation." *Postgraduate Med*. 1975;57:55.

Bhaskaram C, Reddy V. "Cell-mediated immunity in iron- and vitamin-deficient children." *BMJ*. 1975;3:522.

Blair SN, Kohl HW, Paffenbarger RS, et al. "Physical fitness and all-cause mortality." *JAMA*. 1989;262:2395-2401.

Blake DR, et al. "Hypoxic-reperfusion injury in the inflamed human joint." *Lancet*. 1989 (Feb 11):289-293.

Blankenhorn DH, Kramsch DM. "Reversal of atherosis and sclerosis. The two components of atherosclerosis." *Circulation*. 1989;79:1-15.

Block G. "Vitamin C and cancer prevention: the epidemiologic evidence." *Am J Clin Nutr*. 1991;53:270S-282S.

Bohigian MD, presenter. "Dietary fiber and health." Information Report of the Council on Scientific Affairs. AMA. 1988; Apr:1-14.

Bordella A. "Personal observations." International Bioenergetic Conference. Belgium. 1986.

Bordia AK. "Effect of garlic on blood lipids in patients with coronary heart disease." *Am J Clin Nutr*. 1981;34:2100.

Bordia AK, et al. "Essential oil of garlic on blood lipids and fibrinolytic activity in patients with coronary artery disease." *Atherosclerosis*. 1977;28:155.

Borish ET, Prior WA. "Cigarette smoking, free radicals, and free radical DNA damage. In:Cross CE, moderator, Oxygen radicals and human disease. *Ann Int Med*. 1987;107:526-545.

Boxer LA, Watanabe AM, et al. "Correction of leukocyte function in Chediak-Higashi syndrome by ascorbate." *NEJM*. 1976;295:1041-45.

Bray GA. "The energetics of obesity." Twenty-Ninth Annual Meeting of the AC Sports Med. May, 1982.

Brownlee S. "Alzheimer's, is there hope?" *U.S. News and World Reports*. 1991; Aug 12:40-49.

Bulrum RR, Clifford CK, Lanza E. "NCl dietary guidelines: rationale." *Am J Clin Nutr.* 1988;48:888-95.

Burkitt DP, Walker ARP, Painter NS. "Dietary fiber and disease." *JAMA.* 1974;229:1068.

Burkitt DP. "Some disease characteristic of modern western civilization." *BMJ.* 1973;1:274.

Burton GW, Ingold KU. "Beta-carotene: an unusual type of lipid antioxidant." *Science.* 1984;224:569-573.

Camaione DN, Sinatra ST. "Beneficial effects of exercise and current concepts in adult fitness." *CT Med.* 1981;45(10):620-25.

Castell WP. "Cardiovascular disease in women." *Am J Obstet Gynecol.* 1988;158:1153-60.

Chandra RJ, et al. "Vitamins for the elderly." *The Lancet.* 1993;340:1124-1127.

Chihara G, et al. "Fractionation and purification of the polysaccharides with marked antitumor activity, especially lentinan, from LENTINUS EDODES (Berk.) Sing. (an edible mushroom)." *Cancer Res.* 30,1970; 2776-81.

Colditz GA, Hankinson SE, et al. "The use of Estrogens and Progestins and the risk of breast cancer in postmenopausal women." *The New Engl J of Med.* 1995;332:1589-1593.

Cooper KH. "Coronary combat." *Modern Maturity.* Dec 1988-Jan 1989:78-84.

Connett JR, Kuller IH, Kjelberg, MO, et al. "Relationship between carotenoid and cancer: the MRFIT study." *Cancer.* 1989;64:126-134.

Conrad CC. "The President's council on physical fitness and sports. *Am J Sports Med.* 1981;9:199-202.

Cosgrove DM. "Coronary artery surgery in women." *CVR&R.* Sept 1994;54-59.

Cleary-Merker L. "Childhood sexual abuse as an antecedent to obesity." *The Bariatrician, AM J Bariatric Med.* Spring, 1991;17-22.

Costill DL, et al. "Effects of caffeine ingestion on metabolism and exercise performance." *Medicine and Science in Sports.* 1978;10(3):155-58.

Cox IM. "Magnesium Therapy Improves Symptoms of Chronic Fatigue Syndrome." *Lancet.* Southampton, UK;1991,337:757-60.

Cummings JH, et al. "Colonic response to dietary fiber from carrot, cabbage, apple, bran and guar gum." *Lancet.* January 7, 1978;5-8.

D'Agostino RB, Belanger AJ, Kannel WB. "Relations of Low Diastolic Blood Pressure to Coronary Heart Disease Death in Presence of Myocardial Infarction: the Framingham Study." *BMJ.* August 17, 1991;303:385-89.

Davis KJA, et al. "Free radical and tissue damage produced by exercise." *Biochem, Biophys Res. Comm.* 1982;107:1178-1205.

Delver E, Pence B. "Effects of dietary selenium levels on UV-induced skin cancer and epidermal antioxidant status." *FASEB J.* 1993;7:A290.

Donoghue S. "The correlation between physical fitness, absenteeism, and work performance." *Can J Pub Health.* 1977;69:201-203.

Dyckner T, Wester PO. "Potassium/magnesium depletion in patients with cardiovascular disease." *Am J of Med.* March 1987;62:11-17.

Enstrom JE, Kanim LE, Klein ME. "Vitamin C intake and mortality among a sample of the United States' population." *Epidemiology.* 1992;3:194-202.

Esterbauer H., et al. "Role of Vitamin E in preventing the oxidation of low-density lipoprotein." *Am J Clin Nutr.* 1991;53:314S-321S.

Facchinetti F, Borella P, Sances G, et al. "Oral magnesium successfully relieves premenstrual mood changes." *Obstetrics & Gynecology.* August 1991;78:2:177-81.

Fardy PS, et al. "An assessment of the influence of habitual physical activity, prior sport participation, smoking habits and aging upon indices of cardiovascular fitness: preliminary report of a cross-sectional and retrospective study." *J Sports Med Phys Fit.* 1976;16:77-90.

Felson DT, Zhang Y, et al. "The effect of postmenopausal Estrogen therapy on bone density in elderly women." *The New Engl J of Medicine.* 1993;329:1141-1146.

"Fish Oil." *The Medical Letter.* January 11, 1991:4.

Folkers K, Langsjoen P, et al. "Lovastatin decreases Co Enzyme Q10 levels in humans." *Proc Natl Acad Sci.* 1990;87:8931-8934.

Folkins DH, et al. "Psychological fitness as a function of physical fitness." *Arch Phys Med Rehabil.* 1972;53:503-8.

Foster WR, Burton BT. "Health implications of obesity." *Ann Int Med.* 1985;103:1024-30.

Frambach DA and Rick EB. Letter to the editor regarding "Zinc supplementation and anemia." *JAMA.* February 20, 1991;265(7):879.

Frankel EN, Kanner J, German JB, et al. "Inhibition of oxidation of human low-density lipoprotein by phenolic substances in red wine." *The Lancet.* 1993;341:454-456.

Gaziano JM, Manson JE, et al. "Beta-carotene therapy for chronic stable angina." *Circulation.* 1990;82:111-201.

Gey KF, et al. "Inverse correlation between plasma, Vitamin E and mortality from ischemic heart disease in cross-cultural epidemiology." *Am J Clin Nutr.* 1991;53:326S-344S.

Gey KF, Puska P. "Plasma vitamins E and A inversely correlated to mortality from ischemic heart disease in cross-cultural epidemiology." *Ann N Y Acad Sci.* 1989;570:268-282.

Giles TD. "Magnesium deficiency: an important cardiovascular risk factor." *Advances in Cardiology.* 1990;1(5).

Giles TD, Chobanian MD. "Magnesium deficiency: a new cardiovascular risk factor in sudden cardiac death." A Symposium. 1990.

"Girth and Death." Metropolitan Life Ins Co. 1939.

Gloth FM III, et al. "Can vitamin D deficiency produce an unusual pain syndrome?" *Arch Intern Med.* August 1991;151:1662-64.

Goldschmidt MG. "Dyslipidemia and ischemic heart disease mortality among men and women with diabetes. *Circulation.* 1994:89:991-997.

Goldsmith M. "Will exercise keep women away from oncologists or obstetricians?" *JAMA.* 1988;259(12):1769-70.

Gorsky RD, Koplan JP, et al. "Relative risks and benefits of long-term Estrogen Replacement Therapy: a decision analysis." *Obstet Gynecol.* 1994;83:161-166.

Gotto AM Jr chairman. "Atherosclerosis, a decade in perspective." Highlights of symposium sponsored by Baylor College of Medicine. Winter 1991.

Greenberg SM, Frishman WH. "Co Enzyme Q10: A new drug for myocardial ischemia?" *The Medical Clinics of North America.* 1988;72(1):243-258.

Greenberg SM, Frishman WH. "Co Enzyme Q10: A new drug for cardiovascular disease." *Journal of Clinical Pharmacology.* 1990;30:596-608.

Greiser EM, Maschewski-Schneider U, Tempel G, Helmert U. "Smoking, medication found to increase cholesterol levels." *Cardiology World News.* 1991; Sept:26-27.

Grundy SM. "Cholesterol and coronary heart disease, future directions." *JAMA.* 1990;264(23):3053-59.

Grundy SM. "Comparison of monounsaturated fatty acids and carbohydrates for lowering plasma cholesterol." *NEJM.* March 20, 1986;314(12):745-48.

Grundy SM. "High serum cholesterol: treatment by diet." *Cardiology Board Review.* 1989;6(3):32-8.

Haber JB, Heaton KW, Murphy D, Burroughs LF. "Depletion and disruption of dietary fiber: effect on satiety, plasma, glucose and serum insulin." *Lancet.* 1977;2:679.

Halevy O, Sklan D. "Inhibition of arachidonic acid oxidation by beta-carotene, retinol and alpha-tocopherol." *Biochem Biophys Acta.* 1987;918:304-307.

Hankinson SE, Stampfer MJ. "All that glitters is not beta carotene." *JAMA.* 1994;272(18):1455-1456.

Harman D. "Free radicals: aging and disease." In:Cross CE, moderator, Oxygen radicals and human disease. *Ann Int Med.* 1987;526-545.

"Harvard Heart Letter." Harvard Medical School. 1991;2(1):1-7.

Henderson BE, Ross RK, et al. "Estrogen use and cardiovascular disease." *Am J Obstet Gynecol.* 1986;154:1181-86.

Hennekens CH. Personal communication at Hartford Cardiovascular Symposium. 1991.

Hennekens CH, et al. "Final report on the aspirin component of the ongoing physicians' health study." *NEJM.* 1989;321:129-35.

Hennekens CH, Gaziano, JM. "Antioxidants and heart disease: epidemiology and clinical evidence." *Clin Card.* 1993 Apr Suppl 1(16);1-15.

Herbert J. "The age of Dehydroepiandrosterone." *The Lancet.* 1995; 345:1193-94.

Herold KC and Herold BC. Letter to the editor regarding "Benefits and risks of exercise." *JAMA.* June 3, 1983;249:21.

Hertog MGL, et al. "Dietary antioxidant flavonoids and risk of coronary heart disease: The Zutphen Elderly Study." *The Lancet.* 1993;342(8878):1007-1011.

Hodis HN, et al. "Serial coronary angiographic evidence that antioxidant vitamin intake reduces progression of coronary artery atherosclerosis." *Jama.* 1995:273:1849-1854.

"How Risky is Physical Exercise?" *Harvard Heart Letter.* May, 1994;4(9).

Huag A. *Composition and Properties of Alginates, Report No. 30.* Trondheim: Norw Seaweed Res Inst, 1964.

Hunter DJ, Manson JE, Colditz GA, et al. "A prospective study of the intake of vitamin C, E, and A and the risk of breast cancer." *NEJM.* 1993;329(4):234-240.

Jackson R, Scragg R, Beaglehole R. "Alcohol consumption and risk of coronary heart disease." *BMJ.* 1991;303:211.

Jacques PF, Chylack Jr LT. "Epidemiological evidence of a role for the antioxidant vitamins and carotenoids in cataract prevention." *Am J Clin Nutr.* 1991;53:3525-3555.

Jacques PF, Chylack Jr. LT, McGandy Jr. RB, et al. "Antioxidant status in persons with and without senile cataract." *Arch Ophth.* 1988b;106:337-340.

Jain RC, et al. "Onion and blood fibrinolytic activity." *BMJ.* 1969;258:514.

Jancin B. "Exercise study may point to hormones as the breast cancer culprit." *Family Practice News.* Nov, 1994;5.

Jewett SL, Eddy LJ, Hochstein P. "Is the antioxidation of catecholamines involved in ischemia-reperfusion injury?" 1989;6:185-188.

Jialal I. "Can vitamins slow the atherosclerotic process? Presented at the AHA 19th Science Writer's Forum, TX. January, 1992.

Jialal I, Fuller CJ. "Oxidized LDL and antioxidants." *Clin Card.* 1993 Apr Suppl 1(16);1-9.

Jialal I, Norkus EP, Cristol L, Grundy SM. "Beta carotene inhibits the oxidative modification of low-density lipoprotein." *Biochem Biophys Acta.* 1991;1086;134-138.

Jialal I, Vega GL, Grundy SM. "Physiologic levels of ascorbate inhibit the oxidative modification of low-density lipoprotein." *Atherosclerosis.* 1990;82:185-191.

Jialal I, Grundy SM. "Vitamin E inhibits LDL oxidation; may help prevent atherosclerosis." *J Lipid Res.* 1992;33:899-906.

Kamikawa T, Kobayashi A, Yamashita T, et al. "Effects of Co Enzyme Q10 on exercise tolerance in chronic stable angina pectoris." *Am J Card.* 1985;56(4):247-251.

Kannel WB, Wilson P. "Risk factors that attenuate the female coronary disease advantage." *Arch Intern Med.* 1995:155:57-61.

Kanter MM, Nolte LA, et al. "Effects of an antioxidant vitamin mixture on lipid peroxidation at rest and postexercise." *J Appl Physiol.* 1993;74(2):965-969.

Kaplan JR, Manuck SB, Clarkson TB, et al. "Social status, environment, and atherosclerosis in cynomolgus monkeys." *Arteriosclerosis.* 1982;2(5):359-68.

Kardinaal AF, Kok FJ, et al. "Antioxidants in adipose tissue and risk of myocardial infarction." *Lancet.* 1991;337:1-5.

Kennedy SH. "Vitamin supplements win new-found respect." *Mod Med.* 1992;60:15-18.

Keys A, et al. "The diet and 15-year death rate in the seven countries study." *Am J Epid.* December 1986;124(6):903-15.

Kok FJ, Martin RF, Mervyn L, et al. "Selenium, cancer foe." *Better Nutrition for Today's Living.* November, 1990

Koplan JP, Powell KE, Silkes RK, et al. "An epidemiological study of the benefits and risks of running." *JAMA* 1982;248(23):3118-21.

Korthuis RJ, Granger DN. "Reactive oxygen metabolites, neutrophils, and the pathogenesis of ischemic-tissue/reperfusion." *Clin Card.* 1993 Apr Suppl 1(16);1-19.

Kirby RW, et al. "Oat-bran intake selectively lowers serum low-density lipoprotein cholesterol concentrations of hypercholesterolemic men." *Am J Clin Nutr.* May 1981;34:824-29.

Lanza E, Jones Y, Block G, Kessler L. "Dietary fiber intake in the US population." *Am J Clin Nutr.* 1987;46:790-97.

Lau BHS, et al. "Allium sativum (garlic) and atherosclerosis: a review." *Nutr Res.* 1983;3:119-28.

Lauer MS, Anderson KM, Kannel WB, et al. "The impact of obesity on left ventricular mass and geometry. The Framingham heart study." *JAMA.* July 10, 1991;266(2):231-36.

Leaf A, Weber PC. "Cardiovascular effects of n-3 fatty acids: an update." *NEJM.* 1988;318:549-57.

Leibovitz B, Hu ML, Tappel AL. "Dietary supplements of Vitamin E, Beta Carotene, Co Enzyme Q10 and Selenium protect tissues against lipid peroxidation in rat tissue slices." *J Nutr.* 1990;120:97-104.

Lobstein DD, et al. "Depression as a powerful discriminator between physically active and sedentary middle-aged men." *J Psychosom Res.* 1983;27:69-76.

Lockwood K, Moesgaard S, et al. "Partial and complete regression of breast cancer in patients in relation to dosage of Co Enzyme Q10." *Biochem and Biophys Res Comm.* 1994;199:1504-08.

Lowe TW. "Cardiovascular disease and pregnancy: maternal cardiac disease: the obstetrician's viewpoint." *CVR&R* May, 1995;40-45.

Lutter LD. "Running athlete in office practice." *Foot and Ankle.* 1982;3(1):53-59.

McKeigue P. "Trans fatty acids and coronary heart disease: weighing the evidence against hardened fat." *The Lancet.* 1995;345:269-270.

MacNeil Lehrer Report. "Eat smart." September 16, 1991.

Manetta A, Fuchtner C. "The role of B-carotene in cancer chemoprevention." *Drug Therapy.* July, 1992;55-60.

Manson JE, Buring JE, Satterfield S, Hennekens CH. "Baseline characteristics of participants in the Physicians' Health Study: a randomized trial of aspirin and beta-carotene in U.S. physicians." *Am J Prev Med.* May-June, 1991;7(3):150-154.

Maresh CM, Sheckley BG, Allen GJ, Camaione DN, Sinatra ST. "Middle-age male distance runners: physiological and psychological profiles." *J Sports Med Phys Fit.* 31:461-469.

Marx JL. "Oxygen free radicals linked to many diseases." *Science.* 1987;235:529-531.

Matthew K, et al. "Influence of the perimenopause on cardiovascular risk factors and symptoms of middle-aged healthy women." *Arch Intern Med.* 1994;154:2349-2355.

Mauer I, Bernhard A, Zierz S. "Co Enzyme Q10 and respiratory chain enzyme activities in hypertrophied human left ventricles with aortic valve stenosis." *Am J of Cardiology.* August 15, 1990;66:504-05.

McBarron J. "Bariatrics." *The Bariatrician, Am J Bariatric Med.* Spring, 1991:9-16.

McCord JM. "Oxygen-derived free radicals in postischemic tissue injury." *NEJM.* 1985;312(3):159-163.

Mehta J, Yang B, Nichols W. "Free radicals, antioxidants, and coronary heart disease." *J Myocardial Ischemia.* 1993;5(8):31-41.

Metropolitan Life Insurance Company: 1983 Metropolitan Height and Weight Table. Reprinted courtesy of Metropolitan Life Insurance Company.

Metz R. "Obesity: an eclectic review." *Hosp Pract.* 1987;22(2)152.

Michaelis L. "Fundamental principles in oxido-reductions." *Biol Bull.* 1949;92, 2939, 1489.

Millane TA, Ward De, Camm AJ, "Is hypomagnesemia arrhythmogenic?" *Clinical Cardiology.* 1992;15:103-108.

Montano CB. "Recognition and treatment of depression in a primary care setting." *J Clin Psych.* 1994;55:19-34.

Morris DL, et al. "Serum carotenoids and coronary heart disease." *JAMA.* 1994;272:1439-1441.

Morris JN, Heady JA, Raffle PAB, et al. "Coronary heart disease and physical activity of work." *Lancet.* 1953;2:1053.

Morris JN, Kogan A, Patterson DC, et al. "Incidence and prediction of ischemic heart disease in London busmen." *Lancet.* 1966;2:553.

"Multiple risk factor intervention trial." *JAMA.* 1982;248:1465-77.

National Heart, Lung, and Blood Institute, National Institute of Health, US Department of Health and Human Services. "National cholesterol education program, report of the expert panel in population strategies for blood cholesterol reduction: executive summary." *Arch of Int Med.* June, 1991;151:1071-84.

Nerem RM, Levesque MJ, Cornhill JF, et al. "Social environment as a factor in diet-induced atherosclerosis." *Science.* 1980;208:1475.

"Nutritional Trends." *Internal Medicine News.* 1991; July 15-31:30.

Ornish D, et al. "Can lifestyle changes reverse coronary heart disease? The lifestyle heart trial." *Lancet.* 1990;336:129-33.

"Pectin may reduce cholesterol, colon cancer incidence." *Cardiology World News.* 1991; Sept:8.

Pomare EW, Heaton KW. "Alteration of bile salt metabolism by dietary fiber (bran)." *BMJ.* 1973;4:262.

Prescott L. "Symposium: magnesium in clinical medicine and therapeutics. Wide range of diseases linked to low magnesium levels." *Intrn Med World Rpt.* June 15,30, 1991:7.

Proctor PH and Reynolds ES. "Free radicals and disease in man." *Physiol Chem Phys.* 1984;16,175.

Psyllium and rice bran: more obscure than oat bran - but they lower cholesterol, too." *Mayo Clin Nutr Lett.* 1990;3(7):1-2.

Quintanilha AT. "Effects of physical exercise and/or Vitamin E on tissue oxidative metabolism." *Biochem Soc Trans.* 1984;12:403-404.

Ravussin E, Lillioja S, Knowler WC, et al. "Reduced rate of energy expenditure as a risk factor for body-weight gain." *NEJM.* 1988;318:467-72.

Rayssiguier Y, Gueux E, Bussiere L, et al. "Dietary magnesium affects susceptibility of lipoproteins in tissues to peroxidation in rats." *J Am Col N.* 1993;12:133-137.

Renaud S, de Lorgeril M. "Wine, alcohol, platelets and the french paradox for coronary heart disease." *The Lancet.* 1992;339:1523-1526.

Riemersma RA, Wood DA, MacIntyre CC, et al. Abstract:"Risk of angina rises with low vitamin E, C, and carotene intake." *Modern Medicine.* 1991;59:68.

Rimm EB, et al. "Vitamin E consumption and the risk of coronary disease in men." *New Engl J Med.* 1993;328:1450-1456.

Risch H, et al. "Dietary fat intake and risk of epithelial ovarian cancer." *J of the Natl Canc Inst.* 1994;86(18):1409-1415.

Roberts SB, Savage J, Coward WA, et al. "Energy expenditure and intake in infants born to lean and overweight mothers." *NEJM.* 1988;318:461-66.

Roberts TL, et al. "Trans isomers of oleic and linoleic acids in adipose tissue and sudden cardiac death." *The Lancet.* 1995;345:278-282.

Roubenoff, RA. "Nutritional risk factors in cardiovascular disease, part 18 Omega-3 fatty acids and coronary heart disease." *Choices in Cardiology.* 1990;4(6):297-98.

Roubenoff RA. "Nutritional risk factors in cardiovascular disease, part 21, Maintaining adequate calcium intake on low-fat diets." *Choices in Cardiology.* 1991.

Roubenoff RA. "Nutritional risk factors in cardiovascular disease, part 22, Dietary guidelines for healthy American adults." *Choices in Cardiology.* 1991;5(4):165-66.

Sastre J, et al. "Exhaustive physical exercise causes oxidation of glutathione status in blood: prevention by antioxidant administration." *Amer J Physiol.* 1992;R992-995.

Seddon JM, et al. "Dietary carotenoids, vitamins A, C, and E, and advanced age-related macular generation." *JAMA.* 1994;272(18):1413-1420.

Shapiro B. "Personal observations." International Bioenergetic Conference. Miami, 1992.

Sheffy BE, Schultz RD. "Influence of vitamin E and selenium on immune response mechanisms." *Fed Proc.* 1979;38:2139-43.

Shimomura Y, et al. "Protective effect of Co Enzyme Q10 on exercise-induced muscular injury." *Biochem Biophys Res Commun.* 1991;176:349-355.

Shirlow MJ, et al. "A study of caffeine consumption and symptoms; indigestion, palpitations, tremor, headache and insomnia." *Int J Epid.* June 1985;14(2):239-48.

Siegel AJ. "New insights about obesity and exercise." *Your Patient and Fitness.* 1988;2(6):6-13.

Simon-Schnass I, Pabst H. "Influence of Vitamin E on physical performance." *Int J Vitam Nutr Res.* 1988;58:49-54.

Sinatra ST. "Stress - a cardiologists point of view." *Postgraduate Med.* 1984;76:231-34.

Sinatra ST. "Stress and the heart - behavioral interaction and plan for strategy." *CT Med.* 1984;48:81-86.

Sinatra ST, et al. "Effects of continuous passive motion, walking, and a placebo intervention on physical and psychological well-being." *J Cardiopul Rehab.* August 1990;10(8)279-86.

Sinatra ST, Chawla S. "Aortic dissection associated with anger, suppressed rage, and cute emotional stress." *J Cardiopul Rehab.* 1986;6(5).

Sinatra ST, Feitell LA. "The heart and mental stress, real and imagined." *Lancet.* 1985;223-223.

Sinatra ST, Graham S. "Healing the heart - Surrendering to Love Meditation." 1989.

Sinatra ST, Hatch H. "Healing the heart." *New England Heart Center.* 1986.

Sinatra ST, Hatch H. "Physiological and psychological profiles of participants in a six day Healing the Heart seminar." Unpublished data. 1987.

Sinatra ST, Lowen A. "Heartbreak and heart disease - the origin and essence of coronary prone behavior." *British Hol Med.* 1987;2:169-171.

Sirtori CR, et al. "Controlled evaluation of fat intake in the Mediterranean diet: comparative activities of olive oil and corn oil on plasma lipids and platelets in high-risk patients." *Am J Clin Nutr.* 1986; 44:635-42.

Sismann G, et al. ILIB Advisory Board. "Focus on diet and exercise." *Lipid Digest.* 1988; 1(2):1-6.

Smith JB, Ingerman CM, and Silver MJ. "Malondialdehyde formation as an indicator of prostaglandin production by human platelets." *J Lab Clin Med.* 1976;88,167.

Snider, Mike. "Doctors urge lowering dietary fat to 25%." *USA Today.* 1991.

Soma MR, Peoletti R. "Lipids and menopause." *CVR&R.* May, 1995;10-11.

Southorn PA. "Free radicals in medicine. 1. Chemical nature and biologic reactions." *Mayo Clin Proc.* 1988;63:381-389.

Sperduto R. "Macular degeneration." *Arch of Ophth.* January, 1993;111:104-109.

Spiller GA, Gates JE. "Effect of diets high in monounsaturated fats, plant proteins and complex carbohydrates on serum lipoproteins in hypercholesterolemic humans." *Internation Symposium on Drugs Affecting Lipid Metabolism.* Nov 8-11, 1989.

Spinsi A, et al. "Interactions between ubiquinones and phospholipid bilayers spin-label study." *Arch Biochem Biophys.* 1978;190:454-462.

Stampfer MJ, et al. "Vitamin E consumption and the risk of coronary disease in women." *NEJM.* 1993;328:1444-1449.

Stanford JL, et al. "Combined Estrogen and Progestin hormone replacement therapy in relation to risk of breast cancer in middle-aged women." *Jama.* 1995;274:137-142.

Starkebaum G and Harlan JM. "Endothelial cell injury due to copper-catalyzed hydrogen peroxide generation from homocysteine." *J Clin Invest.* 1986;77:1370-1376.

Steen SN, Oppliger RA, Brownell KD. "Metabolic effects of repeated weight loss and regain in adolescent wrestlers." *JAMA.* 1988;260(1): 47-50.

Steinberg D, et al. "Mechanisms of disease beyond Cholesterol modifications of low-density lipoprotein that increases its atherogenicity." *NEJM.* 1989;320(14):915-924.

Swain JF, Rouse IL, Curley CB, Sacks FM. "Comparison of the effects of oat bran and low-fiber wheat on serum lipoprotein levels and blood pressure." *NEJM.* 1990;322:147-52.

Subak-Sharpe GJ, Hammock DA, "The Family Circle Pocket Nutrition Counter." *Family Circle Magazine.* 1991.

Tanaka J, Tominaga R, Yoshitoshi M, et al. "Co Enzyme Q10: "The prophylactic effect on low cardiac output following cardiac valve replacement." *The Annals of Thoracic Surgery.* 1982;33:145-151.

Tappel A. "Vitamin E spares the parts of the cell and tissues from free radical damage." *Nutrition Today.* 1973;8:4.

Teas J. "The consumption of seaweed as a protective factor in the etiology of breast cancer." *Med Hypotheses.* 1981;7:(5)601-13.

Thompson PD, Funk EJ, Carleton RA, et al. "Incidence of death during jogging in Rhode Island from 1975-1980." *JAMA.* 1982;247(18):2535-38.

"Twelve weeks to a healthier diet." *Choices in Cardiology.* 1991;5(4):167-68.

Ulbricht TL. "Coronary heart disease: seven dietary factors." *Lancet.* 1991;338:985-992.

Vallance S. "Relationship between ascorbic acid and serum proteins of the immune system." *BMJ.* 1977;2:437-38.

VanCamp SP. "The Hazards of exercise." *Your Patient and Fitness.* 1987;1(4):18-21.

Verlangieri AJ, Bush MJ. "Effects of d-a-tocopherol supplementation on experimentally induced primate atherosclerosis." *J Am Coll Nutr.* 1992;11:131-138.

Wald NJ, Thompson SG, Densen JW, et al. "Corpus and cervical cancer: a nutritional comparison." *Am J Obstet & Gyn.* 1985;153:775-779.

Walker ARP, Burkitt DP. "Colonic cancer: hypotheses of causation, dietary prophylaxis and future research." *Am J Clin Nutr.* 1976(1978)31:910.

Warshafsky S, et al. "Effects of garlic on total serum cholesterol: a meta-analysis." *Annals of Internal Medicine.* October, 1993;119(7)Part I:599-605.

Weiner MA. "Cholesterol in foods rich in omega-3 fatty acids." *NEJM.* 1986;315:833.

Weisburger, JH. "Nutritional approach to cancer prevention with emphasis on vitamins, antioxidants, and carotenoids." *Am J Clin Nutr.* 1991;53:226S-37S.

Weiss SJ, LoBuglio AF. "Phagocyte generated oxygen metabolite and cellular injury." *Lab Invest.* 1982;47:5-18.

Whang R. "Magnesium deficiency: Pathogenesis, prevalence, and clinical implications." *Am J of Med.* March 20, 1987;82:24-29.

Wilber, JF. "Neuropeptides, appetite regulation, and human obesity." *JAMA.* 1991;266(2):257-58.

Willett WC, Manson JE, Stampfer MJ, et al. "Weight, weight change, and coronary heart disease in women: risk within the 'normal' weight range." *JAMA.* 1995;273(6):461-465.

Wynder EL, Shigematsu T. "Environmental factors of cancer of the colon and rectum." *Cancer.* 1967;20:1520.

Wyshak G, Frisch RE. "Carbonated beverage, dietary calcium, the dietary calcium/phosphorus ratio, and bone fractures in girls and boys." *Jnl of Adolescent Health.* 1994;15:210-215.

INDEX

A Cardiologist's Prescription for

OPTIMUM HEALTH

is available at special quantity discounts. For details
regarding quantity purchases, contact:

Special Markets
The Lincoln-Bradley Publishing Group
Creative Living, Inc.
P.O. Box 808
Gatlinburg, TN 37738

423/436-4150

• • • • • • • • • • • • • •

Other books by Lincoln-Bradley that emphasize guidelines
and suggestions for *Winning Lifestyles* include:

A STRATEGY FOR WINNING
In Business • In Sports • In Family • In Life
(ISBN 1-879111-75-6)
by Carl Mays, with a Foreword by Lou Holtz
(272-page hardcover, $21.95)

WINNING THOUGHTS
(ISBN 1-879111-23-3)
by Carl Mays
(96-page softcover, $5.95)

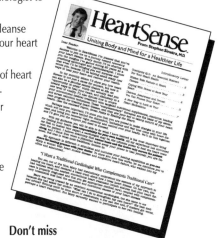

About The Author

DR. STEPHEN T. SINATRA, M.D., F.A.C.C., is board certified in Internal Medicine and Cardiology. He is Chief of Cardiology and Director of Medical Education at Manchester Memorial Hospital in Manchester, CT.

With his own line of vitamins, minerals and nutrients sold through his health food store in Manchester, Dr. Sinatra practices what he preaches.

He has special expertise in utilizing behavior modification and emotional release as tools for healthy living. Trained in Gestalt and Bioenergetic psychotherapy, he is a Certified Bioenergetic Analyst.

Editor of the monthly Phillips' *HeartSense* newsletter, Dr. Sinatra is a much sought-after speaker for medical conventions and anti-aging conferences.

His first book with Lincoln-Bradley, *LOSE TO WIN*, was a featured selection of the *Doubleday Book Club*.